INTRACELLULAR BACTERIAL VACCINE VECTORS

INTRACELLULAR BACTERIAL VACCINE VECTORS

IMMUNOLOGY, CELL BIOLOGY, AND GENETICS

Edited by

YVONNE PATERSON, PH.D.
University of Pennsylvania Medical Center
Department of Microbiology
Philadelphia, PA

WILEY-LISS

A JOHN WILEY & SONS, INC., PUBLICATION

New York • Chichester • Weinheim • Brisbane • Singapore • Toronto

This book is printed on acid-free paper. ♾

While the authors, editors and publisher believe that drug selection and dosage and the specification and usage of equipment and devices, as set forth in this book, are in accord with current recommendations and practice at the time of publication, they accept no legal responsibility for any errors or omissions, and make no warranty, expressed or implied, with respect to material contained herein. In view of ongoing research, equipment modifications, changes in governmental regulations and the constant flow of information relating to drug therapy, drug reactions, and the use of equipment and devices, the reader is urged to review and evaluate the information provided in the package insert or instructions for each drug, piece of equipment, or device for, among other things, any changes in instructions or indication of dosage or usage and for added warnings and precautions.

For ordering and customer service, call 1-800-CALL-WILEY.

Library of Congress Cataloging-in-Publication Data:

Intracellular bacterial vaccine vectors : immunology, cell biology, and genetics / edited by Yvonne Paterson.
p. cm.
Includes index.
ISBN 0-471-17278-2 (cloth : alk. paper)
1. Bacterial vaccines. I. Paterson, Yvonne, 1941– .
[DNLM: 1. Bacterial Vaccines. 2. Vaccines, DNA. 3. Immunity, Cellular. 4. Immunity, Mucosal. 5. Antigens, Bacterial—immunology. WC 200 I615 1999]
QR189.5.B33I56 1999
615′.372—dc21
DNLM/DLC
for Library of Congress 98-47838
CIP

Printed in the United States of America.

10 9 8 7 6 5 4 3 2 1

CONTENTS

PREFACE

Two centuries have elapsed since Edward Jenner published "An inquiry into the causes and effects of the *variolae vaccinae*, or cow pox" which introduced the first live vaccine into Europe. The vaccinia vaccine ultimately led to the eradication of Small Pox from 1967 to 1977 which was perhaps the most remarkable triumph of public health policy in the history of human-kind. Indeed, the 20th century will be commemorated as the period when the potential of Jenner's dream was realized by various public health programs aimed at universal vaccination in childhood. Thus, in the western world at least, childhood scourges such as diphtheria, type B *Hemophilus influenzae*, polio, measles, mumps, and rubella have been virtually eliminated.

Many vaccine strategies have been developed in the past few decades. These include pathogens killed with heat or chemical treatment and live attenuated pathogens that are avirulent but still induce protective immunity. More recently, sub-unit vaccines in which an immunogenic protein usually prepared by recombinant DNA technology, or carbohydrate, from the pathogen of interest, is used as an immunogen. Why, then, the need to use live recombinant bacterial vectors as a vaccine strategy? This book attempts to explain the immune basis for the burgeoning interest in this group of intracellular parasites as vaccine vectors for those diseases for which prior approaches have either failed to provide an efficacious vaccine or for which a live attenuated autologous vaccine is considered too risky.

HIV is the obvious example of a modern plague that has thus far been recalcitrant to vaccine development but there are also many "older" diseases for which there is still no optimal vaccine including, but certainly not restricted to, influenza, tuberculosis, herpes simplex virus and malaria. In Part I we will describe in detail how intracellular bacteria induce strong cell mediated immunity at mucosal surfaces. Since this is the site of infection of most pathogens it is hoped that by harnessing these vectors to deliver antigen, they will provide protective immunity where other approaches have failed.

Cellular immunity has been shown to play a significant role in controlling many viral infections. The primary antigens of intact virus exposed to the humoral immune system are the envelope glycoproteins. The mutation rate of these genes for viruses such as influenza, rhinovirus and HIV, however, is very high and viral escape mutants emerge which evade the humoral immune response. A low rate of mutation in the genes that code for viral core proteins is a major advantage in vaccines aimed at enhancing the cellular arm of the immune response to viruses which have mechanisms for avoiding humoral immune responses. In contrast to humoral responses that are very strain-specific, cell mediated immunity is often broadly cross-reactive because it is easily invoked by viral core proteins that are more conserved. Intracellular bacteria are extraordinary agents for promoting cell-mediated responses. A further advantage of using a live vector is that this results in long lasting immunity which cannot be induced with killed preparations or soluble protein and adjuvant. Indeed in the past few years it has become apparent that in the absence of the early burst of innate immunity that accompanies infection by live microbes the immune response to an inert antigen may become indolent.

When putting together a volume that focuses on intracellular bacteria as vaccine vectors I was mindful of the fact that interested readers may come from varied fields and may not necessarily be familiar with the fundamental microbiology and immunology of these vectors. I have, therefore, provided an introductory chapter that compares and contrasts various aspects of the life-styles and immunology of these organisms. The main body of the book is divided into two parts. In Part I the basic cell biology and immunology of each of these vectors is covered in addition to aspects of the pathogenicity, life cycle, and epidemiology of the organisms. Special consideration is given to the specifics of mucosal immunity since all of these organisms encounter the host at mucosal surfaces. It is hoped that this will prepare the reader for Part II of the book, that deals with their potential as vaccine vectors. In Part II we describe genetic methods for the expression of foreign antigens in these bacteria, studies that have used these bacteria as vaccine vectors and practical limitations and safety concerns with their use.

The authors of the chapters of this book are international experts who have not only made fundamental contributions to understanding the host defense to these bacteria but also recognize their utility as novel vaccines for other diseases. It is important that I thank them for their scholarly contributions to this volume. I am also grateful to the editorial staff of John Wiley for their patient assistance in its production and to my research coordinator Gayle Viale for her editorial help and her artistic rendition of Figures 1, Chapters 1 and 3.

YVONNE PATERSON
Philadelphia, PA

CONTRIBUTORS

ANNA ALDOVINI, M.D., Assistant Professor, Department of Medicine, Children's Hospital and Department of Pediatrics, Harvard Medical School, Boston, Massachusetts

TOBY K. EISENSTEIN, Ph.D., Professor, Department of Microbiology and Immunology, Temple University School of Medicine, Philadelphia, Pennsylvania

DAVID HONE, Ph.D., Associate Professor, Divisions of Vaccine Research and Basic Science, Institute of Human Virology, University of Maryland, Baltimore, Maryland

GEORGE K. LEWIS, Ph.D., Professor, Divisions of Vaccine Research and Basic Science, Institute of Human Virology, University of Maryland, Baltimore, Maryland

ERIC G. PAMER, M.D., Associate Professor, Infectious Diseases Section, Department of Internal Medicine, Section of Immunobiology, Yale University School of Medicine, New Haven, Connecticut

DAVID W. PASCUAL, Ph.D., Assistant Professor, Veterinary Molecular Biology Laboratory, Agricultural Experimental Station, Montana State University, Bozeman, Montana

YVONNE PATERSON, Ph.D., Professor, Department of Microbiology, University of Pennsylvania School of Medicine, Philadelphia, Pennsylvania

MOHAMMED T. SHATA, M.D., Ph.D., Divisions of Vaccine Research and Basic Science, Institute of Human Virology, University of Maryland, Baltimore, Maryland

JELLE E. R. THOLE, Ph.D., Senior Scientist, Division of Immunological and Infectious Diseases, TNO Prevention and Health, Leiden, The Netherlands

SUJATA VIJH, Ph.D., Infectious Disease Section, Department of Internal Medicine, Section of Immunobiology, Yale University School of Medicine, New Haven, Connecticut

LARRY M. WEISKIRCH, Ph.D., Department of Microbiology, University of Pennsylvania, Philadelphia, Pennsylvania

DOUGLAS B. YOUNG, Ph.D., Fleming Professor of Medical Microbiology, Imperial College School of Medicine at St. Mary's, London, England

RICHARD YOUNG, Ph.D., Member, Whitehead Institute for Biomedical Research and Professor, Department of Biology, Massachusetts Institute of Technology, Nine Cambridge Center, Cambridge, Massachusetts

CHAPTER 1

THE RELATIONSHIP BETWEEN INTRACELLULAR BACTERIAL LIFE-STYLES AND IMMUNE RESPONSIVENESS TO BACTERIAL DELIVERED ANTIGENS

YVONNE PATERSON

1.1 INTRODUCTION

This volume brings together recent advances in recombinant intracellular bacterial vectors in vaccine research. It reviews in detail approaches that exploit three different bacterial vectors, *Listeria*, *Salmonella*, and bacillus Calmette-Guérin (BCG) (the vaccine strain of *Mycobacteria bovis*). Recent developments in the use of *Shigella* as a vaccine vector are described in Chapter 6. Part I of this book (Chapters 2 through 4) covers the cell biology and host immune responses of these bacteria. Part II (Chapters 5 through 7) describes how they may be harnessed as vaccine vectors to present passenger antigens to the immune system. This chapter introduces similar mechanisms by which this group of bacteria invade and colonize host cells and the

Abbreviations: AIDS, acquired immunodeficiency syndrome; β2-M, β2-microglobulin; BALT, bronchial-associated lymphoid tissue; BCG, *Mycobacterium bovis* bacillus Calmette-Guérin; CTL, cytotoxic T lymphocyte; ER, endoplasmic reticulum; GALT, gut-associated lymphoid tissue; GI, gastrointestinal; HIV, human immunodeficiency virus; hsp, heat shock protein; IEL, intraepithelial lymphocyte; IFN-γ, interferon-γ IL, interleukin; GALT, gut-associated lymphoid tissue; i.n., intranasal; i.p., intraperitoneal; i.v., intravenous; LLO, listeriolysin O; LPS, lipopolysaccharide; MHC, major histocompatibility complex; NK, natural killer; p.o., per os; SOD, superoxide dismutase; TCR, T-cell receptor; Th, T helper; TNF, tumor necrosis factor.

Intracellular Bacterial Vaccine Vectors, Edited by Yvonne Paterson.
ISBN 0-471-17278-2

arms of the host's immune system that are activated by such infection. Differences in the antigen-processing pathways that are accessible by intracellular bacteria, and how these impact on their efficacy as vaccine vectors, are also discussed. We also review recent advances that explore features of antigen processing of bacteria and bacterial products peripheral to the main focus of the rest of this volume.

1.2 ROLE OF THE MACROPHAGE AND PHAGOLYSOSOME IN INTRACELLULAR BACTERIAL INFECTIONS

Key to understanding the potential of intracellular bacteria as carriers of passenger antigens to the immune system is a knowledge of their cellular localization and mechanisms for inducing immunity. Their potency as vaccine vectors for cell-mediated immunity is dependent on the techniques they have evolved to escape humoral immune responses by sequestration in phagocytic cells. All the bacteria discussed naturally invade the host at mucosal surfaces, usually the gut mucosa, in the case of *Listeria*, *Salmonella*, and *Shigella*, and the lung mucosa in the case of *Mycobacteria*. Thus, their first struggle with the immune system is most likely to be with phagocytic cells in the Peyer's patches or draining lymph nodes or alveolar macrophages in the case of infection at bronchial surfaces. The burst of innate immunity that precedes the adaptive mucosal immune response must be overcome for a successful infection to take place. In order to survive the hostile environment of the phagosome, intracellular bacteria secrete a variety of virulence factors that modify phagolysosomal microbicidal mechanisms such as defensins, reactive oxygen and nitrogen intermediates, and lysosomal enzymes that are active at acid pH. Some mechanisms are common to many intracellular bacteria. Superoxide dismutase (SOD) and catalase, for example, are common virulence factors that act to neutralize the bactericidal activity of reactive oxygen intermediates; SOD converts superoxide to hydrogen peroxide which is then broken down by catalase. The production of antibiotic polypeptides, called defensins, by the host cell is stimulated by phagocytosis of bacteria. The *S. typhimurium* phoP locus is believed to control the expression of a virulence factor that acts against these agents by an unknown mechanism (1). Indeed, the precise mechanisms of many virulence genes are unknown, but there are indeed a staggering number that testify to the ingenuity of these bacteria in adapting to life inside the cell.

Other methods enable intracellular bacteria to survive inside the host cell. One cunning ploy used by *M. tuberculosis* (2) and *S. typhimurium* (3) takes the form of preventing acidification of the phagosome by inhibition of phagosome–lysosome fusion, thereby constructing an innocuous vacuole within which the bacteria can live and replicate. *Mycobacteria* that live and replicate in phagosomes have developed a waxy cell wall that is resistant to lysosomal enzymes and inhibits macrophage activation (4). *Salmonella* virulence factors encoded in the *phoP* locus induce the formation of spacious vacuoles from phagosomes that allow bacterial persistence and growth in these organelles (5). Perhaps the most extraordinary strategy for avoiding destruction in the phagolysosome is that displayed by a small group of intracellular bacteria, including *Listeria* and *Shigella*, which have evolved virulence factors that allow them to escape this vacuole and live in the less hostile environment of the cell cytoplasm (6,7). Indeed, the life-styles of the intracellular bacteria that are currently under investigation as vaccine vectors largely differ by this feature and may be divided into those that persist in a phagosomal compartment and adapt the phagosome for this purpose (*Salmonella* and *Mycobacteria*) and those that escape from this compartment to live in the cytoplasm of the cell in which they harness the host cell actin to further their passage into neighboring cells (*Listeria* and *Shigella*). Details of the cell biology of these events will be found in Part I, but these major differences are highlighted in Figure 1.1.

1.3 COUNTERIMMUNE MECHANISMS

The immune system has not stood idly by while these organisms have evolved ways to evade recognition and elimination. The uptake of bacteria by macrophages results in activation events that promote changes not only in the microbicidal properties of the phagolysosomal compartment but also in the antigen-presenting function of these cells to the adaptive arm of the immune system. Bacterial phagocytosis, usually mediated by binding to complement or mannose-binding receptors, stimulates macrophages to secrete a variety of humoral factors. These include chemokines that recruit new cells to the site of infection, inflammatory cytokines that increase vascular permeability, autocrines that promote the expression of major histocompatibility complex (MHC) molecules and molecules associated with antigen processing, and lymphokines that act to promote cell mediated

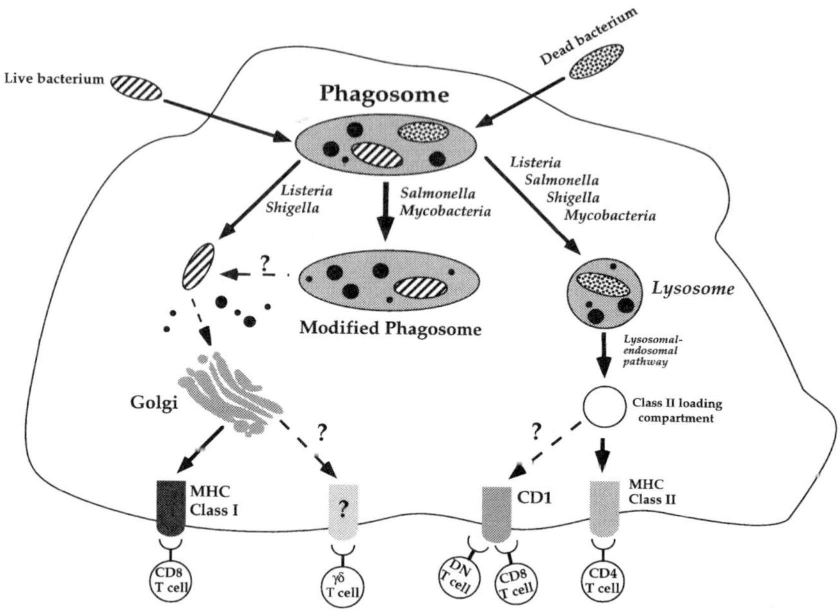

Figure 1.1 Bacterial vector-mediated delivery of recombinant antigens for recognition by T cells. Live and dead bacteria can be phagocytosed by antigen-presenting cells. Dead bacteria remain exclusively in the phagolysosomal vacuole and are targeted to the major histocompatibility complex (MHC) class II pathway for antigen presentation. Live bacteria are either destroyed within the phagosome or, in the case of *Listeria* and *Shigella* some may escape into the cytoplasm of the cell. *Salmonella* and *Mycobacteria* can modify this compartment so that they can continue to grow and persist within the vacuole. Fusion of the phagosome with lysosomes directs antigen released by dying bacteria into the endosomal pathway, where peptides may be loaded onto MHC class II molecules. In the cytosolic compartment, *Listeria* and *Shigella* replicate; any protein they secrete can be processed by proteosomes into peptides that will be transported to the endoplasmic reticulum for loading onto MHC class I molecules in the Golgi apparatus. *Salmonella* and *Mycobacteria* are also capable of accessing this pathway of antigen presentation by unknown mechanisms. It is also unclear as to how bacterial cell wall components are loaded on to CD1 molecules for recognition by $CD8^+$ and $CD4^-CD8^-$ (DN) T cells, but the class II loading compartment has been implicated in this process. Both $\alpha\beta$ and $\gamma\delta$ cells can recognize antigens presented by CD1. Finally the ligand and antigen for most $\gamma\delta$ T cells is still largely unknown, but peptides bound to heat shock proteins as part of the peptide chaperone function of the MHC class I pathway may be involved.

immunity. A key lymphokine in this process is interleukin-12 (IL-12). Macrophages are stimulated by intracellular bacteria to release IL-12. This in turn acts on natural killer (NK) cells to release interferon-γ, (IFN-γ) that further activates macrophages and promotes the destruction of the intracellular bacterium. Indeed, the production of IFN-γ by NK cells, promoted by IL-12, has been shown to be a key factor in early host defense mechanisms against *Salmonella*, *Mycobacteria*, and *Listeria* (8). In addition to its potent effects on innate immunity, IFN-γ helps drive the burgeoning antigen-specific $CD4^+$ T-cell response to the Th1 phenotype required to generate $CD8^+$ T cells and clear bacterial infection through adaptive cell-mediated immunity.

The precise events that result in IL-12 synthesis and secretion on phagocytosis of bacteria are unknown but presumably require the interaction of a bacterial product or products with phagosomal receptors. In vitro studies have verified that macrophages can be induced to release IL-12 or express IL-12 genes when exposed to live *Salmonella* (9), *Listeria* (10), or *Mycobacteria* (11–13). Some bacterial products have been implicated as IL-12-stimulating molecules. Macrophage secretion of IL-12 in vitro can be induced by lipopolysaccharide (LPS) from gram-negative bacteria such as *Salmonella*, mycobacterial heat shock proteins, and secreted listerial antigens, including listeriolysin O (LLO) (10). Bacterial cell wall components such as trehalose dimycolate, a glycolipid component of mycobacterial cell walls (14), and lipoteichoic acid, a surface glycolipid of gram-positive bacteria such as *Listeria* (15) upregulate IL-12 p40 gene expression in cultured macrophages. By contrast, soluble purified protein derivative from *Mycobacteria* was unable to stimulate IL-12 secretion by human monocytes although, when coupled to latex particles, it can stimulate IL-12 production by lung macrophages (16). Killed bacteria can also elicit IL-12 synthesis in cultured macrophages (8,9,17). However, the levels of expression are very much lower, in general, than those induced by living organisms (8,9,18) and production of effective levels of IL-12 in vivo appears to require immunization with living organisms (9). Indeed, it has long been known that heat-killed *Mycobacteria* (19), *Listeria* (20,21), and *Salmonella* (22–24) are far less competent than live vaccines in inducing protection against challenge with virulent bacteria. In the case of *Listeria*, it has been shown that this inefficacy may be reversed by supplementing the heat-killed bacterial immunogen with recombinant IL-12 (25).

The cytokine-driven activation of macrophages that occurs early in infection will fail to kill those intracellular bacteria such as *L. monocytogenes* and *Shigella* that have retreated into the cytoplasm of the cell. However, their escape from phagosomal destruction does not render them invisible to the immune system. Indeed, their presence in the cytosol facilitates the generation of $CD8^+$ CTL T cells that detect and lyse-infected cells. T cells of this phenotype recognize antigenic peptides bound to MHC class I molecules. Generation of these peptides takes place in the cytosol of the cell and they are loaded onto MHC class I after transport to the endoplasmic reticulum (ER) by specialized chaperone molecules. Thus, bacterial virulence factors secreted by these bacteria into the cytosol become a potent source of peptides for the generation of CTL. $CD8^+$ cells are essential for the clearance of listerial infections and CTL have been found that are specific for many of the secreted listerial virulence factors required for phagosomal lysis and cell-to-cell spread (26). These findings are reviewed in detail in Chapter 4. The ability of *Listeria* and *Shigella* to target the MHC class I pathway of antigen processing has been a driving force in the exploitation of these bacteria as vaccine vectors (27,28). Attempts have even been made to modify intracellular bacterial vectors such as BCG to provide them with this facility. Recombinant BCG strains were constructed that secreted a hemolytic fusion protein containing LLO (29), in an effort to obtain better access to the class I pathway of antigen processing. However, the secretion of LLO did not allow the bacteria to escape from the phagosomal compartment, although it did enhance the presentation of co-phagocytosed soluble protein to $CD8^+$ T cells, suggesting that the release of LLO into the phagosome somehow improved the passage of antigen into the MHC class I pathway (29).

In addition to the common adaptive immune responses that generally result from viral and bacterial infections (i.e., $CD4^+$ T cells, $CD8^+$ T cells, and antibody responses), there are specific immune mechanisms that have developed to fight invasion by this group of bacteria at the site of infection. These intracellular bacteria are profound inducers of a specialized group of T cells that are particularly frequent at mucosal surfaces and use the γ and δ T-cell receptor genes. Curiously, $\gamma\delta$ T cells that frequent epithelial surfaces, the mucosal epithelia and the skin, use a limited number of T-cell receptor genes at each site (30,31). Thus murine skin and vaginal epithelia are inhabited by specific monoclonal populations of $\gamma\delta$ T cells, while the intestinal epithelium uses a unique $V\gamma$ but a more diverse array of $V\delta$ genes. Lung $\gamma\delta$ T-cell populations are oligoclonal but still show a restricted V gene usage. These cells clearly play a role in controlling infection to intracellular bacteria and may be of extra thymic origin (31,32). In the case of *M. tuberculosis*, they are the largest component of peripheral blood T cells in exposed, uninfected individuals (33,34) and clear changes in the $\gamma\delta$ T-cell repertoire are detected in the lungs of patients with active pulmonary infection (35). $\gamma\delta$ T cells are also frequently found in *M. leprae*-induced tuberculous skin lesions (36). The abundant variety of T cells that recognize mycobacterial antigens are described in detail in Chapter 2.

The influx of $\gamma\delta$ T cells to the site of infection also occurs in murine listerial infections in the peritoneal cavity (32,37) and in the intestine (38). In the initial immune response, they are a potent source of IFN-γ and TNF-α (38,39) that may be required to activate NK cells early in infection (39). In this regard, they provide an important link between components of the adaptive and innate immune response. They have also been identified in peripheral blood of humans infected with *L. monocytogenes* (40). $\gamma\delta$ T cells may also play a role early in *Salmonella* infections in the peritoneum after i.p. infection (41). Their generation is thought to be driven by IL-15, rather than by IL-2, as is the case for conventional $\alpha\beta$ T cells (42). However, $\gamma\delta$ T cells are not as important as $\alpha\beta$ T cells in the invasion of *S. dublin* through the intestinal cell wall and into the Peyer's patches (43) or in resisting infection by the aroA$^-$ mutant *S. typhimurium* (44) or *S. choleraesuis* (45) when delivered orally. Thus, although $\gamma\delta$ T cells are abundant at mucosal surfaces, the level of their importance in natural *Salmonella* infections remains largely unknown.

Exactly what antigen(s) are recognized by $\gamma\delta$ T cells is also quite enigmatic but, given their appearance early in immune responses at sights of primary infection, host stress proteins such as heat shock proteins have come under close scrutiny as ligands for $\gamma\delta$ TCR (46). However, other protein antigens of listerial (47,48) and mycobacterial (49) origin have also been shown to stimulate $\gamma\delta$ T cells; nonprotein mycobacterial antigens have also been implicated as recognition molecules (50). In addition, the molecular nature of such recognition is still not clearly understood. $\gamma\delta$ T cells probably do not recognize processed antigen in the context of conventional class I or II MHC (51). Indeed, the nonclassical MHC class I antigens have been implicated in their recognition (52,53) and $\gamma\delta$ T cells are represented among the different T-cell types that recognize mycobacterial lipoglycans in the context of CD1b molecules (54). Whatever the precise nature of the antigens that stimulate $\gamma\delta$ T cell generation and maintenance, intracellular bacteria are potent inducers of this subset, which appear to play a role in immunity at mucosal surfaces.

1.4 EXPLOITING CURRENT CONCEPTS OF IMMUNE DEFENSE FOR VACCINOLOGY

The ability of intracellular bacteria to drive the $CD4^+$ T-cell response toward a Th1 response makes them attractive candidates for vaccine vectors for those diseases in which cell-mediated immunity is more effective than humoral responses. Murine viral infections that clearly require Th1 responses for clearance include murine hepatitis virus (55), Rous sarcoma virus (RSV) (56), vaccinia (57), and a murine form of acquired immunodeficiency syndrome (AIDS) (58) caused by infection with the retrovirus LP-BM5. Less is known about the cytokine requirements for viral clearance and control of human infections, but one that has come under such scrutiny is human immunodeficiency virus (HIV). Although somewhat controversial it has been suggested that the humoral immune response, far from being beneficial or even ineffective in HIV infection, may actually be harmful because it impairs the ability of the host to mount a protective cellular immune response (59–61). This thesis is supported by other disease models. Thus, it has long been known (62) that either the humoral or cell-mediated arm predominates in the immune response to infectious agents, particularly pathogens such as *Leishmania major* and *M. leprae* (63), resulting in either resistance or susceptibility to the disease. It has been shown that the decline in T-cell proliferation and IL-2 production that accompanies the progression of disease in HIV^+ individuals is accompanied by a concomitant increase in B-cell activity (61,64,65). These data suggest two important advantages in using intracellular bacteria as vaccine vectors for HIV antigens. One is that they can effectively introduce passenger antigens to the MHC class I pathway for the generation of $CD8^+$ T cells, particularly for the intracytoplasmic vectors, *Shigella* and *Listeria*. Second is their ability to provide the cytokine milieu required to promote the maturation of $CD8^+$ responses via Th1 $CD4^+$ T cells.

The Th1/Th2 dichotomy in vivo is largely regulated by IL-10 and IL-12 (66,67). The lack of Th2 cells and therefore of IL-4 production, in infections with intracellular bacteria suggests that these vectors would be defective in promoting a vigorous B-cell response. Antibodies are likely to be ineffective in clearing systemic infections of intracellular bacteria that are sequestered in cells and inaccessible to direct binding. Thus only antibodies that fix complement are produced in immune responses driven by Th1 cells; these are IgG2a and IgG3 in mice. However, both BCG and *Salmonella* are known to produce B-cell responses at mucosal surfaces in the form of the secreted immunoglobulin IgA. Thus, although oral administration of *Salmonella* elicits a classical Th1 type response, it also promotes the abundant secretion of mucosal IgA (68). It is now thought that a third Th phenotype Th3 (69) may exist in mucosally associated lymphoid tissue that secretes a cytokine profile required for B-cell switching to the production of IgA. TGF-β has been implicated in this process (70,71). It has also been suggested that cytokine-producing $CD8^+$ T cells in Peyer's patches may provide help in immunoglobulin secretion at mucosal surfaces (72).

The most crucial requirement for any vaccine is the induction of memory lymphocytes in lymphoid tissue that has immediate access to the site of infection. With few exceptions, these sites are mucosal surfaces in the bronchial, gastrointestinal (GI) and genital tract. For this reason, those bacteria that naturally infect through the GI tract have been exploited as oral vaccine vectors for inducing mucosal immunity. The paradigm for this purpose is *Salmonella* because the capacity of *Salmonella* to induce neutralizing IgA responses at the site of infection was recognized early in the field of vaccinology (73,74). Chapter 3 reviews the role of the mucosal immune system in host defense against *Salmonella* infection and reconsiders the importance of humoral responses in this process in the light of more recent work on cell-mediated responses in the gut.

Surprisingly, comparatively little is known about the mucosal immune response to *L. monocytogenes*. *Listeria* has been used as a standard to study murine cell-mediated immunity to infection for the past two decades (75), but almost all these studies have delivered the organism by the parenteral route, despite the fact that the natural route of infection is oral. During the past 5 years, an attempt has been made to redress this omission, oral administration of *L. monocytogenes* has been shown to result in an increase of intraepithelial and lamina propria lymphocytes in the intestine in addition to an increase of lymphocytes in the liver (76) with extrathymic T cells being induced before thymus-derived cells. This finding suggests that adaptive immunity plays a key role in anti-*Listeria* mucosal immunity. Perhaps the most serious effort to investigate immunity to *Listeria* invasion through the intestinal route has been made by Kauffmann's group (47). These investigators have shown particular interest in the role of $\gamma\delta$ intraepithelial lymphocytes in mucosal immunity against *Listeria*, as we have discussed above, because this group of lymphocytes appear to make up about 40% of the total $CD3^+$ T cells in the Peyer's patches of *L. monocytogenes* in infected mice (47). However, whether the other 60% of "conventional" $CD3^+$ cells in gut-associated lymphoid tissue (GALT) play a role in preventing the invasion of listeriae, although the gut is still largely unknown. Kaufmann and colleagues have attempted to address the issue of the induction of $CD8^+$ T cells in mice challenged with *Listeria* p.o., using mice that lack the ability to express the β2-microglobulin (β2-M) gene (38). This defect prevents the cell surface expression of those molecules that require β2-M to correctly fold and egress to the cell surface; these include MHC class I and CD1 (Fig. 1.1). The lack of MHC class I-expressing cells in the thymus results in the loss of the thymus-derived $CD8^+$ T-cell compartment of the immune system. Most intraepithelial lymphocytes (IEL) (>80%) are $CD8^+$ T cells (77), but the site of maturation of some of these is thought to be extrathymic and may be in situ. Thus, β2-M-deficient mice will lack thymus-derived $CD8^+$ T cells in the gut but will have a full complement of $\gamma\delta$ T cells and those $\alpha\beta$ T cells that develop exclusively in the gut. Oral listeriosis was shown to increase the number of IFN-γ-secreting $\alpha\beta$ IEL by two- to three-fold in both β2-M-negative and β2-M-positive (normal) mice but, although $\gamma\delta$ IEL were also increased by this extent in normal mice, they were increased by 10-fold in β2-M-negative mice, suggesting that the activation of this group of cells may be suppressed by cells expressing MHC class I molecules.

Even less is known about whether listerial infection through the gut results in IgA secretion by GALT. Invasion of most intracellular bacteria is probably by the route shown in Figure 2.1, with M cells acting as the conduit for the entry of bacteria into Peyer's patch germinal centers. The dogma associated with immunity to *L. monocytogenes* is that antibody responses play little role in either the protection or clearance of the bacterium (75). However, this wisdom has been derived exclusively from studies in which *L. monocytogenes* has been administered i.v. or i.p. It has been propagated by the elucidation of the life cycle of the bacterium, which highlights its ability to spread from cell to cell, and from macrophages into nonphagocytic cells, thus evading interaction with antibodies. This is also true of *Shigella* (7), and there is a wealth of evidence that secreted IgA is induced by *Shigella* and plays a key role in protective immunity to this organism (78–80). In addition, *Listeria* is a facultative intracellular bacterium and in the nutritional and cozy environment at the gut surface, many bacteria may well remain extracellular and susceptible to IgA binding. Indeed, the expression of virulence factors such as LLO required to invade cells is suppressed by nutrients that are in abundance in the gut, such as iron (81). *L. monocytogenes* mutants that lack LLO are unable to invade through the gut wall and into Peyer's patches (82), attesting to the crucial role of the regulation of these factors by the extracellular environment in the life style adopted by the bacterium. Further evidence that *Listeria* may well induce a humoral response at the gut surface is provided by studies in domestic animals in which *Listeria* has been delivered orally (83–85) and in humans who have acquired the organism from contaminated food (86,87). The studies in domestic animals suggest that *Listeria* is not only competent to induce a systemic humoral response (83–85) when delivered orally, but that this response may be protective against subsequent oral challenge (83). Indeed, the presence of serum antibodies to the virulence factor LLO is used as an indicator of prior oral exposure to *L. monocytogenes* (84,87).

Mycobacteria do not normally infect through the gut, although *M. avium* invasion through intestinal surfaces can cause serious opportunistic infections in immunocompromised individuals (88) and infection of the GALT, lungs, and spleen of germfree mice (89). However, the constitution of the mucosal immune system is such that immune lymphocytes are thought to express specific receptors, allowing them to traffic between the germinal centers and providing protection at different mucosal surfaces (90–92). Thus, the ability to induce immunity in GALT or bronchial-associated lymphoid tissue (BALT) may provide immunity at other mucosal surfaces such as the genital tract. It should be noted that the precise extent of this intercommunication, and the most appropriate site of immunization for induction of mucosal immunity in the reproductive tract is still largely undefined (93). However, the intranasal route of immunization has been shown in some instances to induce secreted IgA at the bronchial, intestinal, and vaginal surfaces (94). BCG immunization at the nasal surface induces immunity in BALT that may be transferable to other mucosal surfaces. This possibility has been exploited in a live BCG vaccine that expressed the outer-surface protein A antigen from *B. burgdorfei* the causative agent of Lyme disease (95). A single nasal immunization with this vaccine induced a long-lived systemic humoral IgG response and a secretory IgA response that was distributed throughout the mucosal immune system at both proximal (lung) and distal (vagina and lamina propria) sites (95). By contrast, oral immunization by BCG induced only low levels of IgA in GALT and no detectable response at other mucosal sites. Intranasal immunization has also been used to deliver a recombinant BCG-measles virus nucleoprotein vaccine to provide protection at bronchiolar surfaces (96). Finally, the ability of BCG to induce Th1 responses in BALT in mice (97,98) has been exploited to reverse allergen-induced airway eosinophilia in mice by i.n. immunization with BCG (99).

1.5 INERT BACTERIAL PRODUCTS AS ANTIGEN VECTORS

Live bacteria are more potent immunostimulators than are dead bacteria. Nevertheless, knowledge of bacterial virulence factors and their role in the life cycles of the organisms has suggested new purposes for these bacterial products. The listerial virulence factor LLO, which facilitates the destruction of the phagolysosomal membrane and the escape of the bacterium into the cell cytosol, has been used to target inert molecules into this cellular compartment by co-encapsulation into liposomes (100). These particles are taken up by phagocytosis whereupon their contents are released into the phagosome. The inclusion of LLO in the liposomes ensures their entry into the cytosol. The obvious utility for this technique is to target antigens to the class I pathway for antigen processing but it could be applied to targeting any drug to the cytosolic compartment.

Heat shock proteins (hsp) are produced by intracellular bacteria in response to the stress of the phagolysosomal compartment. They are highly immunogenic within the context of an active infection and appear to activate both adaptive and innate immunity (101). The adjuvant properties of hsp70 from *Mycobacteria* have been explored for promoting immunity toward a passenger protein antigen. HIV p24 was either physically mixed with hsp70 or covalently conjugated to hsp70. The conjugated HIVp24/hsp70 was found to induce potent humoral and cellular immunity in the absence of any other adjuvant (102). Covalent coupling appeared to be required to induce good immune responses for this protein antigen (102), although mycobacterial hsp70 is effective at delivering unconjugated peptides to the immune system (103). Curiously, conjugation of hsp70 to soluble protein antigens appears to promote the entry of these soluble antigens into the endogenous MHC class I antigen processing of a foreign antigen for the induction of CTL (104). The ability of live intracellular bacteria to enter the endogenous pathway of antigen processing will be reviewed in Part I of this volume. However, there is growing evidence that inert particles and nonintracellular bacteria are not inept at inducing CTL, despite no obvious way to reach the appropriate compartment. Heat shock proteins of mammalian (105,106) and bacterial (102) origin have been found to be effective carriers of passenger antigens to this arm of the immune response. A clue to the possible mechanisms of uptake of these exogenous antigenic particles into the cytosol was provided by studies in which protein antigens were coupled to beaded particles. Such particulate antigens are eagerly phagocytosed by macrophages (107) or dendritic cells (108) and appear to pass from the phagolysosomal compartment into the cytosol of the cell. Whether this passage is a passive leaking of the antigen from one compartment to the other or requires active transport is still unknown, but it does appear to require that the antigen is in particulate form (109). However, given that some intracellular bacteria that are contained within the phagosome, and that are unable to escape into the cytoplasm of the cell, do induce potent CTL responses it seems likely that there is an active mechanism for transport of bacterial antigens across the phagolysosomal pathway that can be accessed by phagocytosed particulate antigens. The antigens may be presented covalently coupled to beaded supports as described above or as recombinant proteins expressed by free-living bacteria such as *Escherichia coli* (110,111).

1.6 INTRACELLULAR BACTERIA AS VECTORS FOR DNA VACCINES

This book covers the development of intracellular bacteria as vaccine vectors for foreign antigenic proteins. However, the facility with which this group of bacteria enter into, and persist in, phagocytic cells has not escaped the attention of investigators with interests in DNA vaccines. The bacteria themselves may be used to target DNA vaccines to professional antigen-presenting cells (APCs). The delivery of bacterial plasmids to the cytoplasm of the cell, where they are transcribed to antigenic proteins competent to induce strong cell-mediated immunity, has been achieved using *Shigella* (28), *Salmonella* (112), and *Listeria* (113) vectors. The development of rationally attenuated mutants of *Listeria* that remain competent to escape into the cytoplasm of the cell (113–115) will aid in the utilization of *Listeria* for this purpose in addition to providing safe vectors for passenger protein antigens. Such mutants have already been developed for *Salmonella* (see Chapters 3 and 6) and for *Shigella* (116,117) because these organisms are, themselves, serious pathogens for which avirulent mutants have been exhaustively explored as autologous vaccines.

1.7 CONCLUDING REMARKS

A revision of thinking in the requirements for cell-mediated immune responses has led to the rediscovery of the role of innate immunity in boosting and maintaining strong cell mediated immunity (118). The immune system has evolved specifically to deal with pathogens. It is not surprising, therefore, that the most potent immune responses may be those that are directed against these infectious particles. Live recombinant bacterial vectors are a powerful way of harnessing this evolutionary learning for the development of more potent vaccines against those infections that have been recalcitrant to more conventional vaccine development such as malaria, HIV, and leprosy. In addition, they may also be used as delivery systems for the immune modulators of innate and cell-mediated immunity (see discussion in Chapter 5). Of course, there are always safety concerns with the use of pathogenic organisms for vaccine vectors; however, avirulent mutant strains of these bacteria, which are still protective, are available for use as carriers of passenger antigens. Indeed, BCG, a strain of mycobacteria that is not pathogenic in humans, has been used for decades as a safe, live vaccine against tuberculosis in many areas of the world (119). In addition to stimulating innate immunity, intracellular bacteria are excellent carriers of antigens to appropriate antigen-presenting cells similar to live attenuated viral vectors. However, these bacteria have some safety advantages over many viral vectors. Bacteria have not evolved mechanisms to downregulate adaptive immunity, as do many viral vaccine vectors such as vaccinia and advenovirus (120), and, unlike viruses, bacterial vectors are susceptible to a wide range of antibiotics which may be used for patients who may have adverse effects.

Several hurdles remain to be overcome before recombinant versions of these bacteria will be suitable for use as vaccines. Pre-existing immunity can prevent effective boosting by means of a vector that has already been widely used as a vaccine, such as BCG. However, even in the case of *Salmonella* and *L. monocytogenes*, which have not been used previously in vaccine development, there may have been appreciable exposure to these organisms in the general population (121,122). Clinical trials using recombinant listerial vectors have not yet been conducted, and only limited trials with *Salmonella* have been performed (see Chapter 6). Therefore, how much these factors will impact on the use of these vectors will become more apparent when this promising group of vaccine vectors emerge from the laboratory and into the clinical setting.

1.8 REFERENCES

1. Groisman, E. A., C. Parra-Lopez, M. Salcedo, C. J. Lipps, and F. Heffron. 1992. Resistance to host antimicrobial peptides is necessary for *Salmonella* virulence. *Proc. Natl. Acad. Sci. USA 89*:11939.
2. Sturgill-Koszycki, S., P. H. Schlesinger, P. Chakraborty, P. L. Haddix, H. L. Collins, A. K. Fok, R. D. Allen, S. L. Gluck, J. Heuser, and D. G. Russell. 1994. Lack of acidification in *Mycobacterium* phagosomes produced by exclusion of the vesicular proton-ATPase. *Science 263*:678.
3. Buchmeier, N. A., and F. Heffron. 1991. Inhibition of macrophage phagosome–lysosome fusion by *Salmonella typhimurium*. *Infect. Immun. 59*:2232.
4. Britton, W. J., P. W. Roche, and N. Winter. 1994. Mechanisms of persistence of mycobacteria. *Trends Microbiol. 2*:284.
5. Alpuche-Aranda, C. M., E. L. Racoosin, J. A. Swanson, and S. I. Miller. 1994. *Salmonella* stimulate macrophage macropinocytosis and persist within spacious phagosomes. *J. Exp. Med. 179*:601.
6. Portnoy, D. A., T. Chakraborty, W. Goebel, and P. Cossart. 1992. Molecular determinants of *Listeria monocytogenes* pathogenesis. *Infect. Immun. 60*:1263.
7. Southwick, F. S., and D. L. Purich. 1998. *Listeria* and *Shigella* actin-based motility in host cells. *Trans. Am. Clin. Climatol. Assoc. 109*:160.
8. Biron, C. A., and R. T. Gazzinelli. 1995. Effects of IL-12 on immune responses to microbial infections: a key mediator in regulating disease outcome. *Curr. Opin. Immunol. 7*:485.
9. Chong, C., K. L. Bost, and J. D. Clements. 1996. Differential production of IL-12 mRNA by murine macrophages in response to viable or killed *Salmonella* spp. *Infect. Immun. 64*:1154.
10. Skeen, M. J., M. A. Miller, T. M. Shinnick, and H. K. Ziegler. 1996.

Regulation of murine macrophage IL-12 production. Activation of macrophages *in vivo*, restimulation *in vitro*, and modulation by other cytokines. *J. Immunol. 156*:1196.

11. Sieling, P. A., X. H. Wang, M. K. Gately, J. L. Oliveros, T. McHugh, P. F. Barnes, S. F. Wolf, L. Golkar, M. Yamamura, Y. Yogi, K. Uyemura, T. H. Rea, and R. L. Modlin. 1994. IL-12 regulates T helper type 1 cytokine responses in human infectious disease. *J. Immunol. 153*:3639.
12. Cooper, A. M., A. D. Roberts, E. R. Rhoades, J. E. Callahan, D. M. Getzy, and I. M. Orme. 1995. The role of IL-12 in acquired immunity to *Mycobacterium tuberculosis* infection. *Immunology 84*:423.
13. Fulton, S. A., J. M. Johnsen, S. F. Wolf, D. S. Sieburth, and W. H. Boom. 1996. Interleukin-12 production by human monocytes infected with *Mycobacterium tuberculosis*: role of phagocytosis. *Infect. Immun. 64*:2523.
14. Oswald, I. P., C. M. Dozois, J. F. Petit, and G. Lemaire. 1997. Interleukin-12 synthesis is a required step in trehalose dimycolate-induced activation of mouse peritoneal macrophages. *Infect. Immun. 65*:1364.
15. Cleveland, M. G., J. D. Gorham, T. L. Murphy, E. Tuomanen, and K. M. Murphy. 1996. Lipoteichoic acid preparations of gram-positive bacteria induce IL-12 through a CD14-dependent pathway. *Infect. Immun. 64*:1906.
16. Chensue, S. W., K. S. Warmington, J. H. Ruth, P. S. Sanghi, P. Lincoln, and S. L. Kunkel. 1996. Role of monocyte chemoattractant protein-1 (MCP-1) in Th1 (mycobacterial) and Th2 (schistosomal) antigen-induced granuloma formation: relationship to local inflammation, Th cell expression, and IL-12 production. *J. Immunol. 157*:4602.
17. Hsieh, C. S., S. E. Macatonia, C. S. Tripp, S. F. Wolf, A. O'Garra, and K. M. Murphy. 1993. Development of TH1 $CD4^+$ T cells through IL-12 produced by *Listeria*-induced macrophages. *Science 260*:547.
18. Song, F., G. Matsuzaki, M. Mitsuyama, and K. Nomoto. 1996. Differential effects of viable and killed bacteria on IL-12 expression of macrophages. *J. Immunol. 156*:2979.
19. Orme, I. 1988. Induction of nonspecific acquired resistance and delayed-type hypersensitivity, but not specific acquired resistance, in mice inoculated with killed mycobacterial vaccines. *Infect. Immun. 56*:3310.
20. von Koenig, C. H., H. Finger, and H. Hof. 1982. Failure of killed *Listeria monocytogenes* vaccine to produce protective immunity. *Nature 297*:233.
21. Koga, T., M. Mitsuyama, T. Handa, T. Yayama, K. Muramori, and K.

Nomoto. 1987. Induction by killed *Listeria monocytogenes* of effector T cells mediating delayed-type hypersensitivity but not protection in mice. *Immunology 62*:241.

22. Nickol, A. D. and P. F. Bonventre. 1981. Acquired immunity against mouse typhoid: genetic restriction and comparative efficacy of ribosomal and conventional vaccines. *J. Med. Microbiol. 14*:419.
23. Kita, E., M. Emoto, K. Yasui, K. Yasui, N. Katsui, K. Nishi, and S. Kashiba. 1986. Cellular aspects of the longer-lasting immunity against mouse typhoid infection afforded by the live-cell and ribosomal vaccines. *Immunology 57*:431.
24. Mukkur, T. K., G. H. McDowell, B. A. Stocker, and A. K. Lascelles. 1987. Protection against experimental salmonellosis in mice and sheep by immunization with aromatic-dependent *Salmonella typhimurium. J. Med. Microbiol. 24*:11.
25. Miller, M. A., M. J. Skeen, and H. K. Ziegler. 1995. Nonviable bacterial antigens administered with IL-12 generate antigen-specific T cell responses and protective immunity against *Listeria monocytogenes. J. Immunol. 155*:4817.
26. Pamer, E. G., A. J. Sijts, M. S. Villanueva, D. H. Busch, and S. Vijh. 1997. MHC class I antigen processing of *Listeria monocytogenes* proteins: implications for dominant and subdominant CTL responses. *Immunol. Rev. 158*:129.
27. Weiskirch, L. M., and Y. Paterson. 1997. *Listeria monocytogenes*: a potent vaccine vector for neoplastic and infectious disease. *Immunol. Rev. 158*:159.
28. Sizemore, D. R., A. A. Branstrom, and J. C. Sadoff. 1995. Attenuated *Shigella* as a DNA delivery vehicle for DNA-mediated immunization. *Science 270*:299.
29. Hess, J., D. Miko, A. Catic, V. Lehmensiek, D. G. Russell, S. H. Kaufmann 1998. *Mycobacterium bovis* Bacille Calmette-Guérin strains secreting listeriolysin of Listeria monocytogenes. *Proc. Natl. Acad. Sci. USA 95*:5299.
30. Allison, J. P. and W. L. Havran. 1991. The immunobiology of T cells with invariant $\gamma\delta$ antigen receptors. *Annu. Rev. Immunol. 9*:679.
31. Haas, W., P. Pereira, and S. Tonegawa. 1993. Gamma/delta cells. *Annu. Rev. Immunol. 11*:637.
32. Ohtsuka, K., K. Sato, H. Watanable, M. Kimura, H. Asakura, and T. Abo. 1995. Unique order of the lymphocyte subset induction in the liver and intestine of mice during *Listeria monocytogenes* infection. *Cell Immunol. 161*:112.
33. Kabelitz, D., A. Bender, S. Schondelmaier, B. Schoel, and S. H. Kaufmann. 1990. A large fraction of human peripheral blood $\gamma\delta^+$ T cells

is activated by *Mycobacterium tuberculosis* but not by its 65-kD heat shock protein. *J. Exp. Med. 171*:667.

34. Kabelitz, D., A. Bender, T. Prospero, S. Wesselborg, O. Janssen, and K. Pechhold. 1991. The primary response of human $\gamma\delta^+$ T cells to *Mycobacterium tuberculosis* is restricted to Vγ9-bearing cells. *J . Exp. Med. 173*:1331.
35. Li, B., M. D. Rossman, T. Imir, A. F. Oner-Eyuboglu, C. W. Lee, R. Biancaniello, and S. R. Carding. 1996. Disease-specific changes in $\gamma\delta$ T cell repertoire and function in patients with pulmonary tuberculosis. *J. Immunol. 157*:4222.
36. Modlin, R. L., C. Pirmez, F. M. Hofman, V. Torigian, K. Uyemura, T. H. Rea, B. R. Bloom and M. B. Brenner. 1989. Lymphocytes bearing antigen-specific $\gamma\delta$ T cell receptors accumulate in human infectious disease lesions. *Nature 339*:544.
37. Kimura, Y., S. Tomida, Y. Matsumoto, K. Hiromatsu, and Y. Yoshikai. 1996. Evidence for the early recruitment of T-cell receptor $\gamma\delta^+$ T cells during rat listeriosis. *Immunology 87*:21.
38. Emoto, M., O. Neuhaus, Y. Emoto, and S. H. Kaufmann. 1996. Influence of beta 2-microglobulin expression on γ interferon secretion and target cell lysis by intraepithelial lymphocytes during intestinal *Listeria monocytogenes* infection. *Infect. Immun. 64*:569.
39. Ladel, C. H., C. Blum, and S. H. Kaufmann. 1996. Control of natural killer cell-mediated innate resistance against the intracellular pathogen *Listeria monocytogenes* by $\gamma\delta$ T lymphocytes. *Infect. Immun. 64*:1744.
40. Jouen-Beades, F., E. Paris, C. Dieulois, J. F. Lemeland, V. Barre-Dezelus, S. Marret, G. Humbert, J. Leroy, and F. Tron. 1997. *In vivo* and *in vitro* activation and expansion of $\gamma\delta$ T cells during *Listeria monocytogenes* infection in humans. *Infect. Immun. 65*:4267.
41. Emoto, M., H. Danbara, and Y. Yoshikai. 1992. Induction of $\gamma\delta$ T cells in murine salmonellosis by an avirulent but not by a virulent strain of *Salmonella choleraesuis. J. Exp. Med. 176*:363.
42. Nishimura, H., K. Hiromatsu, N. Kobayashi, K. H. Grabstein, R. Paxton, K. Sugamura, J. A. Bluestone, and Y. Yoshikai. 1996. IL-15 is a novel growth factor for murine $\gamma\delta$ T cells induced by *Salmonella* infection. *J. Immunol. 156*:663.
43. Weintraub, B. C., L. Eckmann, S. Okamoto, M. Hense, S. M. Hedrick, and J. Fierer. 1997. Role of $\alpha\beta$ and $\gamma\delta$ T cells in the host response to *Salmonella* infection as demonstrated in T cell receptor-deficient mice of defined Ity genotypes. *Infect. Immun. 65*:2306.
44. Hess, J., C. Ladel, D. Miko, and S. H. Kaufmann. 1996. *Salmonella typhimurium* aroA-infection in gene-targeted immunodeficient mice:

major role of CD4$^+$ TCR-$\alpha\beta$ cells and IFN-γ in bacterial clearance independent of intracellular location. *J. Immunol. 156*:3321.

45. Emoto, M., H. Nishimura, T. Sakai, K. Hiromatsu, H. Gomi, S . Itohara, and Y. Yoshikai. 1995. Mice deficient in $\gamma\delta$ T cells are resistant to lethal infection with *Salmonella choleraesuis. Infect. Immun. 63*:3736.
46. Born, W. K., R. L. O'Brien, and R. L. Modlin. 1991. Antigen specificity of $\gamma\delta$ T lymphocytes. *FASEB J. 5*:2699.
47. Yamamoto, S., F. Russ, H. C. Teixeira, P. Conradt, and S. H. Kaufmann. 1993. *Listeria monocytogenes*-induced γ interferon secretion by intestinal intraepithelial $\gamma\delta$ T lymphocytes. *Infect. Immun. 61*:2154.
48. Munk, M. E., C. Elser, and S. H. Kaufmann. 1996. Human $\gamma\delta$ T cell response to *Listeria monocytogenes* protein components *in vitro. Immunology 87*:230.
49. Haregewoin, A., G. Soman, R. C. Hom, and R. W. Finberg. 1989. Human $\gamma\delta^+$ T cells respond to mycobacterial heat-shock protein. *Nature 340*:309.
50. Constant, P., F. Davodeau, M.-A. Peyrat, Y. Poquet, G. Puzo, M. Bonneville, and J.-J. Fournié. 1994. Stimulation of human $\gamma\delta$ T cells by nonpeptidic mycobacterial ligands. *Science 264*:267.
51. Schild, H., N. Mavaddat, C. Litzenberger, E. W. Ehrich, M. M. Davis, J. A. Bluestone, L. Matis, R. K. Draper, and Y.-H., Chien. 1994. The nature of major histocompatibility complex recognition by $\gamma\delta$ T cells. *Cell 76*:29.
52. Bonneville, M., K. Ito, E. G. Krecko, S. Itohara, D. Kappes, I. Ishida, O. Kanagawa, C. A. Janeway, D. B. Murphy, and S. Tonegawa. 1989. Recognition of a self major histocompatibility complex TL region product by $\gamma\delta$ T cell receptors. *Proc. Natl. Acad. Sci. USA 86*:5928.
53. Vidovic, D., M. Roglic, K. McKune, S. Guerder, C . MacKay, and Z. Dembic. 1989. Qa-1 restricted recognition of foreign antigen by a $\gamma\delta$ T cell hybridoma. *Nature 340*:646.
54. Porcelli, S. A., and R. L. Modlin. 1995. CD1 and the expanding universe of T cell antigens. *J. Immunol. 155*:3709.
55. Schijns, V. E., C. M. Wierda, M. van Hoeij, and M. C. Horzinek. 1996. Exacerbated viral hepatitis in IFN-γ receptor-deficient mice is not suppressed by IL-12. *J. Immunol. 157*:815.
56. Fischer, J. E., J. E. Johnson, R. K. Kuli-Zade, T. R. Johnson, S. Aung, R. A. Parker, and B. S. Graham. 1997. Overexpression of IL-4 delays virus clearance in mice infected with respiratory syncytial virus. *J. Virol. 71*:8672.
57. Sharma, D. P., A. J. Ramsay, D. J. Maguire, M. S. Rolph, and I. A. Ramshaw. 1996. Interleukin-4 mediates down regulation of antiviral

cytokine expression and cytotoxic T-lymphocyte responses and exacerbates vaccinia virus infection in vivo. *J. Virol. 70*:7103.

58. Kanagawa, O., B. A. Vaupel, S. Gayama, G. Koehler, and M. Kopf. 1993. Resistance of mice deficient in IL-4 to retrovirus induced immunodeficiency syndrome (MAIDS). *Science 262*:240.
59. Salk, J., P. A. Bretscher, P. L. Salk, M. Clerici, and G. M. Shearer. 1993. A strategy for prophylactic vaccination against HIV. *Science 260*:1270.
60. Atlan, H., M. J. Gersten, P. L. Salk, and J. Salk. 1993. Can AIDS be prevented by T-cell vaccination? *Immunol. Today 14*:200.
61. Clerici, M., and G. M. Shearer. 1993. A Th1 → Th2 switch is a critical step in the etiology of HIV infection. *Immunol. Today 14*:107.
62. Parrish, C. R. 1972. The relationship between humoral and cellular immunity. *Transplant Rev. 13*:35.
63. Scott, P., and S. H. Kaufmann. 1991 The role of T-cell subsets and cytokines in the regulation of infection. *Immunol. Today 12*:346.
64. Lucey, D. R., S. A. McGuire, M. Clerici, K. Hall, J. Benton, C. A. Butzin, W. W. Ward, G. Shearer, R. N. Boswell, and C. W. Hendrix. 1991. Comparison of spinal fluid β2-microglobulin levels with CD4$^+$ T cell count, in vitro T helper cell function, and spinal fluid IgG parameters in 163 neurologically normal adults infected with the HIV-1. *J. Infect. Dis. 163*:971.
65. Clerici, M., F. T. Hakim, D. J. Venzon, S. Blatt, C. W. Hendrix, T. A. Wynn, and G. M. Shearer. 1993. Changes in IL-2 and IL-4 production in asymptomatic, human immunodeficiency virus-seropositive individuals. *J. Clin. Invest. 91*:759.
66. Trinchieri, G. 1995. The two faces of IL-12: a pro-inflammatory cytokine and a key immunoregulatory molecule produced by antigen presenting cells. *Ciba Found. Symp. 195*:203.
67. Rennick, D. M., M. M. Fort, and N. J. Davidson. 1997. Studies with IL-10 −/− mice: an overview. *J. Leukoc. Biol. 61*:389.
68. Yamamoto, M., J. L. Vancott, N. Okahashi, M. Marinaro, H. Kiyono, K. Fujihashi, R. J. Jackson, S. N. Chatfield, H. Bluethmann, and J. R. McGhee. 1996. The role of Th1 and Th2 cells for mucosal IgA responses. *Ann. NY Acad. Sci. 778*:64.
69. Fukaura, H., S. C. Kent, M. J. Pietrusewicz, S. J. Khoury, H. L. Weiner, and D. A. Hafler. 1996. Induction of circulating myelin basic protein and proteolipid protein-specific TGF-β1-secreting Th3 T cells by oral administration of myelin in multiple sclerosis patients. *J. Clin. Invest. 98*:70.
70. Mayer, L. 1997. Local and systemic regulation of mucosal immunity. *Aliment. Pharmacol. Ther. 3*:81.
71. Kim, P. H., L. Eckmann, W. J. Lee, W. Han, and M. F. Kagnoff.

1998. Cholera toxin and cholera toxin B subunit induce IgA switching through the action of TGF-beta 1. *J. Immunol. 160*:1198.

72. Lagoo, A. S., J. H. Eldridge, S. Lagoo-Deenadaylan, C. A. Black, B. U. Ridwan, K. J. Hardy, J. R. McGhee, and K. W. Beagley. 1994. Peyer's Patch $CD8^+$ memory T cells secrete T helper type 1 and type 2 cytokines and provide help for immunoglobulin secretion. *Eur. J. Immunol. 24*:3087.
73. Collins, F. M., G. B. Mackaness, and R. V. Blanden. 1966. Infection-immunity in experimental salmonellosis. *J. Exp. Med. 124*:601.
74. Eddie, D. S., M. L. Schulkind, and J. B. Robbins. 1971. The isolation and biologic activities of purified secretory IgA and IgG anti-*Salmonella typhimurium* "O" antibodies from rabbit intestinal fluid and colostrum. *J. Immunol. 106*:181.
75. Unanue, E. R. 1997. Why listerosis? A perspective on cellular immunity to infection. *Immunol. Rev. 158*:5.
76. Ohtsuka, K., K. Sato, H. Watanabe, M. Kimura, H. Asakura, and T. Abo. 1995. Unique order of the lymphocyte subset induction in the liver and intestine of mice during Listeria monocytogenes infection. *Cell. Immunol. 161*:112.
77. Guy-Grand, D., and P. Vassalli. 1993. Gut intra-epithelial lymphocytes. *Curr. Opin. Immunol. 5*:247.
78. Keren, D. F., R. A. McDonald, J. S. Wassef, L. R. Armstrong, and J. E. Brown. 1989. The enteric immune response to *Shigella* antigens. *Curr. Top. Microbiol. Immunol 146*:213.
79. Islam, D., B. Veress, P. K. Bardhan, A. A. Lindberg, and B. Christensson. 1997. Quantitative assessment of IgG and IgA subclass producing cells in rectal mucosa during shigellosis. *J. Clin. Pathol. 50*:513.
80. Phalipon, A., M. Kaufmann, P. Michetti, J. M. Cavaillon, M. Huerre, P. Sansonetti, and J. P. Kraehenbuhl. 1995. Monoclonal immunoglobulin A antibody directed against serotype-specific epitope of *Shigella flexneri* lipopolysaccharide protects against murine experimental shigellosis. *J. Exp. Med. 182*:769.
81. Cossart, P., and J. Mengaud. 1989. *Listeria monocytogenes.* A model system for the molecular study of intracellular parasitism. *Mol. Biol. Med. 6*:463.
82. Pron, B., C. Boumaila, F. Jaubert, S. Sarnacki, J.-P. Monnet, P. Berche, and J.-L. Gaillard. 1998. Comprehensive study of the intestinal stage of listeriosis in a rat ligated ileal loop system. *Infect. Immun. 66*:747.
83. Miettinen, A., and J. Husu. 1991. Antibodies to listeriolysin O reflect the acquired resistance to *Listeria monocytogenes* in experimentally infected goats. *FEMS Microbiol. Lett. 61*:81.
84. Lhopital, S., J. Marly, P. Pardon, and P. Berche. 1993. Kinetics of anti-

body production against listeriolysin O in sheep with listeriosis. *J. Clin. Microbiol. 31*:1537.

85. Belen-Lopez, M., V. Briones, J. F. Fernandez-Garayzabal, J. A. Vazquez-Boland, J. A. Garcia, M. M. Blanco, G. Suarez, and L. Dominguez. 1993. Serological response in rabbits to *Listeria monocytogenes* after oral or intragastic inoculation. *FEMS Immunol. Med. Microbiol. 7*:131.
86. Grenningloh, R., A. Darji, J. Wehland, T. Chakraborty, and S. Weiss. 1997. Listeriolysin and IrpA are major protein targets of the human humoral response against *Listeria monocytogenes. Infect. Immun. 65*:3976.
87. Salamina, G., E. Dalle Donne, A. Niccolini, G. Poda, D. Cesaroni, M. Bucci, R. Fini, M. Maldini, A. Schuchat, B. Swaminathan, W. Bibb, J. Rocourt, N. Blinkin, and S. Salmaso. 1996. A foodborne outbreak of gastroenteritis involving *Listeria monocytogenes. Epidemiol. Infect. 117*:429.
88. Cooper, A. M., R. Apelberg, and I. M. Orme. 1998. Immunopathogenesis of *Mycobacterium avium* infection. *Front. Biosci. 3*:E141.
89. Collins, F. M., and R. W. Stokes. 1987. *Mycobacterium avium*-complex infections in normal and immunodeficient mice. *Tubercle 68*:127.
90. Shaw, S. K., and M. B. Brenner. 1995. The beta 7 integrins in mucosal homing and retention. *Semin. Immunol. 7*:335.
91. Brandtzaeg, P., I. N. Farstad, G. Haraldsen, and F. L. Jahnsen. 1998. Cellular and molecular mechanisms for induction of mucosal immunity. *Dev. Biol. Stand. 92*:93.
92. Mallett, C. P., T. L. Hale, R. W. Kaminski, T. Larsen, N. Orr, D. Cohen, G. H. Lowell. 1995. Intranasal or intragastric immunization with proteosome-*Shigella* lipopolysaccharide vaccines protects against lethal pneumonia in a murine model of *Shigella* infection. *Infect. Immun. 63*:2382.
93. Brandtzaeg, P. 1997. Mucosal immunity in the female genital tract. *J. Reprod. Immunol. 36*:23.
94. VanCott, T. C., R. W. Kaminski, J. R. Mascola, V. S. Kalyanaraman, N. M. Wassef, C. R. Alving, J. T. Ulrich, G. H. Lowell, and D. L. Birx. 1998. HIV-1 neutralizing antibodies in the genital and respiratory tracts of mice intranasally immunized with oligomeric gp160. *J. Immunol. 160*:2000.
95. Langermann, S., S. Palaszynski, A. Sadziene, C. K. Stover, and S. Koenig. 1994. Systemic and mucosal immunity induced by BCG vector expressing outer-surface protein A of *Borrelia burgdorferi. Nature 372*:552.
96. Zhu, Y. D., G. Fennelly, C. Miller, R. Tarara, I. Saxe, B. Bloom, and M. McChesney. 1997. Recombinant bacilli Calmette-Guérin expressing

the measles virus nucleoprotein protects infant rhesus macaques from measles virus pneumonia. *J. Infect. Dis. 176*:1445.

97. Erb, K. J., J. Kirman, B. Delahunt, W. Chen, and G. Le Gros. 1998. IL-4, IL-5, and IL-10 are not required for the control of *M. bovis*-BCG infection in mice. *Immunol. Cell. Biol. 76*:41.
98. Boom, W. H. 1996. The role of T-cell subsets in *Mycobacterium tuberculosis* infection. *Infect. Agents Dis. 5*:73.
99. Erb, K. J., J. W. Holloway, A. Sobeck, H. Moll, and G. Le Gros. 1998. Infection of mice with *Mycobacterium bovis*-baccilus Calmette-Guérin (BCG) suppresses allergen-induced airway eosinophilia. *J. Exp. Med. 187*:561.
100. Lee, K.-D., Y.-K. Oh, D. A. Portnoy, and J. A. Swanson. 1996. Delivery of macromolecules into cytosol using liposomes containing hemolysin from *Listeria monocytogenes. J. Biol. Chem. 271*:7249.
101. Young, R. A. 1990. Stress proteins and immunology. *Annu. Rev. Immunol. 8*:401.
102. Suzue, K., and R. A. Young. 1996. Adjuvant-free hsp70 fusion protein system elicits humoral and cellular immune responses to HIV-1 p24. *J. Immunol. 156*:873.
103. Roman, E. and C. Moreno. 1996. Synthetic peptides non-covalently bound to bacterial hsp 70 elicit peptide-specific T cell responses *in vivo. Immunology 88*:487.
104. Suzue, K., X. Zhou, H. Eisen, and R. A. Young. 1997. Heat shock fusion proteins as vehicles for antigen delivery into the major histocompatibility complex class I presentation pathway. *Proc. Natl. Acad. Sci. USA 94*:13146.
105. Srivastava, P. K., and H. Udono. 1994. Heat shock protein-peptide complexes in cancer immunotherapy. *Curr. Opin. Immunol. 6*:728.
106. Ciupitu, A.-M., M. Petersson, C. L. O'Donnell, K. Williams, S. Jindal, R. Kiessling, and R. M. Welsh. 1998. Immunization with a lymphocytic choriomeningitis virus peptide mixed with heat shock protein 70 results in protective antiviral immunity and specific cytotoxic T lymphocytes. *J. Exp. Med. 187*:685.
107. Kovacsovics-Bankowski, M., and K. L. Rock. 1995. A phagosome-to-cytosol pathway for exogenous antigens presented on MHC class I molecules. *Science 267*:243.
108. Shen, Z., G. Reznikoff, G. Dranoff, and K. L. Rock. 1997. Cloned dendritic cells can present exogenous antigens on both MHC class I and class II molecules. *J. Immunol. 158*:2723.
109. Oh, Y.-K., C. V. Harding, and J. A. Swanson. 1997. The efficiency of antigen delivery from macrophage phagosomes into cytoplasm for MHC class I-restricted antigen presentation. *Vaccine 15*:511.

110. Wick, M. J., J. D. Pfeifer, K. A. Findlay, C. V. Harding, and S. J. Normark. 1993. Compartmentalization of defined epitopes expressed in *Escherichia coli* has only a minor influence on efficiency of phagocytic processing for presentation by class I and class II major histocompatibility complex molecules to T cells. *Infect. Immun. 61*:4848.

111. Pfeifer, J. D., M. J. Wick, R. L. Roberts, K. Findlay, S. J. Normark, and C. V. Harding. 1993. Phagocytic processing of bacterial antigens for class I MHC presentation to T cells. *Nature 361*:359.

112. Darji, A., C. A. Guzman, B. Gerstel, P. Wachholz, K. N. Timmis, J. Wehland, T. Chakraborty, and S. Weiss. 1997. Oral somatic transgene vaccination using attenuated *S. typhimurium. Cell 91*:765.

113. Dietrich, G., A. Bubert, I. Gentschev, Z. Sokolovic, A. Simm, A. Catic, S. H. E. Kauffmann, J. Hess, A. A. Szalay, and W. Goebel. 1998. Delivery of antigen encoding plasmid DNA into the cytosol of macrophages by attenuated suicide *Listeria monocytogenes. Nat. Biotechnol. 16*:181.

114. Kocks, C., E. Goulin, M. Tabouret, P. Berche, H. Ohayon, and P. Cossart. 1992. *L. monocytogenes*-induced actin assembly requires the actA gene product, a surface protein. *Cell 68*:521.

115. Thompson, R. J., H. G. A. Bouwer, D. A. Portnoy, and F. R. Frankel. 1998. Pathogenicity and immunogenicity of a D-alanine-requiring strain of *Listeria monocytogenes. Infect. Immun. 66*:3552.

116. Kotloff, K. L., F. Noriega, G. A. Losonsky, M. B. Sztein, S. S. Wasserman, J. P. Nataro, and M. M. Levine. 1996. Safety, immunogenicity, and transmissibility in humans of CVD 1203, a live oral *Shigella flexineri* 2a vaccine candidate attenuated by deletions in *aroA* and *virG. Infect. Immun. 64*:4542.

117. Noriega, F. R., J. Y. Wang, G. Losonsky, D. R. Maneval, D. M. Hone, and M. M. Levine. 1994. Construction and characterization of attenuated delta aroA delta virG *Shigella flexneri* 2a strain CVD 1203, a prototype live oral vaccine. *Infect. Immun. 62*:5168.

118. Matzinger, P. 1994. Tolerance, danger and the extended family. *Annu. Rev. Immunol. 12*:991.

119. Colditz, G. A., T. F. Brewer, C. S. Berkey, M. E. Wilson, E. Burdick, H. V. Fineberg, and F. Mosteller. 1994. Efficacy of BCG vaccine in the prevention of tuberculosis. Meta-analysis of the published literature. *JAMA 271*:698.

120. Spriggs, M. K. 1996. One step ahead of the game: viral immunomodulatory molecules. *Annu. Rev. Immunol. 14*:101.

121. Gomez, T. M., Y. Motarjemi, S. Miyagawa, F. K. Kaferstein, and K. Stohr. 1997. Foodborne salmonellosis. *World Health Stat. Q. 50*:81.

122. Schuchat, A., B. Swaminathan, and C. V. Broome. 1991. Epidemiology of human listeriosis. *Clin. Microbiol. Rev. 4*:169.

PART I

THE BIOLOGY AND IMMUNOLOGY OF INTRACELLULAR BACTERIAL VECTORS

CHAPTER 2

THE IMMUNE RESPONSE TO MYCOBACTERIA

DOUGLAS B. YOUNG AND JELLE E. R. THOLE

2.1 INTRODUCTION

Mycobacteria are consummate immunologists. The outcome of mycobacterial infection is critically dependent on the immune response of the host, not only in terms of resistance or disease, but also in terms of the clinical manifestations of disease. Infection with *Mycobacterium leprae* can give rise to a broad spectrum of disease, for example, with quite distinct clinical symptoms in leprosy patients with strong or weak immune responses. Patients who fail to mount a cell-mediated immune response to *M. leprae* develop multibacillary lepromatous leprosy, while patients with an intact immune response can suffer from the tuberculoid form of the disease, characterized by immune-mediated neuropathy, but with few detectable bacteria. Similarly, the predominant localized pulmonary form of tuberculosis is often replaced by a more disseminated disease in immunocompromised individuals, and disease due to other mycobacterial species is largely restricted to individuals with some form of immune deficiency. Underlying these clinical manifestations is a complex and intimate series of interactions between mycobacteria and many different com-

Abbreviations: ATP, adenosine triphosphate; cAMP, cyclic adenosine monophosphate; BCG, bacille Calmette-Guérin; CR, complement receptor; ELISA, enzyme-linked immunosorbent assay; HIV, human immunodeficiency virus; IFN, interferon; Ig, immunoglobulin; IL, interleukin; LAM, lipoarabinomannan; LAMP, lysosome-associated membrane protein; MHC, major histocompatibility complex; M., mycobacterium; NK, natural killer; SOD, superoxide dismutase; TCR, T-cell receptor; TGF, transforming growth factor; TNF, tumor necrosis factor; V, variable region.

Intracellular Bacterial Vaccine Vectors, Edited by Yvonne Paterson.
ISBN 0-471-17278-2

ponents of the immune response. In most infected people, these interactions combine in a delicate balance that provides protection against disease; differing clinical symptoms arise from disruption of this balance. Pathogenic mycobacteria have evolved a life-style that is intimately bound up with the immune response of their mammalian host; the study of mycobacterial immunity, in addition to its obvious importance in relation to mycobacterial disease, provides an opportunity to gain insight into fundamental immune processes from a microbial perspective. It is attractive to think that we will eventually learn to manipulate the immune system as effectively as a mycobacterium. This chapter summarizes the various interactions between mycobacteria and host cells, with a view to understanding their relative contributions to protection and disease.

2.2 MYCOBACTERIA AND THE MACROPHAGE

Mycobacteria typically enter the body in the form of aerosolized droplets, initiating infection in the lung (or perhaps nasal mucosa in the case of leprosy). Alveolar macrophages represent their first serious encounter with the immune system (1). Macrophages play a pivotal role in the biology of mycobacterial infection. During a protective immune response, they are probably the key effector cells responsible for killing of mycobacteria (2), yet they provide an environment for mycobacterial replication during progressive infection. Many investigators have studied survival and death of mycobacteria in macrophages, recording a diversity of observations that most probably reflects the diversity of macrophage populations in terms of differentiation and activation (3). The most common bactericidal pathway involves engulfment in a phagosome, which is made toxic by acidification, generation of short-lived oxygen and nitrogen radicals, and exposure to hydrolytic enzymes released by lysosomal fusion (4). In general, there is agreement that reactive nitrogen intermediates play an important role in killing of mycobacteria by murine macrophage populations (5–7) and that this activity is enhanced in macrophages exposed to a combination of cytokines, including interferon-γ (IFN-γ) and tumor necrosis factor-α (TNF-α) (8,9). Induction of reactive nitrogen is not observed in blood monocyte-derived human macrophages, although it has been demonstrated in human alveolar macrophages (10), providing a possible explanation for the difficulties encountered during attempts to demonstrate mycobacterial killing by such cells. Treatment of human macrophages with vitamin D metabolites appears to enhance antimycobacterial activity, whereas the addition of IFN-γ had little (and, in some cases, a deleterious) effect on mycobacterial killing in vitro (11,12). Other technical aspects of macrophage culture conditions may also be important; using monocyte-derived macrophages from human peripheral blood, it was found that only the nonadherent population was able to kill nonpathogenic *Mycobacterium smegmatis*, for example (13). An intriguing alternative pathway for mycobacterial killing has been observed in macrophage cultures treated with exogenous adenosine triphosphate (ATP) (14). This triggers programmed cell death—*apoptosis*—of the macrophage by a mechanism that also results in killing of intracellular BCG.

Mycobacteria have evolved two different strategies to cope with the bactericidal activities of macrophages. The first strategy relies on an inherent resistance to harsh environments and a wide range of physiological insults. In large part, this resistance is mediated by the unusual cell wall of mycobacteria (15) (Fig. 2.1). Mycobacteria have a remarkably thick cell wall structure comprising, in addition to a conventional peptidoglycan, a carbohydrate arabinogalactan matrix covalently attached to a set of branched long-chain fatty acids, termed mycolic acids. They also synthesize a series of noncovalently associated lipids and glycolipids that are thought to intercalate with the mycolic acids to form a waxy outer membrane structure. This highly impermeable cell wall provides a defensive barrier against toxic solutes and hydrolytic enzymes encountered within host cells (15). Modifications to the mycolic acid side chains confer an additional line of defense against free radicals. The introduction of cyclopropane groups in mycolic acids of *M. smegmatis*, using a cloned *M. tuberculosis* enzyme, for example, resulted in an increase in resistance to hydrogen peroxide (16). Mycobacteria also express enzymes capable of detoxifying oxygen radicals; superoxide dismutase (SOD) and catalase have been most widely studied (17,18), although other peroxidases are probably important as well (19). Transcriptionally mediated adaptation to changing environments within the host is a widely accepted paradigm for bacterial infection (20); it is interesting to consider whether mycobacterial survival is similarly mediated by alterations in gene expression. Upregulation of stress, or heat shock, proteins might contribute to intracellular survival (21), for example, and the attenuation of *M. bovis* as a result of alteration of a sigma subunit of RNA polymerase suggests a role for transcription in the

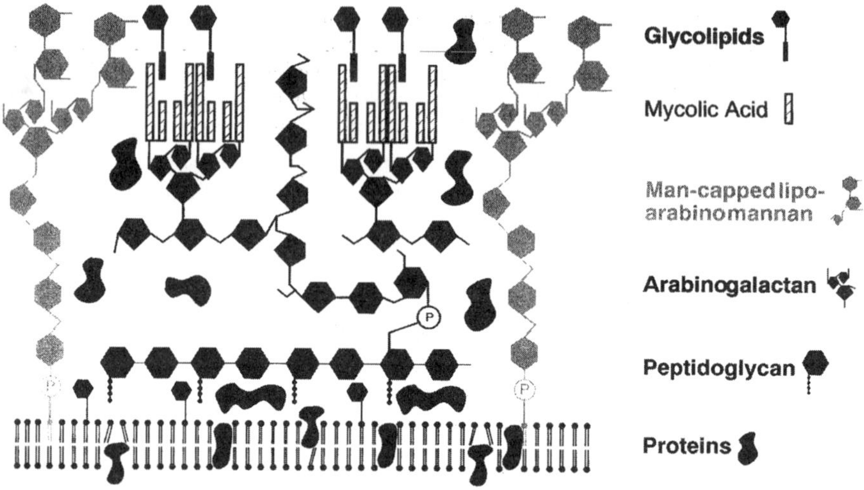

Figure 2.1 Schematic representation of the cell wall of *Mycobacterium tuberculosis*. Reprinted with permission of the American Society of Microbiology from Besra and Chatterjee, in "Tuberculosis-Pathogenesis, Protection and Control" page 297, ASM Press, Washington, DC.

regulation of virulence (22). Against this, however, is the unexpected finding that *M. tuberculosis* has dispensed with the OxyR regulatory system (23). OxyR is commonly used by bacteria to regulate induction of catalase and other enzymes in response to exposure to hydrogen peroxide. As a "professional" pathogen, *M. tuberculosis* may simply have elected to synthesize such enzymes at constitutively high levels, rather than risk their absence at a critical juncture in their predominantly hostile life-style.

A second strategy to circumvent macrophage killing involves occupation of a phagocytic compartment that is segregated from the conventional endosomal–lysosomal pathway (24). While there is undoubtedly variation between different macrophage populations, several experimental approaches have indicated that live mycobacteria are able to isolate themselves in an unusual phagosome that resists acidification and lysosome fusion. Reports have differed in the extent to which the mycobacterial phagosome interacts with endocytic pathways; Sturgill-Koszycki et al. (25) found that the phagosome accumulates normal amounts of lysosome-associated membrane protein (LAMP); others found reduced amounts of LAMP (26,27) and Hasan et al. reported LAMP to be completely excluded from the phagosome

(28). Again, these differences may relate to heterogeneity amongst macrophages. There is agreement, however, that only live mycobacteria are found in this compartment; mycobacteria killed before phagocytosis are processed by the normal endosomal–lysosomal route. The factors that determine entry into this unusual phagosome are unknown. Live mycobacteria might engage some specific receptor on the surface of the macrophage, activating a signal transduction mechanism that affects endosomal trafficking. A broad range of receptors have been implicated in mycobacterial cell entry, including complement receptors CR1, CR3, and CR4; the mannose-binding receptor; surfactant protein A; CD14; and laminin-α2 (29–33). Potential mycobacterial ligands include a family of fibronectin-binding proteins, a haemagglutinin, and an RGD-containing peptide (34–36). Alternatively, some function expressed by the internalized mycobacterium might modify phagosome maturation. The release of small molecules from metabolically active bacteria could be involved—ammonia and cyclicadenosine monophosphate (cAMP) have been suggested (37,38). Cell-surface or secreted mycobacterial proteins that interact with key host molecules within the phagosome would represent a further potentially exciting area for research. Again, in this context, the idea that such proteins might be subject to differential expression—being produced only within the intracellular environment—provides an important stimulus for research.

While the macrophage clearly plays a central role in the biology of mycobacterial infection, other cell types may also play a transient or sustained part in the process of infection. For example, neutrophils may provide short-term accommodation for intracellular mycobacteria and have been suggested to possess some antimycobacterial activity (39). *M. leprae* is found inside many different cell types in vivo, and the ability of these bacteria to enter Schwann cells of the peripheral nervous system is fundamental to the pathology of leprosy (33,40). *M. tuberculosis* is also taken up by a wide range of non-professional phagocytes cultured in vitro, although intracellular bacteria are found only in macrophages in vivo (41). Filley and Rook (42) have suggested that although other cells may take up *M. tuberculosis* during infection, such cells are rendered particularly susceptible to TNF-α-mediated cytotoxicity and may therefore be rapidly killed at the site of the lesion. There is little information as to possible interactions between mycobacteria and dendritic cells; potentially, these cells could play an important role in spread of mycobacteria through the body, as well as in antigen presentation (43).

2.3 PROCESSING OF MYCOBACTERIAL ANTIGENS

The ability of macrophages to restrict mycobacterial growth is dependent on T-cell-mediated activation, which is in turn dependent on the presentation of mycobacterial peptides for T-cell stimulation. Mycobacterial antigens are processed by different pathways, resulting in presentation within the context of cell surface proteins belonging to members of the class I and II major histocompatibility complex and of mycobacterial (glyco)lipids in the context of CD1 molecules (44). It is unclear how mycobacterial proteins or peptides present in the segregated phagosome are able to enter these different antigen-processing pathways. Observations based on cell culture systems suggest that human macrophages infected with live mycobacteria gradually lose their ability to present antigens for T-cell stimulation via MHC class II molecules (45). This observation is compatible with the presence of live mycobacteria in a compartment that is segregated from an "endocytic" MHC class II loading compartment. On the other hand, the critical dependence of bacillus Calmette-Guérin (BCG) vaccine efficacy on bacterial viability, demonstrates the importance of live mycobacteria in immune priming in vivo (46). Viability seems a prerequisite for MHC class I processing, as recent experiments using mouse macrophages indicate that only live mycobacteria facilitate processing of antigens through the class I pathway (47). The processing and presentation pathway of antigens via CD1 molecules is largely undefined, however the recent observation that CD1 molecules are co-localized in the MHC class II loading compartment suggests similarity to the class II pathway (48). Potential pathways for processing of mycobacterial antigens can be envisaged in three general categories (Fig. 2.2). First, antigens may be able to leave the mycobacterial phagosome in such a way that they are able to enter compartments involved in loading of class I and II molecules. Alternatively, mycobacteria may move to other intracellular compartments; escape into the cytoplasm provides a potential route for class I processing, for example, while incorporation into the normal endosomal–lysosomal pathway would confer entry into the class II and CD1 pathway. A third possibility is that the infected macrophage is not primarily the antigen-presenting cell (APC) but that antigens synthesized by extracellular bacteria, or released after the death of an infected cell, are taken up and processed by adjacent APCs. Experimental testing of these different possible pathways might provide important insights into mycobacterial immunogenicity.

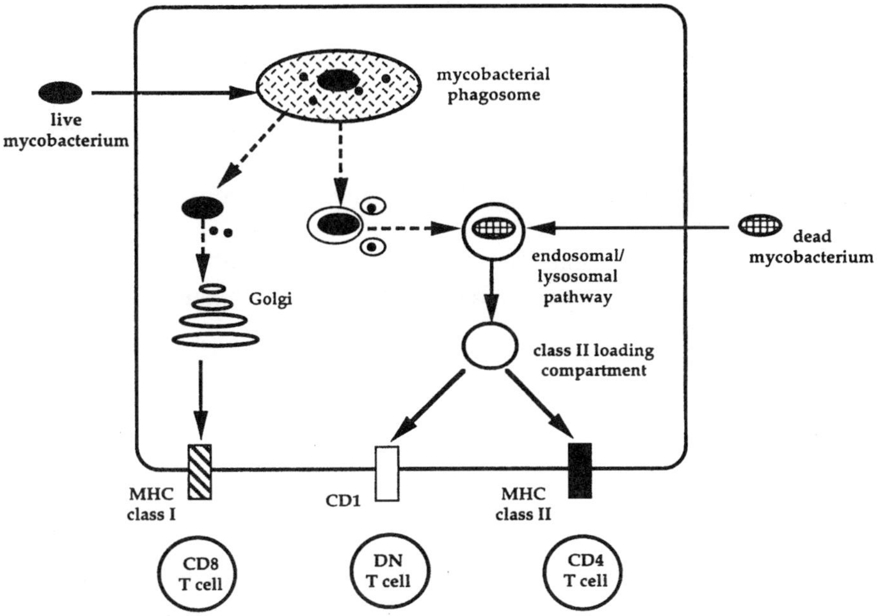

Figure 2.2 Mycobacteria–macrophage interactions and antigen processing. After phagocytosis, live mycobacteria occupy an unusual phagosome that is segregated from the ensosomal/lysosomal pathway. For immune recognition, whole mycobacteria, or individual antigens, have to enter different intracellular compartments to allow processing and presentation to T cell subsets as indicated (the mechanism of antigen presentation to $\gamma\delta$ T cells is unknown). Alternatively, antigens produced by extracellular mycobacteria, or released by lysis of infected macrophages, may be recycled for presentation by separate, uninfected cells.

Considerable effort has been invested in identifying the targets of the immune response to mycobacteria. An array of biochemical and recombinant DNA techniques have been used to characterize a diverse range of mycobacterial proteins involved in stimulation of antibody and cellular immune responses (for reviews, see refs. 49 and 50). The best characterized antigens can be separated into three general categories (Table 2.1). Various proteins have been described as being "immunodominant" by different researchers, although the diversity of the T-cell and antibody repertoires between different individuals makes it difficult to formulate an accurate hierarchy in immunodominance. Proteins belonging to the highly conserved heat shock families—hsp60 and hsp70—are prominent components of mycobacterial cell extracts and are often targets of both antibody and T-cell responses (21). Such antigens were found to be particularly immunodominant during early attempts to generate monoclonal antibodies against mycobacterial proteins in BALB/c mice. The high degree of sequence conservation among such proteins has stimulated discussion as to their possible role in autoimmune responses (51). While mycobacterial hsp60 has been shown to modulate responses in animal models of autoimmunity, it is clear that the bulk of the immune response to these proteins in patients with mycobacterial disease is directed toward antigenic determinants that are not shared with the corresponding self proteins (52). A second class of proteins of particular interest are those that are secreted from live mycobacteria. It can be reasoned that these proteins may become available for immune recognition at the early stages of an infection—before release of cytoplasmic proteins from killed bacteria—and may therefore trigger an early protective immune response (53,54). Particular attention has been given to the antigen 85 complex, a family of proteins known to function as mycolate transferase enzymes involved in the biosynthesis of cell wall components (55). Another important secreted antigen is a low molecular weight protein termed ESAT6 (56). Interestingly, the gene encoding ESAT6 is absent from BCG (57). Finally, a third set of proteins are synthesized as cell-associated lipoproteins (58). Some members of this class have a proteolytically sensitive site near the N-terminus, allowing them to be released into the culture medium as soluble secreted antigens. Proteolysis is regulated by the presence or absence of O-linked sugars on threonine residues within the cleavage site (59). In addition to protein antigens, cell wall molecules such as lipoarabinomannan (LAM) and mycolic acids have recently been identified as dominant targets of antibody and cell-mediated immune responses to mycobacteria. Both molecules seem to be frequent targets for double-negative T cells (that lack both the CD4 and the CD8 co-ligand) and $CD8^+$ T cells that recognize antigens in the context of CD1 molecules on the surface of antigen presenting cells (44,60–62). The importance of nonprotein antigens is further highlighted by the finding that phosphorylated nucleotide derivative stimulates a dominant subset of T cells carrying a $\gamma\delta$ T-cell receptor (63,64). It is possible that the different classes of antigen differ in their access to different antigen-processing pathways and may therefore differ in their recognition by the various T-cell subsets activated by mycobacterial infection.

TABLE 2.1 Protein Antigens from *M. tuberculosis*[a]

Antigen	Mycobacterial Function Description	Mol. Wt. (kDa)
	I. Major Cytoplasmic Proteins	
hsp70/DnaK	Molecular chaperone Member of conserved heat shock protein family	70
hsp60/GroEL	Molecular chaperone Member of conserved heat shock protein family (*M. tuberculosis* has two genes belonging to the *GroEL* family)	65
SOD	Superoxide dismutase (SOD can also be detected in early culture filtrates)	23
16 kDa	Major protein in stationary phase cultures Some homology to α-crystallin family	16
hsp10/GroES	Molecular chaperone Member of conserved heat shock protein family	10
	II. Culture Filtrate Proteins	
apa	Proline-rich glycoprotein	45
antigen 85	A set of related proteins mycolyl transferase activities (also described as fibronectin-binding proteins)	30/31
MPT64	Secreted protein—absent from some strains of BCG	24
MPT70	An immunodominant antigen in *M. bovis*	18
ESAT6	Major secreted antigen—absent from all strains of BCG	6
	III. Lipoproteins	
PstS	Binding protein, involved in phosphate transport	18
MPT83	An acylated homologue of MPT70	6
19 kDa	Glycosylated lipoprotein	19

[a]A large number of mycobacterial proteins have been identified as targets of antibody and cell-mediated immune responses. A selection of the best characterized antigens is shown, with proteins grouped according to their subcellular location. (For further details, see reviews by Young *et al.*, 1992; Ivanyi and Thole, 1994; Thole *et al.*, 1995.)

2.4 CD4 T-CELL RESPONSES

Antigen recognition by CD4 T cells, and subsequent release of macrophage-activating cytokines such as IFN-γ, represents the central element of the immune response to mycobacteria. The importance of this pathway in human immunity is clearly demonstrated by the enhanced susceptibility to tuberculosis in individuals with a CD4 response compromised by human immunodeficiency virus (HIV) infection (65) and by the observation of lethal mycobacterial infections in a small group of individuals carrying a genetic defect in the gene encoding the IFN-γ receptor (66). Similarly, in experimental animal models, interference with this pathway by either removal or knockout of CD4 T cells or knockout of IFN-γ (67,68) dramatically enhances susceptibility to mycobacterial challenge. In the simplest conceptual model for mycobacterial immunity, one would envisage a direct correlation between the level of IFN-γ production by T cells and the efficiency of mycobacterial killing by macrophages.

In response to activation through their antigen-specific receptor, T cells can produce a variety of cytokines that differ in their effector role. These can be broadly categorized into those that stimulate activation of macrophages—type 1 cytokines, such as IFN-γ, and those that promote B-cell differentiation—type 2 cytokines, such as IL-4 and IL-5. Depending on their cytokine profile, T cells can be divided into type 1 (or Th1) and type 2 (Th2) subsets. Cytokines produced by each T-cell subset tend to inhibit development of the alternative subset, and there is a trend for the immune response to polarize towards one or the other subset. Mycobacteria, like other intracellular bacterial pathogens, stimulate predominantly type 1 responses (69). This is the case for both live and dead mycobacteria and is a reflection of their inherent adjuvant activity. Although the molecular basis remains to be defined, it is probable that mycobacterial cell wall components trigger production of cytokines such as IL-12 that are able to promote T-cell differentiation toward the Th1 phenotype (70). Induction of a Th1 response would seem undesirable from the perspective of the mycobacterium, and one might anticipate some adaptation of the pathogenic strains so as to reduce, or reverse, Th1 immunogenicity. Although there has been no detailed direct comparison of Th1 adjuvanticity of different mycobacterial strains, there is no compelling evidence to suggest that such an adaptation has, in fact, taken place. There is evidence of a generalized reduction in the Th1 response of patients with active tuberculosis, manifested by transient skin-test anergy, and by low levels of IFN-γ production by lymphocytes obtained from peripheral blood or pleural effusions (71). This suppression appears to reflect an increase in production of macrophage products, such as TGF-β, rather than an activation of a Th2 response (72,73). It is unclear whether suppression in these patients reflects some specific property of *M. tuberculosis* or is simply a consequence of the presence of a high antigenic load. Recently, IL-6 produced by mouse macrophages infected by different mycobacteria was also implicated as mediator of suppression (74). Lesions from patients with the lepromatous form of leprosy are characterized by the presence of Th2 cytokines, in contrast to a Th1 bias at the tuberculoid pole of the leprosy spectrum (75). Again, it is unknown whether the existence of a Th2 response actually caused the disease or was in fact a consequence of long-term exposure to high concentrations of antigen. Lepromatous patients have a profound anergy to *M. leprae*, as evidenced by the absence of skin-test responsiveness and T-cell activation. Thus, although there is little doubt that a Th1 response is required for protection against mycobacterial disease, no simple correlation allows a Th1 response to be equated with protection and a Th2 response with disease. Additional factors are important in determining the outcome of mycobacterial infection.

2.5 CD8 T CELLS

There is compelling evidence from murine models that interference with the CD8 T-cell population, by direct CD8 cell depletion or by knockout of the β2-microglobulin gene (76), results in a marked enhancement of susceptibility to *M. tuberculosis*. It is likely that CD8 T cells also have a major influence on the course of mycobacterial infection. As with CD4 cells, there is evidence for type 1 and 2 CD8 subsets, and production of IFN-γ may be an important element of the CD8 cell contribution to antimicrobial immunity (77). In addition, the antigen-specific receptor on CD8 T cells recognizes antigen within the context of class I MHC molecules. Depending on the precise intracellular localization, it may be that some infected cells can be recognized by the presence of class I-associated antigens. Thus, the contribution of CD8 cells might be expressed through their cytotoxic activity (78,79). When a macrophage has failed to kill a phagocytosed mycobacterium, it may be advantageous for the host to kill this cell, making the bacteria available to other more activated phagocytes.

CD8 T cells, with well-established cytotoxic mechanisms for dispatch of virus-infected cells, are clearly suited to this task, although some CD4 T cells might also have analogous function (80). It is probable that immunity to mycobacteria involves the coordinated interaction of multiple cell types in a process involving the recruitment and activation of new macrophages together with the disposal of lethally infected cells.

Characterization of CD8 responses to mycobacterial antigens is less advanced than in the case of CD4 responses. In experimental terms, the properties of the class I processing pathway make it more difficult to analyze CD8, as compared with CD4 responses to a particular protein. Very few attempts have been made to measure human CD8 responses to mycobacteria. Live BCG used either alone or as a delivery system for recombinant antigens can induce a detectable CD8 response both in human cells in vitro or in mice in vivo (79,81). Live *M. tuberculosis* appears to be more efficient in facilitating the class I presentation of an admixed antigen as compared with BCG, indicating that induction of CD8 responses may be related to the ability of mycobacteria to survive inside host cells (47). CD8 responses to mycobacterial antigens have been studied in murine models using synthetic peptides to load target cells, and using viral or nucleic acid vectors to induce responses (82,83). Nucleic acid vaccination has been shown to confer protection against *M. tuberculosis* challenge in mice and is being actively pursued as a strategy for identification of antigens for subunit vaccines. Injection of appropriate nucleic acid constructs induces a broad range of immune responses, with activation of CD8 cells as well as CD4 and antibody responses. This will provide an important technique for studying the role of CD8 cells in mycobacterial infection.

2.6 OTHER T-CELL SUBSETS

Mycobacterial infection activates several other T-cell subsets. Natural killer (NK) cells probably provide an important source of IFN-γ for macrophage activation at the initial stage of infection, for example. Mycobacteria also provide a potent stimulus for T cells with an antigen-specific T-cell receptor (TCR) composed of γ and δ chains (as opposed to the $\alpha\beta$ TCR of most CD4 and CD8 subsets). Two categories of mycobacterial antigen have been shown to stimulate $\gamma\delta$

T cells. The first is a phosphorylated nucleotide derivative, characterized in two separate laboratories and shown to stimulate the dominant $\gamma\delta$ subset present in human peripheral blood (Vγ2/Vδ2) (60,63,64). The second is a peptide from the hsp60 protein antigen, which was shown to stimulate cytokine production by a major subset of murine $\gamma\delta$ T-cell hybridomas (84). The mechanism of antigen recognition by $\gamma\delta$ T cells and the molecular nature of their antigen repertoire remain poorly defined. It is possible that different subsets have $\gamma\delta$ TCRs specific for peptide and nonpeptide antigens. Alternatively, it may be that cell activation requires signaling through multiple receptors and that a cell with a single TCR may be activated by a range of different stimuli in vitro. The functional role of $\gamma\delta$ T cells is also unresolved. On the one hand, cytokine production by $\gamma\delta$ T cells may augment the role of NK cells in providing an early source of IFN-γ for macrophage activation. By contrast, in a murine *Listeria* model, the major effect of removal of $\gamma\delta$ T cells is seen in a failure in regulation of the $\alpha\beta$ response, resulting in excess tissue pathology (85). Therefore, while it is clear that mycobacterial infection stimulates recruitment and activation of $\gamma\delta$ T cells, the functional significance of this response remains to be defined.

Members of a further minor T-cell subset that may express $\alpha\beta$ or $\gamma\delta$ TCR, but neither CD4 nor CD8 co-ligand, have also been shown to respond to mycobacterial antigens. In this case, antigens were recognized within the context of the cell surface protein CD1 as the presenting molecule, and the antigens were identified as lipids and glycolipids (44,61). CD1-restricted responses were triggered by mycolic acids and by lipoarabinomannan (LAM), an important component of the mycobacterial cell wall. Mycobacterial polysaccharides and glycolipids have long been recognized as dominant components of the antibody response (see below), and it would seem advantageous for the T-cell-mediated arm of the immune response also to take advantage of this class of molecule as a signal to recognize the presence of the infecting microbe. As with the $\gamma\delta$ response, the functional role of these CD1-restricted T cells remains to be clarified.

2.7 HUMORAL IMMUNE RESPONSES

While interest in mycobacterial immunogenicity tends to focus on the T-cell response, the potency of mycobacteria in the stimulation of humoral immunity is well established, as evidenced by the inclusion of killed *M. tuberculosis* in complete Freund's adjuvant. The antibody level increases along with the antigen load in patients with progressive mycobacterial infection; a number of attempts have been made to exploit serology as a diagnostic tool for both leprosy and tuberculosis. Serodiagnosis works well for smear-positive tuberculosis and for lepromatous leprosy but has generally failed to replace microscopy in routine practice. Attempts to improve the specificity and sensitivity of serodiagnosis have focused on use of defined antigens in enzyme-linked immunosorbent assay (ELISA) or analogous testing formats. A species-specific phenolic glycolipid provides an excellent antigen for leprosy serology, inducing strong IgM responses in the lepromatous form of the disease (86,87). Low levels of antibody make serology less useful in the case of paucibacillary tuberculoid leprosy, as it is difficult to distinguish responses in patients from similar low levels seen in a percentage of apparently healthy household contacts. Several protein antigens are known to induce species-specific antibody responses in tuberculosis patients, although diversity in the antibody repertoire amongst different individuals generally means that multiple protein antigens have to be combined in order to make a test with high sensitivity at a population level (for a review, see ref. 88). Cell wall components, such as arabinogalactan, induce strong antibody responses and can be used for serological tests in which precise mycobacterial speciation is not required. While the antibody response is generally considered as a "side effect" of mycobacterial infection, it is conceivable that antibodies directed to particular surface components could modulate the course of mycobacterial infection. If, as discussed above, engagement of a specific cell surface receptor plays an important role in directing mycobacterial entry into host cells, for example, such a process could be modulated by appropriate antibody responses. At a more general level, the mycobacterial cell wall offers protection against the action of complement, and there is no evidence that humoral immunity provides protection.

2.8 PROTECTION VERSUS PATHOLOGY

The central issue in development of vaccines against mycobacterial disease, and in considering the use of recombinant mycobacteria to delivery heterologous antigens, lies in the distinction between protective and pathological aspects of mycobacterial immunogenicity. Although high concentrations of some cell wall components can have deleterious biological effects, neither *M. tuberculosis* nor *M. leprae* is known to produce any potent toxin molecules. In each case, disease pathology is thought to be mediated in large part by the action of the immune system itself. It is attractive to suppose that the immune mechanisms associated with pathology will differ from those that mediate protection. However, as discussed above in relation to the CD4 response, while there is some evidence to link Th2 responses with lepromatous leprosy, the more aggressive immunopathology associated with tuberculoid leprosy and tuberculosis appears to be mediated by the same Th1 responses that are required for protection. It seems that, rather than a separate immunological mechanism, pathology is mediated by an unregulated version of the protective immune response. TNF-α serves as a specific illustration. TNF-α is an essential component of the protective immune response, acting in concert with IFN-γ to stimulate macrophage expression of inducible nitric oxide synthase, and thus promoting mycobacterial killing (3,5,89). Infection of macrophages with mycobacteria stimulates TNF-α production, mediated in part by triggering of the CD14 receptor by LAM from the mycobacterial cell wall (90). Interestingly, a structural modification affecting LAM from slow-growing mycobacteria makes it less efficient in stimulation of TNF-α than the corresponding molecule from rapid-growing nonpathogenic species (91). However, during progressive mycobacterial disease, high levels of TNF-α play an important role in pathology, and strategies to reduce TNF-α expression are currently undergoing clinical evaluation in both leprosy and tuberculosis. An important aspect of such interventions, for example, the use of thalidomide (92,93), is that they should reduce TNF-α levels but leave sufficient cytokine to carry out its protective function. Achieving an appropriate balance of different immunological activities may provide the key to protective immunity.

2.9 TOWARD NEW VACCINES

Current attempts to develop improved vaccines for prevention of tuberculosis follow two general strategies. The first strategy involves generation of live attenuated mycobacterial strains that retain full immunogenicity without the ability to cause disease. Recent developments in the field of mycobacterial genetics have made it possible to isolate auxotrophic strains of *M. tuberculosis* that are unable to survive in animals. By analogy with other intracellular bacterial pathogens, this provides a promising route for vaccine development (94,95). Similarly, attenuated BCG auxotrophs are being developed for use as vaccines in immunodeficient individuals at high risk of developing disseminating disease after vaccination with wild-type BCG (96). Several DNA regions have recently been identified that are deleted in BCG as compared with virulent *M. bovis*, detailed study may identify genes that play a role in virulence (57). With the complete genome sequence now available, and with information that will be gathered about the molecular mechanisms underlying mycobacteria–host cell interactions, a new generation of attenuated strains can be envisaged in which specific virulence-associated genes have been inactivated. The second general strategy involves identification of key antigenic determinants of *M. tuberculosis*, and their delivery in the form of a subunit vaccine. Some success has been achieved by immunization with proteins isolated from the culture filtrate of *M. tuberculosis* mixed with appropriate adjuvant (97). An exciting novel development is the use of nucleic acid vaccination to screen for protective antigens. Preliminary results with genes encoding selected mycobacterial antigens has demonstrated the feasibility of the nucleic acid vaccination approach (82,83) and attempts are now under way to screen the entire genome of *M. tuberculosis* to identify optimally protective antigens. While it seems likely that one or both of these strategies will result in the identification of novel vaccine candidates with efficacy in experimental animal models, there are formidable logistical problems associated with the evaluation of tuberculosis vaccine efficacy in humans. It has taken more than 70 years of clinical trials with BCG to establish that its efficacy varies markedly in different geographical areas; its overall contribution to tuberculosis control efforts remains controversial. Evaluation of new vaccine candidates will depend on the identification of suitable correlates of protection—immunological parameters that can be used to give an initial idea of vaccine efficacy. The diversity of the immune response to mycobacteria, and the overlap of protective and pathological responses, imposes considerable problems in identification of appropriate correlates of protection. Progress in disentangling the complex web of cytokines and T-cell subsets will be an essential element for design of correlates of protection. In addition to research directed toward the actual development of novel vaccines, research leading to an improved concept of a protective immune response against tuberculosis is essential.

2.10 REFERENCES

1. Dannenberg, A. M., and G. A. W. Rook. 1994. Pathogenesis of pulmonary tuberculosis: an interplay of tissue-damaging and macrophage-activating immune responses—dual mechanisms that control bacillary multiplication. In: *Tuberculosis. Pathogenesis, Protection, and Control*, edited by Bloom, B. R. Washington, D.C.: ASM Press, p. 459.
2. Mackaness, G. B., and R. V. Blanden. 1967. Cellular immunity. *Prog. Allergy 11*:89.
3. Chan, J., and S. H. E. Kaufmann. 1994. Immune mechanisms of protection. In: *Tuberculosis. Pathogenesis, Protection, and Control*, edited by Bloom, B. R. Washington, D.C.: ASM Press, p. 389.
4. Cohn, Z. A. The fate of bacteria within phagocytic cells. 1963. I. The degradation of isotopically labeled bacteria by polymorphonuclear leucocytes and macrophages. *J. Exp. Med. 117*:27.
5. Chan, J., Y. Xing, R. S. Magliozzo, and B. R. Bloom. 1992. Killing of virulent Mycobacterium tuberculosis by reactive nitrogen intermediates produced by activated murine macrophages. *J. Exp. Med. 175*:1111.
6. Flesch, I. E. A., and S. H. E. Kaufmann. 1991. Mechanisms involved in mycobacterial growth inhibition by gamma interferon-activated bone marrow macrophages: role of reactive nitrogen intermediates. *Infect. Immun. 59*:3213.
7. Denis, M. 1991. Interferon-gamma-treated murine macrophages inhibit growth of tubercle bacilli via the generation of reactive nitrogen intermediates. *Cell. Immunol. 132*:150.
8. Ding, A. H., C. F. Nathan, and D. J. Stuehr. 1988. Release of reactive nitrogen intermediates and reactive oxygen intermediates from mouse peritoneal macrophages. Comparison of activating cytokines and evidence for independent production. *J. Immunol. 141*:2407.
9. Nussler, A. K., and T. R. Billiar. 1993. Inflammation, immunoregulation, and inducible nitric oxide synthase. *J. Leukoc. Biol. 54*:171.
10. Nicholson, S., M. G. Almeida da Boneci, J. R. Lapa da Silva, C. Nathan, Q. W. Xie, R. Mumford, J. R. Weidner, J. Calaycay, J. Geng, N. Boechat, C. Linhares, W. Rom, and J. L. Ho. 1996. Inducible nitric oxide synthase in pulmonary alveolar macrophages from patients with tuberculosis. *J. Exp. Med. 183*:2293.
11. Crowle, A. J., E. J. Ross, and M. H. May. 1987. Inhibition by 1,25$(OH)_2$-vitamin D3 of the multiplication of virulent tubercle bacilli in cultured human macrophages. *Infect. Immun. 55*:2945.
12. Rook, G. A., J. Steele, M. Ainsworth, and B. R. Champion. 1986. Activation of macrophages to inhibit proliferation of *Mycobacterium tuberculosis*: comparison of the effects of recombinant gamma-interferon

on human monocytes and murine peritoneal macrophages. *Immunology* *59*:333.

13. Barker, K., H. Fan, C. Carroll, G. Kaplan, J. Barker, W. Hellmann, and Z. A. Cohn. 1996. Non-adherent cultures of human monocytes kill *Mycobacterium smegmatis*, but adherent cultures do not. *Infect. Immun.* *64*:428.
14. Molloy, A., P. Laochumroonvorapong, and G. Kaplan. 1994. Apoptosis, but not necrosis, of infected monocytes is coupled with killing of intracellular bacillus Calmette-Guérin. *J. Exp. Med. 180*:1499.
15. Brennan, P. J. and H. Nikaido. 1995. The envelope of mycobacteria. *Annu. Rev. Biochem. 64*:29.
16. Yuan, Y., R. E. Lee, G. S. Besra, J. T. Belisle, and C. T. Barry. 1995. Identification of a gene involved in the biosynthesis of cyclopropanated mycolic acids in *Mycobacterium tuberculosis. Proc. Natl. Acad. Sci. USA 92*:6630.
17. Zhang, Y., R. Lathigra, T. Garbe, D. Catty, and D. Young. 1991. Genetic analysis of superoxide dismutase, the 23 kilodalton antigen of *Mycobacterium tuberculosis. Mol. Microbiol. 5*:381.
18. Zhang, Y., B. Heym, B. Allen, D. Young, and S. Cole. 1992. The catalase-peroxidase gene and isoniazid resistance of *Mycobacterium tuberculosis. Nature 358*:591.
19. Sherman, D. R., P. J. Sabo, M. J. Hickey, T. M. Arain, S. L. Morris, C. R. Barry, and C. K. Stover. 1996. Compensatory ahpC gene expression in isoniazid-resistant *Mycobacterium tuberculosis. Science 272*:1641.
20. Finlay, B. B., and S. Falkow. 1989. Common themes in microbial pathogenicity. *Microbiol. Rev. 53*:210.
21. Young, D., R. Lathigra, R. Hendrix, D. Sweetser, and R. A. Young. 1988. Stress proteins are immune targets in leprosy and tuberculosis. *Proc. Natl. Acad. Sci. USA 85*:67.
22. Collins, D. M., R. P. Kawakami, G. W. Lisle, L. Pascopella, B. R. Bloom, and W. R. Jacobs. 1995. Mutation of the principal sigma factor causes loss of virulence in a strain of the *Mycobacterium tuberculosis* complex. *Proc. Natl. Acad. Sci. USA 92*:8036.
23. Sherman, D. R., K. Mdluli, M. J. Hickey, T. M. Arain, S. L. Morris, C. R. Barry, and C. K. Stover. 1995. Disparate responses to oxidative stress in saprophytic and pathogenic mycobacteria. *Proc. Natl. Acad. Sci. USA 92*:6625.
24. Armstrong, J. A. and P. D. A. Hart. 1971. Response of cultured macrophages to *Mycobacterium tuberculosis*, with observations on fusion of lysosomes with phagosomes. *J. Exp. Med. 134*:713.
25. Sturgill-Koszycki, S., P. H. Schlesinger, P. Chakraborty, P. L. Haddix,

H. L. Collins, A. K. Fok, R. D. Allen, S. L. Gluck, J. Heuser, and D. G. Russel. 1994. Lack of acidification in *Mycobacterium* phagosomes produced by exclusion of the vesicular proton-ATPase. *Science 263*:678.

26. Clemens, D. L., and M. A. Horwitz. 1995. Characterization of the *Mycobacterium tuberculosis* phagosome and evidence that phagosomal maturation is inhibited. *J. Exp. Med. 181*:257.

27. Barker, L. P., K. M. George, S. Falkow, and P. L. C. Small. 1997. Differential trafficking of live and dead *Mycobacterium marinum* organisms in macrophages. *Infect. Immun. 65*:1497.

28. Hasan, Z., C. Schlax, L. Kuhn, I. Lefkovits, D. Young, J. Thole, and J. Pieters. 1997. Isolation and characterization of the mycobacterial phagosome: segregation from the endosomal/lysosomal pathway. *Mol. Microbiol. 24*:545.

29. Schlesinger, L. S., C. G. Bellinger-Kawahara, N. R. Payne, and M. A. Horwitz. 1990. Phagocytosis of *Mycobacterium tuberculosis* is mediated by human monocyte complement receptors and complement component C3. *J. Immunol. 144*:2771.

30. Schlesinger, L. S., S. R. Hull, and T. M. Kaufmann. 1994. Binding of the terminal mannosyl units of lipoarabinomannan from a virulent strain of *Mycobacterium tuberculosis* to human macrophages. *J. Immunol. 152*:4070.

31. Peterson, P. K., G. Gekker, S. Hu, W. S. Sheng, Anderson, W. R., R. J. Ulevitch, P. S. Tobias, K. V. Gustafson, T. W. Molitor, and C. C. Chao. 1995. CD14 receptor-mediated uptake of non-opsonized *Mycobacterium tuberculosis* by human microglia. *Infect. Immun. 63*:1598.

32. Gaynor, C. D., F. X. McGormack, D. R. Voelker, S. E. McGowan, and L. S. Schlesinger. 1995. Pulmonary surfactant protein A mediates enhanced phagocytosis of *Mycobacterium tuberculosis* by a direct interaction with human macrophages. *J. Immunol. 155*:5343.

33. Rambukkana, A., J. L. Salzer, P. D. Yurchenko, and E. I. Tuomanen. 1997. Neural targeting of *Mycobacterium leprae* mediated by the G domain of the laminin-alpha2 chain. *Cell 88*:811.

34. Abou-Zeid, C., T. L. Ratliff, H. G. Wiker, M. Harboe, J. Bennedsen, and G. A. W. Rook. 1988. Characterization of fibronectin-binding antigens released by *Mycobacterium tuberculosis* and *Mycobacterium bovis* BCG. *Infect. Immun. 56*:3046.

35. Menozzi, F. D., J. H. Rouse, M. Alavi, M. Laude-Sharp, J. Muller, R. Bisschoff, M. J. Brennan, and C. Locht. 1996. Identification of a heparin-binding haemagglutinin present in mycobacteria. *J. Exp. Med. 184*:993.

36. Arruda, S., G. Bonfim, R. Knights, T. Huima-Byron, and L. W. Riley.

1993. Cloning of an *M. tuberculosis* DNA fragment associated with entry and survival inside cells. *Science 261*:1454.

37. Gordon, A. H., P. D. Hart, and M. R. Young. 1980. Ammonia inhibits phagosome–lysosome fusion in macrophages. *Nature 286*:79.
38. Lowrie, D. B., P. S. Jackett, and N. A. Ratcliffe. 1975. *Mycobacterium microti* may protect itself from intracellular destruction by releasing cyclic AMP into phagosomes. *Nature 254*:600.
39. Brown, A. E., T. J. Holzer, and B. R. Andersen. 1987. Capacity of human neutrophils to kill *Mycobacterium tuberculosis. J. Infect. Dis. 6*:985.
40. Schorey, J. S., Q. Li, D. W. McCourt, M. Bong-Mastek, J. E. Clark-Curtiss, T. L. Ratliff, and E. J. Brown. 1995. A *Mycobacterium leprae* gene encoding a fibronectin binding protein is used for efficient invasion of epithelial cells and Schwann cells. *Infect. Immun. 63*:2652.
41. Rook, G. A. W. and B. R. Bloom. 1994. Mechanisms of pathogenesis in tuberculosis. In *Tuberculosis. Pathogenesis, Protection, and Control.* B. R. Bloom, Ed. ASM Press, Washington, D.C. p. 485.
42. Filley, E. A., and G. A. Rook. 1991. Effect of mycobacteria on sensitivity to the cytotoxic effects of tumor necrosis factor. *Infect. Immun. 59*:2567.
43. Inaba, K., M. Inaba, M. Naito, and R. M. Steinman. 1993. Dendritic cell progenitors phagocytose particulates, including bacillus Calmette-Guérin organisms, and sensitize mice to mycobacterial antigens in vivo. *J. Exp. Med. 178*:47.
44. Beckman, E. M., S. A. Porceli, C. T. Morita, S. M. Behar, S. T. Furlong, and M. B. Brenner. 1994. Recognition of a lipid antigen by CD1-restricted alpha beta+ T cells. *Nature 372*:691.
45. Pancholi, P., A. Mirza, N. Bhardwaj, and R. M. Steinman. 1993. Sequestration from immune $CD4^+$ T cells of mycobacteria growing in human macrophages. *Science 260*:984.
46. Trudeau, E. L. Two experiments in artificial immunity against tuberculosis. *Trans. Natl. Assoc. Study Prev. Tuberc. 1905*:157.
47. Mazzaccaro, R. J., M. Gedde, E. R. Jensen, H. M. van Santen, H. L. Ploegh, K. L. Rock, and B. R. Bloom. 1996. Major histocompatibility class I presentation of soluble antigen facilitated by *Mycobacterium tuberculosis* infection. *Proc. Natl. Acad. Sci. USA 93*:11786.
48. Sugita, M., R. M. Jackman, E. van Donselaar, S. M. Behar, R. A. Rogers, P. J. Peters, M. B. Brenner, and S. A. Porcelli. 1996. Cytoplasmic tail-dependent localization of CD1b antigen-presenting molecules to MIICs. *Science 273*:349.
49. Young, D. B., S. H. E. Kaufmann, P. Hermans, and J. E. R. Thole. 1992. Mycobacterial protein antigens: a compilation. *Mol. Microbiol. 6*:133.
50. Thole, J. E. R., B. Wieles, J. E. Clark-Curtiss, T. H. M. Ottenhoff, and

T. F. Rinke de Wit. 1995. Immunological and functional characterization of *Mycobacterium leprae* protein antigens: an overview. *Mol. Microbiol. 18*:791.

51. van Eden, W. 1991. Heat shock proteins as immunogenic bacterial antigens with the potential to induce and regulate autoimmune arthritis. *Immunol. Rev. 121*:5.
52. Adams, E., A. Basten, S. Rodda, and W. J. Britton. 1997. Human T-cell clones to the 70-kilodalton heat shock protein of *Mycobacterium leprae* define *Mycobacterium*-specific epitopes rather than shared epitopes. *Infect. Immun. 65*:1061.
53. Andersen, P., D. Askgaard, L. Ljungqvist, J. Bennedsen, and I. Heron. 1991. Proteins released from *Mycobacterium tuberculosis* during growth. *Infect. Immun. 59*:1905.
54. Orme, I. M., P. Andersen, and W. H. Boom. 1993. T cell response to *Mycobacterium tuberculosis. J. Infect. Dis. 167*:1481.
55. Belisle, J. T., V. D. Vissa, T. Sievert, K. Takayama, P. J. Brennan, and G. S. Besra. 1997. Role of the major antigen of *M. tuberculosis* in cell wall biogenesis. *Science 276*:1420.
56. Sorensen, A. L., S. Nagai, G. Houen, P. Andersen, and A. B. Andersen. 1995. Purification and characterization of a low-molecular-mass T-cell antigen secreted by *Mycobacterium tuberculosis. Infect. Immun. 63*:1710.
57. Mahairas, G. C., P. J. Sabo, M. J. Hickey, D. C. Singh, and C. K. Stover. 1996. Molecular analysis of genetic differences between *Mycobacterium bovis* BCG and virulent *M. bovis. J. Bacteriol. 178*:1274.
58. Young, D. B., and T. R. Garbe. 1991. Lipoprotein antigens of *Mycobacterium tuberculosis. Res. Microbiol. 142*:55.
59. Herrmann, J. L., P. O'Gaora, A. Gallagher, J. E. R. Thole, and D. B. Young. 1996. Bacterial glycoproteins: a link between glycosylation and proteolytic cleavage of a 19 kDa antigen from *Mycobacterium tuberculosis. EMJO J. 15*:3547.
60. Tanaka, Y., C. T. Morita, Y. Tanaka, E. Nieves, M. B. Brenner, and B. R. Bloom. 1995. Natural and synthetic non-peptide antigens recognized by human gamma delta T cells. *Nature 375*:155.
61. Sieling, P. A., D. Chatterjee, S. A. Porceli, T. I. Prigozy, R. J. Mazzacaro, T. Soriano, B. R. Bloom, M. B. Brenner, M. Kronenberg, P. J. Brennan, and R. L. Modlin. 1995. CD1-restricted T cell recognition of microbial lipoglycan antigens. *Science 269*:227.
62. Moody, D. B., B. B. Rheinhold, M. R. Guy, E. M. Beckman, D. E. Frederique, S. T. Furlong, S. Ye, V. N. Rheinhold, R. L. Modlin, G. R. Besra, and S. A. Porcelli. 1997. Structural requirements for glycolipid antigen recognition by CD1b-restricted T cells. *Science 278*:283.

63. Tanaka, Y., S. Sano, E. Nieves, G. de Libero, D. Rosa, R. Modlin, M. B. Brenner, and C. T. Morita. 1994. Non-peptide ligands for human gamma delta T cells. *Proc. Natl. Acad. Sci. USA 91*:8175.

64. Behr, C., R. Poupot, M. A. Reyrat, Y. Poquet, P. Constant, P. Dubois, M. Bonneville, and J. J. Fournie. 1996. *Plasmodium falciparum* stimuli for human gamma delta T cells are related to phosphorylated antigens of mycobacteria. *Infect. Immun. 64*:2892.

65. De Cock, K. M. 1994. Impact of interaction with HIV. In: *Tuberculosis: Back to the Future*, edited by Porter, J. D. H., and McAdam, K. P. W. J. Chichester: John Wiley & Sons, p. 35.

66. Newport, M. J., C. M. Huxley, S. Huston, C. M. Hawrylowicz, B. A. Oostra, R. Williamson, and M. Levin. 1996. Mutation in the interferon-γ receptor and mycobacterial susceptibility in man. *N. Engl. J. Med. 335*:1941.

67. Cooper, A. M., D. K. Dalton, T. A. Stewart, J. P. Griffin, D. G. Russel, and I. M. Orme. 1993. Disseminated tuberculosis in interferon gamma gene-disrupted mice. *J. Exp. Med. 178*:2243.

68. Flynn, J. L., J. Chan, K. J. Triebold, D. K. Dalton, T. A. Stewart, and B. R. Bloom. 1993. An essential role for interferon gamma in resistance to *Mycobacterium tuberculosis* infection. *J. Exp. Med. 178*:2249.

69. Hsieh, C. S., S. E. Macatonia, C. S. Tripp, S. F. Wolf, A. O'Garra, and K. M. Murphy. 1993. Development of TH1 $CD4^+$ T cells through IL-12 produced by *Listeria*-induced macrophages. *Science 260*:547.

70. Fulton, S. A., J. M. Johnson, S. A. Wolf, D. S. Sieburth, and W. H. Boom. 1996. Interleukin-12 production by human monocytes infected with *Mycobacterium tuberculosis*: role of phagocytosis. *Infect. Immun. 64*:2523.

71. Zhang, M., Y. Lin, D. V. Iyer, J. Gong, J. S. Abrams, and P. F. Barnes. 1995. T-cell cytokine responses in human infection with *Mycobacterium tuberculosis. Infect. Immun. 63*:3231.

72. Toossi, Z., P. Gogate, H. Shiratsuchi, T. Young, and J. J. Ellner. 1995. Enhanced production of TGF-beta by blood monocytes from patients with active tuberculosis and presence of TGF-beta in tuberculosis granulomatous lung lesions. *J. Immunol. 154*:465.

73. Lin, Y., M. Zhang, F. M. Hofman, J. Gong, and P. F. Barnes. 1996. Absence of a prominent Th2 cytokine response in human tuberculosis. *Infect. Immun. 64*:1351.

74. Van Heyningen, T. K., H. Collins, and D. G. Russell. 1997. IL-6 produced by macrophages infected with *Mycobacterium* species suppresses T cell responses. *J. Immunol. 158*:330.

75. Yamamura, M., K. Uyemura, R. J. Deans, K. Weinberg, T. H. Rea,

B. R. Bloom, and R. L. Modlin. 1991. Defining protective responses to pathogens: cytokine profiles in leprosy lesions. *Science 254*:277.

76. Flynn, J. L., M. M. Goldstein, K. J. Triebold, B. Koller, and B. R. Bloom. 1992. Major histocompatibility complex class I-restricted T cells are required for resistance to *Mycobacterium tuberculosis* infection. *Proc. Natl. Acad. Sci. USA 89*:12013.

77. Cooper, A. M., C. D'Souza, A. A. Frank, and I. M. Orme. 1997. The course of *Mycobacterium tuberculosis* infection in the lungs of mice lacking expression of either perforin- or granzyme-mediated cytolytic mechanisms. *Infect. Immun. 65*:1317.

78. Silva, C. L., R. C. Silva, R. C. L. R. Pietro, and D. B. Lowrie. 1994. Protection against tuberculosis by passive transfer with T-cell clones recognizing mycobacterial heat-shock protein 65. *Immunology 83*:341.

79. Turner, J. and H. Dockrell. 1996. Stimulation of human peripheral blood mononuclear cells with live *Mycobacterium bovis* BCG activates cytolytic $CD8^+$ T cells in vitro. *Immunology 8*:339.

80. Ottenhoff, T. H. M. and T. Mutis. 1990. Specific killing of cytotoxic T cells and antigen presenting cells by cytotoxic $CD4^+$ T cell clones. A novel potentially immunoregulatory T-T cell interaction in man. *J. Exp. Med. 171*:2011.

81. Stover, C. K., V. F. de la Cruz, T. R. Fuerst, J. E. Burlein, L. A. Benson, L. T. Bennet, G. P. Bansal, J. F. Young, M. H. Lee, G. F. Hatfull, B. R. Bloom, and W. R. Jacobs. 1991. New use of BCG for recombinant vaccines. *Nature 351*:456.

82. Tascon, R. E., M. J. Colston, S. Tagno, E. Stavropoulous, D. Gregory, and D. B. Lowrie. 1996. Vaccination against tuberculosis by DNA injection. *Nature Med. 2*:888.

83. Huygen, K., J. Content, O. Denis, D. L. Montgomery, A. M. Yawman, R. R. Deck, C. M. deWitt, I. M. Orme, S. Baldwin, C. D'Souza, A. Drowart, E. Lozes, P. Vandenbussche, J.-P. van Vooren, M. A. Liu, and J. B. Ulmer. 1996. Immunogenicity and protective efficacy of a tuberculosis DNA vaccine. *Nature Med. 2*:893.

84. O'Brien, R. L., M. P. Happ, A. Dallas, E. Palmer, R. Kubo, and W. K. Born. 1989. Stimulation of a major subset of lymphocytes expressing T cell receptor gamma delta by an antigen derived from *Mycobacterium tuberculosis. Cell 57*:667.

85. Fu, Y. X., C. E. Roark, K. Kelly, D. Drevets, P. Campbell, R. O'Brien, and W. Born. 1994. Immune protection and control of inflammatory tissue necrosis by gamma delta T cells. *J. Immunol. 153*:3101.

86. Cho, S. N., D. L. Yargihara, S. W. Hunter, R. H. Gelber, and P. J. Brennan. 1983. Serological specificity of phenolic glycolipid-1 from

Mycobacterium leprae and its use in the serodiagnosis of leprosy. *Infect. Immun. 41*:1077.

87. Young, D. B., S. Dissayanake, R. A. Miller, S. R. Khanolkar, and T. M. Buchanan. 1984. Humans respond predominantly with IgM immunoglobulin to the species specific glycolipid of *Mycobacterium leprae. J. Infect. Dis. 149*:870.
88. Ivanyi, J., and J. Thole. Specificity and function of T- and B-cell recognition in tuberculosis. In: *Tuberculosis. Pathogenesis, Protection, and Control*, edited by Bloom, B. R. Washington, D.C.: ASM Press, p. 437.
89. Flynn, J. L., M. M. Goldstein, J. Chan, K. J. Tiebold, K. Pfeffer, C. J. Lowenstein, R. Schreiber, T. W. Mak, and B. R. Bloom. 1995. Tumor necrosis factor-alpha is required in the protective immune response against *Mycobacterium tuberculosis* in mice. *Immunity 2*:561.
90. Zhang, Y., M. Doerfler, T. C. Lee, B. Guilemin, and W. N. Rom. 1993. Mechanisms of stimulation of interleukin-1beta and tumor necrosis factor-alpha by *Mycobacterium tuberculosis* components. *J. Clin. Invest. 91*:2076.
91. Chatterjee, D., A. D. Roberts, K. Lowell, P. J. Brennan, and I. M. Orme. 1992. Structural basis of capacity of lipoarabinomannan to induce secretion of tumor necrosis factor. *Infect. Immun. 60*:1249.
92. Turk, B. E., H. Jiang, and J. O. Liu. 1996. Binding of thalidomide to alpha1-acid glycoprotein may be involved in its inhibition of tumor necrosis factor alpha production. *Proc. Natl. Acad. Sci. USA 93*:7552.
93. Sampaio, E. P., A. L. Moreira, E. N. Sarno, A. M. Malta, and G. Kaplan. 1992. Prolonged treatment with recombinant interferon gamma induces erythema nodosum leprosum in lepromatous leprosy patients. *J. Exp. Med. 175*:1729.
94. McAdam, R. A., T. R. Weisbrod, J. Martin, J. D. Scuderi, A. M. Brown, J. D. Cirillo, B. R. Bloom, and W. R. Jacobs. 1995. In vivo growth characteristics of leucine and methionine auxotrophic mutants of *Mycobacterium bovis* BCG generated by transposon mutagenesis. *Infect. Immun. 63*:1004.
95. Reyrat, J. M., F. X. Berthet, and B. Gicquel. 1995. The urease locus of M. tuberculosis and its utilization for the demonstration of allelic exchange in *M. bovis* BCG. *Proc. Natl. Acad. Sci. USA 92*:8768.
96. Guleria, I., R. M. McAdam, G. Kalpana, W. R. Jacobs, and B. R. Bloom. Auxotrophic vaccines for tuberculosis. *Nature Med. 2*:334.
97. Lindblad, E. R., M. J. Elhay, R. Silva, R. Appelberg, and P. Andersen. 1997. Adjuvant modulation of immune responses to tuberculosis subunit vaccines. *Infect. Immun. 65*:623.

CHAPTER 3

MUCOSAL IMMUNE DEFENSE: THE *Salmonella typhimurium* MODEL

TOBY K. EISENSTEIN

3.1 INTRODUCTION

Before the introduction of the oral polio vaccine, developed by Sabin and field-tested in 1954 (1), all vaccines were administered systemically. Smallpox was given by scarification of the skin, and tetanus and diphtheria toxoids were given by the intramuscular (i.m.) route. Rabies vaccine was originally given subcutaneously (s.c.), but newer formulations are given by the intradermal (i.d.) route. Typhoid vaccination was first begun in 1897, when Wright and Semple (2) prepared heat-killed organisms for administration i.m. to British troops fighting in the Boer War in South Africa. By 1911, in the United States, three

Abbreviations: BALT, bronchial-associated lymphoid tissue; BCG, bacillus Calmette-Guérin; CMI, cell-mediated immunity; Con A, Concanavalin A; CT, cholera toxin; CTL, cytotoxic lymphocyte; DTH, delayed-type hypersensitivity; EBV, Epstein-Barr virus; ELISA, enzyme linked immunosorbent assay; GALT, gut-associated lymphoid tissue; GM-CSF, granulocyte-macrophage colony-stimulating factor; H antigen, flagellar antigen; i.d., intradermal; IEL, intraepithelial lymphocytes; IFN-γ, interferon-γ; IL, interleukin; i.m., intramuscular; iNOS, inducible nitric oxide synthase; i.p., intraperitoneal; i.v., intravenous; KLH, keyhole limpet hemocyanin; LPS, lipopolysaccharide; MAdCAM, mucosal adressin cell adhesion molecule; MBP, myelin basic protein; MLN, mesenteric lymph node; NK, natural killer; NO, nitric oxide; Nramp, natural-resistance-associated macrophage protein; O antigen, surface polysaccharide antigen; PBMC, peripheral blood mononuclear cells; PCR, polymerase chain reaction; pIgR, polymeric immunoglobulin receptor; PMN, polymorphonuclear cells; PP, Peyer's patch; S, Svedberg unit; s.c., subcutaneous; SC, secretory component; sIgA, secretory IgA; SRBC, sheep red blood cells; TCR, T-cell receptor; TD, thoracic duct; TGF-β, transforming growth factor-β; Th, T helper; TNF-α, tumor necrosis factor-α; TT, tetanus toxoid; Vi, virulence antigen = capsular antigen = (α-1,4-2-deoxy-2-N-acetyl galacturonic acid)$_n$.

Intracellular Bacterial Vaccine Vectors, Edited by Yvonne Paterson.
ISBN 0-471-17278-2

doses of heat-killed typhoid vaccine were routinely given to enlistees in the U.S. Army and, by all accounts, this vaccine was effective (3). The vaccine, composed of a systemically injected preparation of heat-killed *Salmonella*, and variant vaccine preparations in which the bacteria were inactivated by alternative methods, have been in continuous use over the course of the twentieth century and are still available today. However, within the past several years, two new vaccines for typhoid fever have been developed and are now commercially marketed—a live, attenuated, oral preparation of *Salmonella typhi* (4), and the other a purified polysaccharide vaccine composed of the Vi, or capsular antigen, or *S. typhi* (5). The existence of these two new vaccines is an outgrowth of intensive research into the mechanisms of host defense to *Salmonella*. A major theme in the literature on host defenses to *Salmonella* over the past 50 years involves trying to assess the relative contribution of cellular versus humoral immunity in resistance to infection with this organism (6–8). The discovery in 1964 that cellular immunity involving T cells and macrophages is important in host defense to *Salmonella* (9–12), and that live, but not nonviable, organisms activate this arm of the immune system, led some investigators to conclude that a live, attenuated vaccine would be more effective than the killed cell formulation (13,14). Parallel advances in immunology that defined the secretory immune system in the intestinal tract provided a scientific rationale for the approach of developing a live oral vaccine.

In 1963 a major conceptual breakthrough occurred in our understanding of host defense. Tomasi and Zigelbaum (15) reported that the mucosal surfaces were bathed predominantly in immunoglobulin of an isotype that was present in only small amounts in serum, termed IgA (15), that had been isolated from serum only a few years previously by Heremans et al. (16). It was demonstrated in secretions that the immunoglobulin was a dimer, with an additional protein piece covalently attached, termed *secretory piece* or *secretory fragment* (17), now called *secretory component* (SC) (18). Later, it was observed that IgA dimers were held together by the J chain, the same protein that maintains IgM as a pentamer (19,20). These observations laid the foundation for studies over the next decades that would explore and delineate the *secretory immune system*. Early experiments on the induction of immune responses in the gastrointestinal tract showed that if given orally, antigen would stimulate the production of IgA in mucosal secretions with little serum immunoglobulin response, whereas system injection of antigen resulted in serum antibody, mostly IgG and IgM and a little serum IgA, but not in secretory IgA (sIgA).

Recognition that the secretory immune response is compartmentalized led to the practical conclusion that optimal IgA production could best be achieved by introduction of antigen via a mucosal route. This implication for vaccine development was the hypothesis that systemic infection would best be prevented by blocking invasion at the mucosal barrier through prior stimulation of mucosal immune responses. Amalgamation of the desirability of vaccination with live organisms and the potential beneficial effects of stimulating mucosal immunity led to the concept that the ideal *Salmonella* vaccine would be an attenuated vaccine strain given orally. In 1980, a live attenuated oral vaccine for typhoid fever was launched in Europe (21). As field trials have shown it to be effective, this first oral bacterial vaccine can be seen as the harbinger of a new era of oral immunization. There is intensive research directed toward development of oral vaccines for cholera, for all types of *Escherichia coli* gastrointestinal illnesses, and for shigellosis.

This chapter is devoted primarily to reviewing the mucosal immune system and experimental work supporting the feasibility and importance of engaging it for host defense against *Salmonella*. However, students of this subject should be mindful of the fact that the demonstration that killed cells of *Salmonella*, or purified Vi antigen, injected i.m., are equally effective in preventing typhoid fever as the present live oral vaccine, shows conclusively that neither secretory immunity nor cellular immunity is necessary for host defense against *S. typhi*. For this organism, apparently multiple strategies will induce resistance. The choice of which vaccine is optimal will undoubtedly be made empirically. A potential disadvantage of live vaccines is that in mice, live, attenuated Salmonella given systemically have been shown to induce a window of immunosuppression to non-*Salmonella* antigens. By contrast, live oral vaccines have many advantages over injectable formulations, including easy and lower cost of administration and the capacity to carry passenger antigens introduced by genetic manipulation (see Chapter 6). The ability to express guest antigens in attenuated *Salmonella* opens the possibility of producing a polyvalent vaccine that could provide protection against several diverse pathogens present in a particular geographic setting. This approach to vaccination is a major advance in vaccine delivery. Implementation of this vision for vaccination has been hindered by gaps in our knowledge of the secretory immune system that impact vaccine development, including the duration of memory and the effect of prior vaccination on efficacy of booster doses, as well as difficulties in the genetic processes involved in expressing and maintaining expression of the passenger antigens. Further, under certain circumstances oral vaccination results in systemic tolerance to the antigen; whether tolerance might result from microbial vaccines is a relatively unexplored point. The results of research on these basic questions will provide information that will allow more sophisticated mobilization of the secretory immune system for mucosal immunization. As demonstrated by this review, however, much of what we have learned about the secretory immune system and its function in host defense to pathogens has arisen from oral infection of animals and humans using vaccine strains of organisms that have potential clinical application. Thus, basic and applied research in the area of oral vaccines has been tightly linked. Current trends suggest that this intertwining of approaches will continue unabated in the foreseeable future.

3.2 THE SECRETORY IMMUNE SYSTEM

3.2.1 Anatomic Structure and Production of sIgA

After the discovery of IgA in mucosal secretions and of a related but smaller molecule component in serum, a number of studies addressed the question of the relationship between immunoglobulin in the two compartments. In contrast to serum, IgA was found to be the predominant immunoglobulin in secretions. The two forms were also shown to be structurally different. Serum IgA was predominantly a monomer (7S) with some dimers (10S), and secretory IgA (11S) contained an additional secretory fragment (18,22). Further, secretory and plasma pools of IgA appeared to originate from anatomically distinct sources, as individuals with the genetic immunodeficiency ataxia-telangiectasia lacked serum IgA but had secretory IgA (23). Evidence for selective transport of IgA from the circulation into the secretory compartment came from studies injecting normal plasma i.v. into agammaglobulinemic patients and showing disproportionate localization of IgA in the saliva (24). Immunization studies also pointed to a compartmentalization of the antibody response. The administration of inactivated polio virus by parenteral injection induced high levels of serum antibody but little antibody in the nasal or duodenal secretions. By contrast, intranasal inoculation of inactivated virus induced a secretory antibody response in the nasopharynx with no antibody in serum (25). Secretory application of live polio virus directly into the colon of children with double-barrel colostomies resulted in detection of only secretory IgA in colonic fluids, whereas the serum response to this artificial local immunization was predominantly IgG and IgM, with little IgA (26). In response to inactivated polio virus injected into the colostomy, no serum response of any isotype was observed, but sIgA was found in the distal colon (26). This was an important study because it showed that the sIgA in the colon must have been locally produced in response to local application of antigen, rather than arising by concentration of IgA from the serum into the intestinal fluids.

A major advance in the understanding of secretory immunity was the recognition of the source of the IgA in secretions as originating from plasma cells lining mucosal tissue (27–31). A conceptual advance of equal proportion was recognition of the process by which the IgA that is produced and secreted by plasma cells in the lamina propria makes its way into the intestinal lumen. The pathway is unique and involves the cooperation of two cell types—epithelial cells and plasma cells—with the plasma cell producing the IgA dimer and the epithelial cell supplying the secretory component (24,31). SC was found to be a cleaved portion of a larger molecule expressed on the basolateral surface of epithelial cells that functions as a polymeric immunoglobulin receptor (pIgR) (32). The process as it is now understood involves the plasma cells, which secrete dimeric IgA with attached joining (or J) chain (19,20,32). The J chain is recognized by the pIgR on the basolateral surface of intestinal epithelial cells. Union of J chain and the pIgR results in binding of the two molecules to form a complex which is internalized. Endocytic vesicles containing IgA move to the apical surface, where exocytosis takes place and a portion of the receptor, the secretory component, is cleaved by a protease (33). The dimeric IgA with part of the secretory component attached, $(IgA)_2SC$, is released into the intestinal lumen. This transport mechanism is also capable of accommodating IgM, owing to the presence of J chain in the pentameric molecule (34). It is quite remarkable that the idea that the protein supplied by the epithelial cells might function to transport the IgA into the secretions was arrived at so early in the history of the field.

There are two subtypes of IgA in secretions, IgA1 and IgA2, which differ by the presence in IgA1 of a 13-amino acid proline-rich stretch in the hinge region (35). The relative concentrations of the two subtypes differ depending on the anatomical location. Most monomeric IgA in serum is IgA1, as are the IgA-positive cells in the bone marrow, spleen, and systemic lymph nodes, whereas in secretions in the intestinal tract, about equal proportions of IgA1 and IgA2 are found (36).

3.2.2 Functions of sIgA

The function of sIgA has been slower to emerge and has been less clear than the function of other immunoglobulins. Skepticism as to whether sIgA has an important role in host defense has been voiced. This view is unlikely, considering the abundance of the immunoglobulin at mucosal surfaces. An estimated 80% of all immunoglobulin-producing immunocytes in the body are in the gut lamina propria (37), with more sIgA secreted every day into the gut lumen than the total daily production of IgG (38). As all mucosal surfaces are bathed in sIgA, evolutionary biology would assert that this effort cannot be for naught. Further, many pathogens which invade at mucosal tissues have proteases which are relatively specific for IgA1. These include the proteases of *Neisseria gonorrhoea* and *N. meningitidis* (39), which were the first to be discovered, as well as a genetically related serine proteinase isolated from *Haemophilus influenzae* (40). Streptococcal species, including *S. pneumoniae*, have metalloproteinases that also cleave IgA1, but are structurally dissimilar from those of *Neisseria* and *Haemophilus* species, and cleave at a different proline–threonine bond (41). It seems unlikely that only pathogens invading at mucosal surfaces would have evolved proteases with such exquisite specificity for sIgA unless they conferred a pathogenic advantage, implying that sIgA must be protective for the host. However, the mechanism by which IgA protects has been elusive. Unlike IgG and IgM, IgA is not associated with inflammatory processes involving phagocytic cells and complement. Neither monomeric nor sIgA triggers complement and subsequent phagocytosis of C3bi-coated particles. The main function of this immunoglobulin seems to be to prevent adherence. Brandtzaeg (42) has deemed its role "immune exclusion," meaning "inhibition of microorganisms, bacterial toxins, and other harmful antigenic material out of the interior of the body." In vitro, human parotid sIgA with specificity for various strains of oral streptococci inhibited their adherence to human buccal epithelial cells (43). sIgA2 may also function by agglutinating bacteria in a non-antigen-specific fashion. It is proposed that exposed mannose residues on truncated carbohydrate residues present in IgA2 but not IgA1 interact with type 1 fimbriae of gram-negative bacteria and cause them to clump (44).

A new function for IgA was recently discovered: intracellular inactivation of viruses in intestinal epithelial cells. In culture, IgA was shown to neutralize Sendai virus in cells transfected with the pIgR gene (45). In vivo studies using IgA specific for a non-surface antigen of the rotavirus showed no protection when given orally but, when administered systemically as a backpack model of hybridoma secretion of immunoglobulin, it blocked viral replication of orally administered virus (46). The interpretation of this study is that the IgA in the circulation was transported via the pIgR into the intestinal epithelial cells; when virus was internalized in endosomes, it was neutralized intracellularly.

3.2.3 Cell Trafficking and Mucosal IgA Responses

The question of the source of the IgA-secreting plasma cells that populate the subepithelial mucosal tissue was a central issue addressed by a number of investigators. Definitive experiments by Craig and Cebra in 1971 (47) showed that cells from rabbit intestine Peyer's patch (PP), when transferred to an irradiated recipient, preferentially repopulated the ileum with IgA-producing cells. By contrast, cells from the peripheral blood or the popliteal lymph node preferentially repopulated the spleen and gave rise to predominantly IgG antibodies. Other cell transfer studies led to the concept that cells from the PP drain into the mesenteric lymph nodes (MLN), and then the thoracic duct (TD), where they are detected as a subpopulation of large dividing cells, which then home to the gut mucosa, where they transform into IgA-secreting plasma cells in the lamina propria (48–50). The cells were precommitted to IgA synthesis by the time they reached the MLN (51). The demonstration that transferred cells from the MLN or TD would populate a fetal intestinal graft, as well as the gut of the recipient, provided additional evidence that there was a homing mechanism to intestinal sites that was antigen independent (50). TD lymphocytes collected from cholera toxin-immunized rats and transferred to normal unimmunized rats were shown to appear in the lamina propria (52).

Evidence pointed to M cells, specialized epithelial cells that overlay PPs, as the site of antigen sampling (Fig. 3.1). Robertson and Cebra (53) showed that immunization of a rabbit ileal loop resulted in appearance of IgA antibodies in a second ileal loop in the same animal only if the immunized loop contained a Peyer's patch. Study of the structure of PPs showed that the patches contain antigen-reactive B cells, T cells, and antigen-presenting cells (APCs), but not IgA-

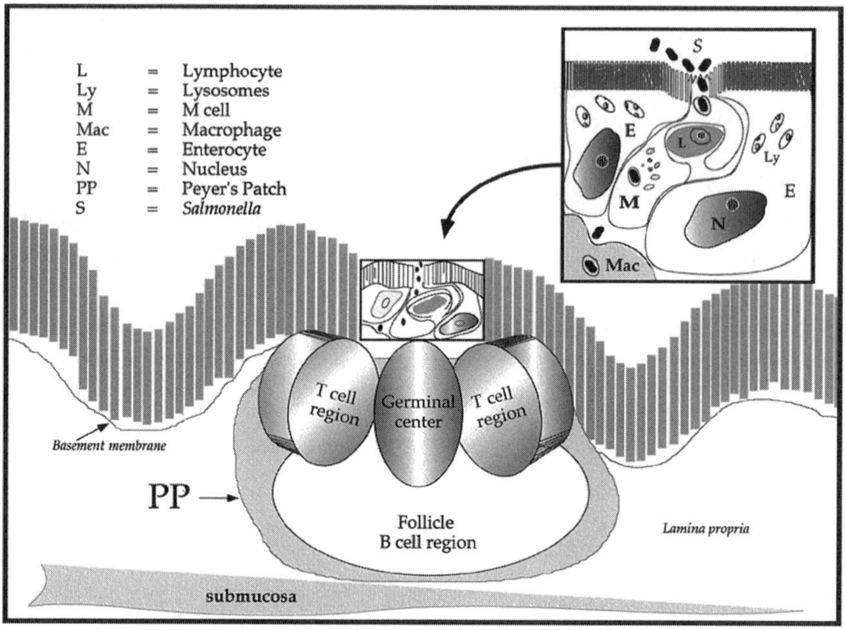

Figure 3.1 *Salmonella* invade from the intestinal lumen through specialized endothelial cells, M cells, that overlay lymphoid follicles in the Peyer's patches. The basolateral surface of the M cell has deep invaginations that form an intraepithelial pocket that contains lymphocytes and macrophages migrating from the underlying PP. From there, they pass through the basement membrane and enter the PP and may be taken up by macrophages for dissemination to other organs.

secreting plasma cells. These findings collectively led to the concept of the gut-associated lymphoid tissue (GALT), where antigen in the intestinal lumen would be taken up by M cells, processed in PP to initiate an immune response, and antigen-reactive cells sent to the MLN to mature and thence to seed the lamina propria via the thoracic duct.

The concept of the secretory immune system was further expanded by the observation that sIgA found in breast milk from developing countries contained antibodies to enteric pathogens endemic to those countries (54,55). In addition, sIgA was found in breast milk after documented clinical infection of the donor with *Salmonella* (56). To explain these findings, it was proposed and proven experimentally that mouse MLN IgA^+ lymphoblasts could home to the lactating mammary gland and give rise to IgA plasma cells in the breast (57). Further, oral immunization of lactating rabbits with dinitrophenylated pneumococci resulted in antibodies in the breast milk (58) and oral immunization of humans with avirulent *E. coli* resulted in antibody-forming cells in colostrum (59). Montgomery showed definitively that the appearance of antibody at the distant site could not be due to movement of antigen from one compartment to the other because animals had high levels of anti-DNP antibodies in the serum that would have absorbed any antigen which leaked into the circulation. In the rabbit, IgA is not transported from serum to milk. Therefore, appearance of IgA in the milk had to be due to movement of IgA-secreting cells (60). Another anatomic site with antigen-processing cells that had homing potential was identified in the bronchial tissue and called bronchial-associated lymphoid tissue (BALT) (61,62). Experiments using irradiated rabbits showed that PP cells could repopulate bronchial lamina propria and cells from the BALT could repopulate the gut (63). Thus, a model of secretory immunity was formulated that proposed that IgA precursor B cells, after encounter with antigen, could traffic from one mucosal site to another (61–63). Other sites of IgA production were subsequently recognized, including the minor salivary glands (64) the cervical uterine glands leading to IgA in the vaginal tract (65), lachrymal glands (66), and nasopharyngeal lymphoid tissue (67). There is good evidence that lymphocyte homing to the mucosal tissues is mediated by interaction of lymphocytes expressing the $\alpha 4\beta 7$ integrin with the mucosal vascular addressin, mucosal addressin cell adhesion molecule (MAdCAM 1) (68,69).

A relatively recent observation has far-reaching implications for the development of vaccines that will stimulate the secretory immune system. Lowell's laboratory reported that intranasal inoculation of *Shigella* antigens resulted in higher levels of IgA in murine lungs that did oral immunization (70). The implication of this finding is that antigens presented at the nasal mucosal surface induce IgA-bearing cells that can populate the respiratory tract. Intranasal vaccination has been shown to be efficacious in developing secretory antibody using a bacillus Calmette-Guérin (BCG) vector for *Borrelia* antigens (71). While influenza vaccines using the i.n. route have been developed (72), the concept that this route would be efficient for inducing antibody in the ileum and colon is novel. The practical advantage of an intranasal route of administration of vaccines designed to stimulate mucosal immunity is the ease of administration. Further, a number of live, attenuated vaccines of enteric pathogens fed to volunteers have produced intestinal symptoms such as cramping and diarrhea. Intranasal administration of the vaccine might induce sIgA without the need to introduce the organism into the portions of the gastrointestinal tract which they normally target, potentially reducing vaccine-associated adverse reactions.

There may seem to be a dichotomy between the studies presented at the beginning of this section and those addressed in the last two paragraphs. The experiments initially cited suggested that local application of antigen produces only a local response at the site of antigen application, and the set of experiments considered later provides evidence that antigen presented at one site can result in IgA at a distant site. These two sets of data are not incompatible. It does appear that the secretory immune response is strongest at the original site of antigen application (73). However, mucosal sites that have specialized tissue for antigen sampling and induction of IgA-secreting cells are centers from which IgA plasmablasts can disseminate. Stimulation of BALT in the bronchial tree or GALT in the intestinal tract can result in a disseminated sIgA response at a distant site. An experiment conducted by Robertson and Cebra (53) is a lynch-pin in this argument, showing that for dissemination to occur, the induction site must have afferent immune processing potential. Thus, antigen presentation at some mucosal sites may be more likely to result in a generalized IgA response than presentation at other sites. In human volunteers fed nonviable *Streptococcus mutans* in gelatin capsules, oral immunization led to sIgA at multiple secretory sites in submandibular, sublingual, and parotid saliva and in tears (74), showing that application of antigen in the intestinal tract can lead to distant mucosal immune responses. Antigen dose and duration of exposure may also be factors in the degree of localization versus dissemination of IgA responses. Alley and associates (75) found that chronic, oral administration of sheep red blood cells to mice resulted in IgA-producing cells in the bone marrow. The hypothesis, that IgA-producing cells traffic through the circulation from a secretory induction site to other sites where sIgA antibody is produced predicts that such IgA committed cells should be detectable in blood (76). Volunteers fed a cholera vaccine composed of whole killed cells and the B subunit of cholera toxin developed peripheral blood lymphocytes, which secreted cholera-specific IgA antibodies (77).

3.2.4 Interconnections Between Serum and Secretory Antibody Compartments

Although the systemic and secretory immune systems appear to be at least partially anatomically distinct, the two compartments still communicate with each other. It was established fairly early in research on the secretory immune system that intraperitoneal priming (systemic) with cholera toxin gave enhanced mucosal responses to the toxin in rats (52). Parenteral priming with cholera toxin/toxoid has also been shown to increase the number of antigen-sensitive B cells in the PP, but duodenal exposure increased the frequency of IgA^+ precursors (78), and the use of PP and MLN cells for fusion leads to increased frequency of IgA^+ hybridomas (79). By contrast, the response to mucosally applied antigen is not necessarily confined to a secretory compartment, especially if the antigen is a live replicating organism. Serum IgM and IgG, as well as monomeric IgA, may be produced. It is presumed that this result is due to leakage of antigen or the microbe into the circulation. Conversely, it is well established in animal models that systemic antibody (IgG or IgM) can transudate from the serum into the intestine. Fubara and Freter (80) demonstrated in mice and rabbits that intravenously passively transferred serum containing anticholera antibody appeared in the gastrointestinal tract of recipients in the absence of a cholera challenge. The movement of serum antibody into secretions in the gastrointestinal tract may be particularly likely to occur in cholera infection, in which the toxin induces massive fluid exudation. Transudation of serum antibodies has been corroborated in humans given parenteral i.m. booster injections of tetanus toxoid. Markedly elevated titers of IgG were found not only in serum, but in saliva and vaginal secretions, as well, implying that the IgG moved from the systemic compartment to the secretory compartment (81). A recent study shows that serum IgG and IgM induced by intraperitoneal immunization with a high-molecular-weight O-polysaccharide of *Pseudomonas* was as effective as oral vaccination in protecting mice against oral challenge with *Pseudomonas* (82). Thus, sIgA may not be necessary for effective protection against all infectious agents that have mucosal routes of entry. Other evidence for movement of antibodies from the circulation to the secretory compartment comes from the recent dramatic experiments from Neutra's laboratory showing that monoclonal sIgA secreted by a hybridoma implanted s.c. in mice finds its way into the intestinal tract (83). Of potential importance in considering the advantages and disadvantages of mucosal immunization is the possibility that leakage of IgA-coated bacteria into the circulation may be detrimental. Griffith showed that IgA1 coating of meningococci could make them resistant to the bactericidal effect of complement-fixing IgG and IgM present in serum (84). In regard to memory T cells, George (85) provided evidence that they can recirculate between the mucosal and the nonmucosal compartments in response to antigenic challenge. Thus, mice immunized with attenuated *Salmonella* by the i.p. route did not produce interferon-γ (IFN-γ) in the PP but, if they were rechallenged by the oral route 4 months later, IFN-γ was seen in the patch.

3.2.5 Origin of B Cells in the Gastrointestinal Tract and Induction of Lymphocyte IgA Production: Role of T Cells in Regulation of IgA Responses

A fundamental question in mucosal immunity is the mechanism by which B lymphocytes are induced to preferentially secrete IgA. Understanding this process would allow intervention and selective up- or downregulation of the secretory IgA response. There is substantial evidence to suggest that the peritoneal cavity of mice is enriched with a type of precursor B cell that can preferentially populate the lamina propria (86,87). The cells express a surface marker previously called CD5, and now designated B-1 (88). These cells are missing in CBA/N mice with X-linked immunodeficiency (89), and the animals have defective mucosal immune responses. Transfer of CD5 B cells from the peritoneal cavity of CBA/N mice without the Xid defect results in normal IgA responses after oral immunization with attenuated *Salmonella* (89).

The mechanism by which plasma cells in the mucosal immune system are induced to secrete primarily IgA, as opposed to other immunoglobulin isotypes has been an area of intensive investigation. The microbial flora have been postulated to play a major role in IgA secretion (90). While it is true that germfree animals do not develop plasma cells in the lamina propria (28,29), IgA production appears to be driven by T-cell-derived cytokines. Indeed, IgA production is highly T-cell dependent, as nude mice have low levels of serum IgA and lack IgA^+ plasma cells in the gastrointestinal tract (91). T-helper cells of both the Th1 and Th2 phenotypes are found in the PPs, as well as in the lamina propria. The patch contains MHC class II-expressing APCs that process and present antigen to $CD4^+$ T cells. There is strong evidence for T cells in the PP with unique capacity to trigger IgA production by B cells (92). T-cell clones that mediate IgA switching have been characterized. The major cytokine mediating the switch in mouse splenocytes and in human splenic and tonsillar B cells to IgA appears to be transforming growth factor-β (TGF-β) (93–95). The demonstration of in vitro TGF-β-driven switching to IgA production by mouse spleen cells requires additional factors such as lipopolysaccharide (LPS) plus IL-2 (96), activated $CD4^+$ T-cell clones plus pokeweed mitogen (97), IL-10 plus anti-CD40 monoclonal antibody presented by cells expressing FcγRII (98), or a combination of anti-IgD plus anti-CD-40 ligand or LPS, plus IL-4 and IL-5 (99). The precise location at which B cells are triggered to switch to IgA is unknown, as is the major cellular source of the TGF-β in the GALT, although the older literature suggests that the switch occurs prior to dissemination of the cells to the mesenteric lymph nodes (51). TGF-β can be made by many cell types, including B and T cells (100). Once the switch has occurred, B cells are induced to become IgA-secreting plasma cells through the action of the Th1 cytokine, IL-2, and by the Th2 cytokines, IL-5 (95,101) and IL-6 (102). Th1 and Th2 $CD4^+$ T cells occur in both the PP and the lamina propria, but Th2 cells predominate in the effector mucosal tissues, including the lamina propria (103). Studies using oral immunization with keyhole limpet hemocyanin (KLH) plus cholera toxin as adjuvant (104) or tetanus toxoid plus cholera toxin (105) have shown the induction of a predominantly Th2 response, with secretion of IL-4 and IL-5, but either zero or low levels of IL-2 or IFN-γ by cells harvested from lamina propria or PP of vaccinated mice. Similarly, in ligated ileal loops, CT alone induced IL-6 and IL-10, but no IFN-γ or Th1-type cytokines (106). Interestingly, when tetanus toxoid was presented as a passenger antigen in an attenuated strain of *Salmonella*, the predominant response in the PP was a Th1 response, even though IgA was induced (107). In ligated ileal loops *S. typhimurium* induced IFN-γ and a Th1 cytokine profile (106). In another approach, it was shown that mice lacking $CD4^+$ cells due to gene-targeting have normal numbers of IgA-bearing cells in the PP and in the lamina propria, but impaired mucosal IgA antibody responses to cholera toxin and failure to be protected against CT-induced diarrhea (108). Another group using mice with an IL-4 gene disruption reported that in mice vaccinated with a mixture of CT and TT, mucosal antibody responses to CT were normal, but responses to TT were impaired (109). In IL-$4^{-/-}$ mice given attenuated Salmonella with a passenger tetanus epitope, normal responses to tetanus toxin were observed. T cells in the gut are also important for natural host defense against enteric bacteria, as nude mice (110), neonatally thymectomized mice (111), or mice depleted of T cells by treatment with monoclonal antibodies (112) show translocation of normal flora or *Salmonella* out of the intestinal tract to the MLN or other extraintestinal sites.

3.2.6 Intraepithelial T Cells

In addition to T cells found in the inductive lymphoid tissue (PP) and in the lamina propria, other classes of T cells are found in the epithelial layer of the gastrointestinal tract between the epithelial cells. These intraepithelial cells (IELs) have complex and somewhat unique phenotypes and their function is currently being dissected. They appear to play a role in IgA responses, but more importantly are probably the site of the gut-associated cellular arm of the immune system. Most of these cells in the mouse are $CD8^+$ (>90%), although some are double positive and also express CD4. Further, many of the $CD8^+$ cells lack the CD8 β-chain, and their CD8 molecules are composed of two α-chains ($CD8\alpha\alpha^+$) (113). IELs show oligoclonality in their $V\beta$ repertoire (114,115). Another oddity is that in addition to $CD8\alpha\alpha^+$ T cells expressing the α/β TCR, IELs are composed of large numbers of T cells expressing the γ/δ TCR, that are either $CD8\alpha\alpha^+$ or $CD4^-CD8^-$, and in the mouse have a restricted repertoire ($V\gamma7$) (116–118). The γ/δ T cells appear to be important in the mucosal immune response, as mice with $TCR\delta^{-/-}$ have reduced frequency of IgA plasma cells in the lamina propria and PPs and make impaired responses to tetanus toxoid administered orally with cholera toxin (119). Studies in nude mice or thymectomized bone marrow-reconstituted mice point to an extrathymic origin of γ/δ IELs (120,121) and of the IEL $CD8\alpha\alpha$ and $CD8\alpha\beta$ subsets bearing α/β T-cell receptors ($TCR\alpha/\beta$) (113,122). Some of these γ/δ and α/β thymic independent IELs display NK markers and have natural killer (NK) toxicity (123), while all $CD3^+$ IEL have cytotoxicity not directed toward NK targets. $CD8\alpha/\beta^+$ IEL have been shown to adoptively transfer resistance to oral infection with *Toxoplasma gondii* through production of IFN-γ (124).

3.2.7 Cross-regulation Between the Systemic and Mucosal Immune Systems and Oral Tolerance

Substantial literature shows cross-regulation between the systemic immune system and the mucosal immune system, and the evidence indicates that it is complex. Most studies report suppression of parenteral immune responses following oral presentation of antigen, a phenomenon that has been termed "oral tolerance" (125). However, some studies show that parenteral immunization can inhibit mucosal immune responses. Pierce (126) reported that prior parenteral immunization of rats suppressed mucosal immune responses to cholera toxin under some conditions.

With regard to oral tolerance, it has been known since the turn of the century that oral administration of antigens can induce systemic immunological tolerance, and feeding of antigens to which patients display allergic reactions has been one approach to allergy desensitization (127). Tolerance can be manifested in the humoral immune system or as an inhibition of delayed-type hypersensitivity (DTH) (128–130). A sound theoretical basis for understanding oral tolerance is not yet fully developed, and the conditions under which tolerance rather than immunity ensues are largely empirically defined. Induction of tolerance may require feeding large amounts of antigen for short terms or administering small doses over long periods of time. Dosages may be critical in the outcome (131). Tolerance may involve induction of anergy (failure to respond immunologically) (132) or active suppression (128,133). Current thinking suggests that tolerance due to active suppression is mediated by secretion of TGF-β by lymphocytes of animals fed using a tolerizing regimen (128). T-cell clones isolated from spleens and MLNs of mice that have been orally tolerized have a Th2 phenotype (secrete IL-10 and IL-4) and produce the immunosuppressive lymphokine, TGF-β (132,133); they have been called Th3 cells (128). In rats, $CD8^+$ clones are also reported to secrete TGF-β and to mediate oral tolerance (134). Even though the mechanisms are incompletely understood, practical application of the phenomenon has been used experimentally in animals and patients to prevent autoimmune disease. Oral feeding of nonobese diabetic mice with human insulin conjugated to cholera toxin B subunit inhibited the spontaneous development of diabetes in these animals (135). Patients with rheumatoid arthritis fed chicken type II collagen for 3 months showed improvement in their symptoms and even complete remission (136). Experimental autoimmune encephalomyelitis, which is induced by injection of myelin basic protein (MBP), can be prevented by feeding of MBP (125,137). This type of laboratory success formed the basis for experimental therapy of patients with multiple sclerosis, which were shown to benefit from feeding of myelin antigens (138). However, contrary results may also occur after oral presentation of antigen, as illustrated by a study in which mice were sensitized to ovalbumin, and subsequent feeding of albumin induced autoimmune diabetes due to activation of cytotoxic T cells (139). While a complete discussion of the current views on oral tolerance is beyond the scope of this review, the possibility that oral presentation of antigen may result in systemic tolerance needs to be considered and evaluated in development of oral vaccines. This potentially undesirable side-effect of oral vaccination has received little attention in the arena of engineering safe vaccines. This phenomenon could be important, because as mentioned in the Introduction, and as is developed further under Systemic Immunity to *Salmonella* (Section 3.3.5), a vaccine strategy that could lead to induction of secretory immunity, with suppression of systemic immunity, would be a poor choice, as systemic immunity has proved to protect against typhoid fever.

3.2.8 Summary of the Role of T Cells in the Gut

Sorting out the complex thymic-dependent and -independent subsets of T cells in the gastrointestinal tract is an ongoing process. Understanding how the various subsets regulate mucosal immunity, and possibly systemic immunity as well, is in an even more primitive state. The demonstration that there are $CD4^+$ cells in the secretory system which exhibit either Th1 or Th2 cytokine profiles suggests that there will be a need to dissect the factors that polarize the immune response of mucosally presented antigens toward one or the other profile. Whether these will be the same or different from the factors identified in the systemic compartment is still to be determined. The apparently dual role of TGF-β in mediating switching to IgA production by B cells and in inducing tolerance has not been clarified. The contribution of cytotoxic T cells and of T cells with NK-like activity to mucosal host defense to various classes of pathogens is presently unknown, as these activities have only recently been defined. These large areas of uncertainty force the vaccine initiatives to proceed largely on the basis of empirical observations of efficacy.

3.3 *SALMONELLA:* INFECTION AND IMMUNITY

3.3.1 Overview

Salmonella comprise a large antigenically diverse group of organisms, with more than a 1,000 serotypes based on variations of surface polysaccharide antigens (O antigens), flagellar antigens (H antigens) and capsular antigens (Vi antigen) (140). The vast majority of bacteria in the genus cause gastroenteritis in humans and have reservoirs in a variety of animals, including farm animals and reptiles (141). Gastroenteritis results from infection of the small intestine after ingestion of Salmonella, and watery diarrhea is the main symptom. The infection usually does not become systemic except in immunocompromised hosts. In contrast, infection with a very limited group of *Salmonella* results in enteric fever, which is a systemic disease. Typhoid fever, caused by *S. typhi* is the prototype. *S. paratyphi* A and B also cause similar but milder syndromes. These organisms differ from the other serotypes of *Salmonella* in that they only infect humans. A few species of *Salmonella*, including *S. cholerasuis*, can also cause a septic syndrome, about which little is known in terms of the source of the organism and mechanism of pathogenicity. Major attention has focused on typhoid fever because in the pre-antibiotic era it was among the major fatal infectious diseases in the world. In developing countries with poor sanitation, typhoid fever continues to be a major cause of morbidity and mortality, with an estimated 12.5 million cases per year (142), and death rates of 15% (143). As noted in the Introduction, risk of typhoid infection was considered such a severe problem for the British military at the turn of the century that Wright developed a typhoid vaccine to protect the troops. There has been an extraordinary amount of research on *Salmonella* host–pathogen interactions during the twentieth century. Since *S. typhi* is a human pathogen and is avirulent for animals except the monkey, it could not be conveniently used in laboratory work. However, it was noted that *S. typhimurium* (literally mouse typhoid) is a naturally occurring pathogen of mice that causes an enteric fever similar to typhoid fever in humans. *S. enteritidis* produces similar systemic symptoms in mice. The model of *S. typhimurium* or *enteritidis* infection in mice was adopted and widely used for pathogenesis, immunity, and vaccine studies of typhoid fever. A potentially confusing aspect of the model is that the same organisms, *S. typhimurium*, and *S. enteritidis*, can infect humans, but in humans they cause gastroenteritis, not enteric fever. Since *S. typhi* has a polysaccharide capsule (α-1,4-2-deoxy-2-N-acetyl galacturonic acid) (144), the virulence (Vi) antigen, and *S. typhimurium* does not, the model is clearly imperfect. Whether the capsule is important in pathogenesis is not yet firmly established, as experimental work with *S. typhi* has been limited. Comparative infectivity of humans and monkeys with strains of *S. typhi* expressing Vi or lacking it showed that Vi does augment virulence (145). Another potentially confounding aspect to infection-immunity studies with *Salmonella* in the mouse is the wide variation in innate susceptibility of outbred and various inbred strains to infection. At least four genes control innate susceptibility (6,146–151), of which only *Ity*, whose gene product is natural resistance-associated macrophage protein (Nramp1) (152), is widely appreciated. Most studies using the mouse model have also employed intravenous or intraperitoneal infection, rather than oral infection. With systemic infection, susceptibility can range from as little as 1 cell i.p. to 10^4 cells. The differences among mouse strains are important because the mechanisms of systemic immunity vary with the innate susceptibility or resistance of the mouse. Thus, killed cells and extracts of Salmonella will protect innately resistant mice but are poorly protective in innately susceptible mice against intraperitoneal challenge (148). Passive serum will protect innately resistant mice against intraperitoneal challenge with *S. typhimurium* but will not protect innately susceptible mice (148). It has been proposed that rather than a single mouse model of typhoid fever, there is a spectrum of models (6). The question has been raised as to which model more closely approximates the human, or whether different geographically isolated populations of humans may also exhibit genetically determined differences in susceptibility and immunizability (6,7). The human would appear to be most similar to the inherently resistant mice, as nonviable vaccines are quite effective, including purified Vi antigen (5,153).

The use of systemic infection, rather than oral infection, in the mouse has been justified in studies examining immune responses, on the theory that the major function of the immune response was to contain dissemination of growth of the organisms once they crossed the gut barrier and gained access to the circulation. Thus, growth in the liver and spleen has been deemed the most important aspect of *Salmonella* infection in need of control. The fact that the killed cell vaccine has efficacy, that it is given systemically, and that it works by inducing antibody to surface antigens suggests that the major control point for arresting the infection is not necessarily at the point of entry in the gut. Antibodies in serum are clearly effective. A practical reason for using parenteral injection of *Salmonella* in studies in mice is the greater uniformity of infection obtained in small groups of animals when organisms are given by injection rather than by feeding. To achieve uniform infection by the oral route, it is necessary to either 1) restrict food intake, as undigested food in the intestinal tract interferes with pathogenesis, or 2) to dose animals with bicarbonate to neutralize stomach acid before infection (154). Also, if inherently resistant mice are used for oral inoculation, the dose necessary to achieve an LD_{50} is quite high, $> 10^6$ (155).

3.3.2 Pathogenesis of *S. typhi* and *S. typhimurium*

From pathological specimens in humans, it was proposed that *S. typhi* infect via the Peyer's patch cells and gain access to the circulation via the mesenteric lymph nodes and then the thoracic duct. From the blood they seed the liver and spleen where they multiply. This general pathway has been substantiated using the chimpanzee (156) given *S. typhi*, and the mouse model of oral infection with *S. typhimurium* (154,157,158). Several studies showed that a significant fraction of an oral inoculum becomes associated with PP within a few hours after introduction into the alimentary tract (157,159,160). The major conduit for the *Salmonella* appears to be the M cells overlaying the PP (Fig. 3.1). In studies using mouse ligated ileal loops *Salmonella* were found to induce membrane ruffling of the M cells, followed by their internalization and subsequent disruption of the architecture of the M cell (161–163). By contrast, *S. typhimurium* introduced into rabbit ligated ileal loops resulted in no cytopathic effect. Instead the organisms transcytosed the M cells (164). Salmonella can also interact with enterocytes, cells of epithelial origin which line the gastric mucosa but are not specialized for antigen sampling. This was first demonstrated in studies by Takeuchi (165) in guinea pigs, who observed that invasion was accompanied by disruption of microvilli, followed by appearance of bacteria in the cytoplasm in membrane-bound vesicles. At the light microscope level, 8 hours after oral inoculation of germfree mice with *S. typhimurium* organisms could be seen in close association with the gastric epithelial cells (166). Morphological observation of the effect of wild-type organisms on tissue culture cells has shown that membrane ruffling is a usual motif before cell penetration (167–172). In polarized epithelial cells in tissue culture, *Salmonella* can also be demonstrated to transcytose from the apical to the basolateral surface (173,174). In a novel model using a layer of human T84 cells that forms tight junctions, *Salmonella* applied to the apical surface were shown to induce migration of human polymorphonuclear cells (PMNs) from the basolateral surface through the tight junctions, apparently due to induction of IL-8 (175). PMNs are prominent in the pathological response to *Salmonella* strains which cause gastroenteritis, as compared with infection with strains such as *S. typhi*, causing enteric fevers.

After *Salmonella* penetrate the epithelial layer of the intestinal tract, there is less known about how they migrate into the circulation. One hypothesis, for which there are data, is that they traffic inside of mononuclear phagocytes. Phagocytic uptake could occur in the PP or in the draining lymph nodes. It has been observed that the majority of *S. typhi* in the blood of patients with typhoid fever is associated with the mononuclear cell fraction (176).

3.3.3 Systemic Immunity to *Salmonella* in Humans

3.3.3.1 Induction of Protective Serum Antibodies by Nonviable Parenteral Vaccines. The history of studies on immunity to typhoid fever stretches throughout the twentieth century, following the formulation and use of the first typhoid vaccine in 1897 by Wright and Semple (2). The vaccine was clearly efficacious as shown by epidemiologic data from the U.S. Army. After adoption of compulsory vaccination in 1911, the attack rate for typhoid fever dropped 14-fold (3). The classic formulation consisted of heat-killed *S. typhi* injected i.m. in three doses at least a week apart. After discovery of the Vi capsular antigen in 1935, acetone-killed cells were used, as this procedure was thought to provide better preservation of the Vi antigen (3). During the 1960s, the World Health Organization (WHO) sponsored a series of large scale, double-blind field trials comparing acetone-killed versus heat-killed cells and other formulations. It was conclusively shown that several of these vaccines offered significant protection that lasted up to 7 years (177–180). A major problem with these systemically injected killed vaccines is their toxicity. Vaccinees may experience soreness at the site of injection, fever, and chills (21). The mechanism of action of these vaccines is by induction of circulating IgM and IgG antibodies to O, H, and Vi antigens (6). Antibody is not regularly found in the feces of vaccinees, suggesting that secretory antibody is not induced by this procedure (181). Purified Vi antigen alone is sufficient to induce protection against typhoid fever, simply by induction of antibodies (5,153). It is of theoretical interest that the presence of antibodies in serum is sufficient to protect against typhoid fever, in spite of the fact that the organisms enter the host via Peyer's patches. Systemic antibody efficacy is probably attributable to reduction of the bacterial burden as organisms pass through the blood on their way to seeding the liver and spleen after leaving the patch. A similar mechanisms is at work in hepatitis B infection, in which vaccine-induced serum antibodies are effective because the organism has a viremic phase before targeting the cells in the liver.

3.3.3.2 Live Versus Nonviable Salmonella Vaccines: Mouse Studies. Complexity in understanding the mechanism of host defense to *S. typhi* arose from several observations in mouse models of typhoid fever using *S. typhimurium* or *S. enteritidis* infection: (1) reports of difficulty in immunizing mice with nonviable vaccines against systemic challenge with these organisms (182,183); (2) reports of difficulty in protecting mice with passive immune serum (182–186); and (3) the discovery of the cellular arm of the immune system and its role in host defense to murine salmonellosis. In 1966, Mackaness, Collins and Blanden at the Trudeau Institute published three seminal papers reporting that killed cells were poorly protective against intravenous challenge with *S. typhimurium*, but that the mice which had been exposed to a sublethal dose of living organisms of the strain showed high levels of resistance (10,11,187). Further, the capacity of the live vaccines to protect, correlated with induction of DTH, which killed vaccines did not induce (188). (DTH was measured by footpad swelling in response to injection of complex protein extracts of *Salmonella*). These studies extended the work of Ushiba who had previously shown that there were two mechanisms of immunity in mouse typhoid, "cellular immunity" and "humoral immunity" (9). The results also supported similar and more extensive studies on the mechanism of protection induced by live *Mycobacteria* and *Listeria* (12,13). Mackaness formulated a brilliant theory that was generalized to apply to all organisms that are facultative intracellular pathogens of macrophages, namely that ultimate resistance depends on activation of macrophages (14). The cellular arm of the immune system, later known as the T-cell arm, provided the antigen-specific memory. Once memory T cells re-engaged the antigen for which they were specifically reactive they secreted molecules into the supernatant which activated the macrophages to an enhanced microbicidal state. The "angry macrophage" was viewed as the most important host defense against pathogens which could parasitize it (14). The development of this theory spurred the research that identified IFN-γ as the major cytokine produced by antigen-activated T cells, and led indirectly to the studies defining the balance between Th1 and Th2 cells as a major determinant in whether immune responses will be primarily cellular (Th1-cell and macrophage) or humoral (Th2) (189). Fortuitously, the mice used by the group at the Trudeau Institute to compare the capacity of viable and nonviable vaccines were inherently hypersusceptible to *Salmonella* infection. It was subsequently demonstrated by Eisenstein and associates that hypersusceptible mice are poorly immunized by nonviable vaccines, while inherently resistant mice are protected to quite high levels (148). Thus, the Trudeau group had concluded that killed *Salmonella* were highly inadequate compared with live cells because they had inadvertently used a mouse that was poorly protected by killed cells. However, because of the enormous import of the theory of cellular immunity, the data impugning the efficacy of nonviable cells quickly permeated the literature. This occurred in spite of the rather extensive literature from a variety of laboratories showing that, in other mouse strains, nonviable vaccines were highly protective (190–193). In fact, Swedish investigators showed that vaccination with purified octasaccharide of the O antigen of *Salmonella* chemically linked to a carrier protein was sufficient to protect mice against 100 LD_{50} doses of virulent organisms (194). Furthermore, several groups showed that passive immune serum raised to killed *Salmonella* confers substantial protection against virulent challenge in inherently resistant mouse strains (190,195). Antiserum to the O-octasaccharide linked to bovine serum albumin (BSA) protected mice against 100 LD_{50} doses (196,197). Eisenstein's group showed that immune serum protected inherently resistant mice, but not inherently hypersusceptible mice (148). Nonetheless, selective reading of the literature gave rise to the generalization promulgated at the Trudeau Institute that only live cells could give maximal protection through a non-antibody-based mechanism (13). Widespread acceptance of the experimental discrediting of killed vaccines, along with their rather marked toxicity in humans, led investigators to look for alternative methods of vaccine development. As described above, developments in understanding mechanisms of immunity to *Salmonella* paralleled the unfolding of knowledge about the secretory immune system. A major conclusion of experimental work in that field suggested that for optimal stimulation of secretory IgA, antigen should be presented at the mucosal surface. A marriage occurred between the concept that the optimal vaccine should be a live attenuated strain and the idea that it should be given orally. However, basic research on the mechanisms of immunity to *Salmonella* continued using systemic routes of infection, and most of our knowledge has actually been gleaned primarily using nonoral inoculations. This literature will be considered before moving to the newer and less explored territory of responses to oral immunization.

3.3.3.3 The Role of T Cells in Systemic Salmonella Immunity. The experiments cited above inferred that the cellular arm of the immune system must play a role in host defense in murine models of *Salmonella* infection using *hypersusceptible* mice based on the observations that 1) the live salmonellae were so much more effective in inducing protective immunity than were killed cells; 2) the living vaccines promoted clearance of challenge organisms from the spleen, which the killed vaccines did not; 3) passive immune serum was not effective in transferring immunity; and 4) development of immunity correlated with the demonstration of a DTH response as assayed in mice by footpad swelling to a *Salmonella* antigen. It is noteworthy that definitive experiments showing that immunity to *Salmonella* could be transferred with T cells from live-cell vaccinated mice were never done by the Trudeau group for *Salmonella* as they were for *Listeria* and *Mycobacteria.* Thus, the evidence for involvement of T cells in defense against *Salmonella* during the late 1960s and early 1970s was largely circumstantial. Experiments carried out during the mid-1970s actually supported a role for B cells as most important in immunity to murine salmonellosis, as immune B cells were reported to be more effective than T cells in transferring adoptive immunity to *Salmonella* (198) and cyclophosphamide, but not antithymocyte serum, sensitized mice to mortality from an attenuated strain of *Salmonella* (199). Some direct evidence for a role for T cells was provided later by Nauciel (200), who showed that depletion of $CD4^+$ cells have a small effect on the ability to eliminate an attenuated strain of *Salmonella*, and by Davies and Kotlarski (201), who reported that anti-CD4 treatment of mice receiving an attenuated strain prevented induction of protective immunity. Several other groups also provided evidence that transfer of immune T-cell-enriched spleen cell fractions could adoptively transfer immunity (7,202–204). These studies did not rule out the possibility that the T cells protected through a helper function that resulted in antibody formation rather than through a cellular immune pathway. Further, Killar and Eisenstein (205,206) showed that protection induced by a live attenuated vaccine could exist in the absence of a (DTH) footpad response. Unlike the case for *Mycobacteria* and *Listeria*, the development of T-cell clones and lines has been slow. It even proved difficult to show that immune mice have T cells that respond to *Salmonella* antigens and to identify *Salmonella* antigens recognized by T cells. Killar and Eisenstein (207) were able to show that peritoneal exudate T cells harvested 2–3 months after vaccination of mice with an attenuated vaccine gave proliferative responses to endotoxin protein and to acetone-killed *Salmonella*, but not to LPS. Kotlarski and associates (208) also observed proliferative responses to *Salmonella* antigens in mice given live vaccines. It was not until 1997 that a T-cell clone was derived which responded to an identifiable *Salmonella* epitope, a flagellar filament protein (209). The clone was isolated from spleen cells of a mouse orally immunized with an attenuated strain of *Salmonella* given 90 days previously. Further, it was shown that spleen cells of immunized mice responded with proliferative responses to the peptide.

Recently, definitive experiments on the role of various types of T cells in innate resistance to *Salmonella* were reported from Kaufmann's laboratory using mice with gene disruptions in different TCRs. It was found that $CD4^+$TCR-α/β cells are necessary for mice to clear attenuated candidate vaccine strains of *Salmonella* given intravenously, but the effect is not manifested until 21 days after infection (210). No effect of depletion of γ/δ T cells on i.v. inoculated *Salmonella* was observed and $CD8^+$ cells were only implicated as playing an auxiliary role in host defense (210).

These studies, using gene disruptions in mice that differentially affect subsets of T cells, as well as the experiments preferentially removing particular subsets of T cells with antibodies, point to $CD4^+$ T cells as the major subset mediating resistance to *Salmonella* infection. This result is in contrast to the conclusion in murine studies of host resistance to *Listeria* infection, in which the $CD8^+$ subset plays an important role (211). Thus, studies in recent years on the mechanisms of cellular immunity to *Salmonella* fail to show direct parallels with T-cell-dependent cellular immune mechanisms in *Listeria*. As $CD4^+$ and not $CD8^+$ cells have been shown to be most important for host defense to *Salmonella* infection, the possibility has not been definitively ruled out that the role of the $CD4^+$ T cells is as helper cells in production of protective antibody, not as effectors of cell-mediated immunity. It is noteworthy that papers from Hormaeche's laboratory (discussed in section 3.3.6.4) describe experiments using oral vaccination and challenge, and report that both T cells and immune serum are necessary for protection (212,213).

3.3.4 Early Events in Immunity to *Salmonella* Infection: Cytokines, NK Cells, and Macrophages

Studies using mice with gene disruptions in the TCR-α/β showed they were sensitized to *Salmonella* infection, but the effect was not manifested until the 21st day postinfection (210). A substantial number of papers in the literature show that recovery from *Salmonella* infection occurs in two stages, an early phase that is T-cell independent and a late phase that requires T cells. This dichotomy was first defined by Hormaeche's laboratory investigating genes governing innate resistance to *Salmonella.* He showed that the genetic mechanism which regulates the early net growth rate of *Salmonella* does not involve a cell-mediated T-cell response (214). O'Brien and Metcalf (215) used nude mice to confirm that early control of *Salmonella* replication is independent of T cells, but that their absence leads to an inability to clear the bacteria and eventual death. Nauciel (200) confirmed these findings and showed the late (day 21) depletion of $CD4^+$ T cells, but not $CD8^+$ cells abrogated protection, but early depletion (day 14) had no effect. NK cells were shown by Schafer and Eisenstein to be induced by a systemically administered live, attenuated vaccine strain of *S. typhimurium,* and to play a role in induction of immunity, as their ablation resulted in failure of the vaccine strain to protect (216). It also appears that in the early stages of infection, macrophages are key in controlling bacterial replication. Removal of macrophages with silica or dextran sulfate sensitized mice to *Salmonella* infection (217,218). Further, Killar and Eisenstein (207) showed that spleen cell fractions rich in macrophages, but not in T cells, could transfer protection from animals vaccinated with live attenuated vaccines at 7 days after infection. The importance of macrophages in the early control of *Salmonella* infection is shown by differences in the ability of macrophages from innately hypersusceptible or innately resistant strains to control bacterial replication (219,220).

Investigation of the contribution of cytokines to systemic infection with *Salmonella* supports the importance of the innate pathway of host resistance which does not depend on T cells. The pathway involves production of IL-12 by infected macrophages, which induces NK cells to produce IFN-γ, in turn activating macrophages to enhanced microbicidal activity (221). In support of this pathway, administration of IFN-γ before i.p. challenge with virulent *Salmonella* has been shown to confer protection (222), and IFN-γ depletion with a monoclonal antibody was found to sensitize mice to infection (223). Innate resistance was shown to be related to higher levels of IFN-γ induced in resistant, compared with susceptible, mouse strains, which in turn was dependent on a macrophage factor (224). The results would be compatible with differences in levels of macrophage-stimulated IL-12 production. Evidence substantiating a role for IL-12 in host defense against *Salmonella* was demonstrated by Hormaeche's group, which showed that anti-IL-12 increased the *Salmonella* burden in mice infected with a virulent strain and partially blocked IFN-γ production (225). Other cytokines have also been shown to play a role in host defense to *Salmonella* infection. Tumor necrosis factor (TNF) protects, and anti-TNF sensitizes, to systemic *Salmonella* infection in mice (223,226). Pretreatment with IL-1 protects resistant but not susceptible mice from systemic infection (227). The studies on TNF and IL-1 were carried out before the discovery of IL-12. Whether either of their effects are related to induction of IL-12 is unknown. A major question pertinent to vaccine development is whether salmonellae induce a Th1 or a Th2 cytokine profile. Mice infected i.p. with *S. dublin* were shown to exhibit a primarily Th1 profile with IFN-γ, TNF-α, granulocyte-macrophage colony-stimulating factor (GM-CSF), IL-1, IL-2, IL-6, IL-10, and IL-12p40, being induced, but not IL-4, IL-5, or TGF-β (228). Interestingly, no difference was found between cytokine profiles examined over a 30-day period for mice expressing the *ity*^{s} versus the *ity*^{r} allele. This result is in contrast to a report showing that splenic macrophages from *ity*^{r} mice exposed in vitro to live *Salmonella* induced greater IFN-γ production in spleen cells than macrophages from *ity*^{s} mice (224).

3.3.5 Attenuated *Salmonella* Vaccines Induce Systemic Immunosuppression in Mice

A potential difficulty with live attenuated vaccines of *Salmonella* is that they have been shown to induce profound immunosuppression in mice. Spleen cells taken from animals seven days after i.p. immunization with a strain of *S. typhimurium* blocked in aromatic synthesis were profoundly suppressed in proliferative responses to Concanavalin A (Con A) and lipopolysaccharide (LPS) (229–231), and in their capacity to mount a primary in vitro plaque-forming response to sheep red blood cells (SRBC) (232). In vivo antibody responses to tetanus toxoid and to SRBCs were also markedly suppressed (233). Immunosuppression was measurable by three days postimmunization, maximal at seven days, and waning by 21 days (229). Eisenstein's laboratory has shown that the immunosuppression is mediated by mature and immature macrophages (232) and that the suppressor factor is nitric oxide (NO) (234). The percent immunosuppression is linearly related to the $\log_{10}$ of the nitrite concentration measured in culture supernatants of spleen cells (235). Further, the degree of immunosuppression is related to the inoculating dose and the bacterial burden in the spleen on day seven (236). IL-12 is crucial for induction of immunosuppression, as administration of antibodies to IL-12 blocks NO production and immunosuppression (237). The interpretation of these results is that if the burden of attenuated *Salmonella* in the spleen exceeds 10^5 organisms, the host mounts an inflammatory response that includes activated macrophages which are making inducible nitric oxide synthase (iNOS) and NO to try to contain the growth of the bacteria. Nitric oxide has not been shown to be directly bactericidal for *Salmonella* (238), but peroxynitrite has salmonellacidal activity (239). Immunosuppression occurs by a "bystander autotoxicity" mechanism in which the NO released by the macrophages results in lymphocyte inactivation (240). Comparison of a panel of *Salmonella* strains with different attenuating lesions showed that many different strains were immunosuppressive (236). For a strain to be immunosuppressive, it had to replicate to approximately 10^5 organisms in the spleen. Interestingly, protective capacity was not correlated with ability to induce immunosuppression. A *pho*P mutant failed to grow, was not immunosuppressive, but gave 100% protection (236). Alternatively, some strains induced suppression, but were not protective (236). Whether immunosuppression will be an undesirable side-effect of attenuated *Salmonella* used as vaccines in humans remains to be determined. In these mouse studies, the attenuated strains were given i.p. whereas in humans they will be given orally. Whether they could cause immunosuppression in the secretory immune system has not been investigated. The possibility exists that if the vaccine were given to an immunocompromised individual, the organisms, although attenuated, might escape into the circulation, reach the spleen, and replicate to sufficient titer to induce immunosuppression. In support of this possibility, vaccinemia has been shown to occur in normal human volunteers in phase I studies with some mutants of the type used for the murine experiments (*aro*A^-) (241). An additional area of uncertainty as to the significance of the immunosuppression work in the mouse is that it has been difficult to demonstrate iNOS induction in human monocytes by cytokines (242).

3.3.6 Immunity to Oral *Salmonella* Infection

3.3.6.1 Early Vaccine Studies Using Oral Challenge. Studies carried out in 1957 before the discovery of the secretory immune system showed that subcutaneous immunization with a sublethal dose of living *Salmonella* could protect mice against oral challenge with *S. paratyphi* C (243). Whether protection was attributable to migration of the live bacteria to the mucosal compartment or to serum antibodies that transudated into the secretory compartment cannot be determined. However, this report is one of the first to show that systemic immunization can protect against oral challenge. The efficacy and therefore the feasibility of oral vaccination with attenuated, temperature-sensitive strains of *S. enteritidis* against oral challenge with a virulent strain of the same serotype was demonstrated in mice by Fahey and Cooper (244). Collins and colleagues (155,158) showed that oral administration with a sublethal dose of a live virulent *Salmonella* strain protected against oral challenge with the virulent strain. Killed cells were found to be less effective, although suboptimal amounts of killed cells were used in some experiments (155). Earlier studies had been carried out in chimpanzees indicating the protective value of oral vaccination of primates (156). Experiments in human volunteers fed enteric tablets containing killed *S. typhi* showed protection against *S. typhi* challenge at levels not different from those of volunteers who had recovered from experimentally induced typhoid fever (245). From a pragmatic point of view, the clear demonstration that oral vaccination is effective indicated that it was possible to vaccinate against *S. typhi* using this route.

3.3.6.2 Role of IgA in Protection Against Oral Salmonella Challenge. Although it might be assumed that antigen introduced orally would have as its main mechanism of immunity induction of sIgA, that is not necessarily the case. Especially with a replicating, inflammation-inducing organism such as *Salmonella*, the possibility is certainly plausible that sufficient organisms might reach the systemic circulation so as to induce systemic immunity, which, as we have already discussed above, is protective, even against an oral challenge. As demonstrated even more definitively with cholera, serum IgM and even IgG antibodies can transudate into the intestinal lumen and confer protection (80). Thus, dissecting out the relative contribution of serum versus secretory antibody was an important and difficult question to answer. A related question was whether sIgA alone is sufficient to protect mice against oral challenge with virulent *Salmonella*. Definitive experiments by Neutra showed that the answer to this latter question is affirmative (83). Her group produced an IgA monoclonal antibody to *S. typhimurium* and implanted the hybridoma cells s.c. into normal mice. Mice passively immunized by secretion of this IgA antibody were protected against oral challenge with virulent *Salmonella*. Interestingly, they were not protected against i.p. challenge. This could be because antibody is not protective in mice with the *ity*^{s} genotype, which makes them hypersusceptible to *Salmonella* infection (148) or because IgA in serum blocks protective and opsonic functions of IgM and IgG (84). The demonstration that IgA alone was protective, since mice that were challenged were naive to *Salmonella*, except for the passive IgA, shows that IgA alone can confer protection against an oral challenge. Similar studies using an IgA monoclonal that recognizes *Shigella* O antigens showed protection against intranasal challenge with *Shigella flexneri* in a murine model (246). The mechanism by which IgA protects against Salmonella appears to be by inhibiting attachment of the microbes to their target cells. Evidence to support this hypothesis was presented by showing that an IgA monoclonal antibody inhibits invasion of a polarized canine kidney epithelial cell line in vitro (247).

3.3.6.3 Cytokine Responses to Oral Salmonella Infection. The parameters of host resistance to oral immunization or challenge with *Salmonella* are just beginning to be elucidated in the mucosal immune system. It has been shown that IFN-γ is induced in PP as early as 6 hours after oral inoculation with a sublethal dose of virulent *Salmonella* and in the mesenteric lymph node by 24 hours (248). Avirulent organisms similarly induce IFN-γ in the PP (85). Further, administration of a monoclonal antibody to IFN-γ sensitized mice to oral infection (248). These studies are consonant with the body of work cited in Section 3.3.4 of this chapter showing the importance of IFN-γ in mice inoculated by various systemic routes. Also, as described above, IL-12 is part of the IFN-γ pathway that leads to macrophage activation, and it has been implicated as an important factor in protection against *Salmonella* given by the oral route. Oral infection with virulent *S. dubin* has been shown to induce IL-12 in mesenteric lymph nodes; anti-IL-12 was shown to sensitize to oral infection; and IL-12 given systemically was protective against oral infection (249). Anti-IL-12 also reduced the protection induced by immunization with a live, attenuated strain of *Salmonella*, when it was given just before oral challenge with the virulent strain (225). The question of whether *Salmonella* induces a Th1 or a Th2 cytokine profile in the gastrointestinal tract has been addressed in recent work. *S. typhimurium* introduced into mouse ligated ileal loops that do not contain Peyer's patches resulted in type 1 cytokines in the exudate fluid, as determined by ELISA, and also by assaying for mRNA for type 1 cytokines in intestinal tissue, as assessed by polymerase chain reaction (PCR) during the first 18 hours after introduction of the microbe (106). The cytokines upregulated included IFN-γ, IL-1, IL-6, IL-10, TNF-α, but not IL-2. In mice immunized with *Salmonella* carrying a fragment of tetanus toxoid as a passenger antigen, purified T cells from Peyer's patches restimulated in vitro with TT produced a Th1 cytokine profile as determined by ELISA, PCR, and ELISPOT techniques (107). IFN-γ and IL-2, but not IL-4 or IL-5 were detected. IL-10 was also induced, as was IL-6 produced by macrophages. Several groups have shown that oral immunization with *Salmonella* results in cytokine induction in the spleen. IFN-γ mRNA was detected by PCR in spleens of mice inoculated orally with *Salmonella* 4 days previously (248). Immunization with live attenuated *Salmonella* by the oral route has been shown to induce mainly an IgG2a serum antibody response, which is indicative of a Th1 response, and also a Th1 cytokine profile in spleen cells stimulated in vitro with whole-cell lysates of *Salmonella* (250).

3.3.6.4 T-Cell Subsets, Antibodies, and Oral Salmonella Infection. There are only a few published reports in which the effect of T cells or passive serum has been examined on *Salmonella* given by the oral route. Depletion of $CD4^+$ or $CD8^+$ cells using systemically administered monoclonal antibodies in mice has been shown to result in increased numbers of organisms cultured from the spleens and liver of mice orally inoculated with *Salmonella*. The results have been interpreted as showing increased translocation of organisms out of the gastrointestinal tract (112). However, an alternative interpretation is that the same number of organisms escaped into the systemic compartment, but they grew better in spleens and livers of T-cell-depleted mice. Other studies have shown that mice selectively depleted of T cells bearing either the γ/δ or α/β TCR by systemic administration of monoclonal antibodies were sensitized to oral Salmonella infection (251). A recent paper of considerable interest comes from Hormaeche's laboratory, in which it was shown that adoptive immunity to oral *Salmonella* challenge required transfer of both immune serum and immune T cells (212). The immune cells for adoptive transfer were pooled from spleens and mesenteric lymph nodes of previously immunized mice. T cells were depleted by administering a combination of anti-CD4 and anti-CD8 to donor mice before cell harvest, and loss of T cells abrogated protection.

3.3.6.5 Oral Typhoid Vaccines. In 1975, Germanier developed an attenuated strain of *S. typhi*, designated Ty21a, by chemical mutagenesis, using nitrosoguanidine (252). The strain was reported to be a *galE* mutant, deficient in UDP-glucose-4-epimerase, rendering it incapable of producing LPS containing O antigen due to the inability to synthesize galactose (253). In preliminary volunteer studies it was shown that Ty21a grown in 0.1% galactose was protective against challenge with virulent *S. typhi*, but in the absence of galactose in the growth medium, protection was not obtained (254). Strains grown in galactose lyse due to the accumulation of galactose-1-phosphate (254). This strain was tested in large scale field trials in school children in Egypt and found to be almost completely effective (4). Subsequent trials during typhoid epidemics in Santiago, Chile, showed wide variations in efficacy with the maximal protection not above 66% (255,256). The formulations used in Egypt and Chile differed, providing a possible explanation for the discrepancy in results (21). Reports of lack of efficacy of the vaccine in European travelers (257) prompted further investigation into the genetic lesion of Ty21a. Silva and associates reported that gal^+ revertants of Ty21a were still avirulent and protective in mice, suggesting that the genetic lesion leading to avirulence is not due to the deficiency in UDP-glucose-4-epimerase, but the precise mechanism was not determined (258). The Ty21a vaccine is currently licensed and in use in many countries.

Demonstration of the feasibility of an oral typhoid vaccine spurred research into producing attenuated strains with defined genetic lesions obtained by molecular genetic manipulation rather than by use of chemical mutagenesis as was done to obtain Ty21a. Hoiseth and Stocker (259) presented the idea of using transposon mutagenesis to disrupt the pathway of aromatic synthesis in *Salmonella* to render the bacteria avirulent. Deficiency in p-aminobenzoic acid and in 2,3-dihydroxybenzoate, compounds that are not available in vertebrate tissue, results in impaired growth in vivo. Prototypic strains with insertions or deletions in the *aro*A gene were shown to be avirulent when given i.p., and to be protective in mice challenged orally or i.p. with virulent *S. typhimurium* (259). In initial trials in humans using genetically manipulated strains of *S. typhi*, a Vi^+ and a Vi^- strain were used, with mutations of *aro*A and *pur*A (the latter causing a requirement for adenine). The double mutation was designed to insure avirulence. While the vaccine proved safe in phase I trials, it was poorly immunogenic (260). Experiments in mice using *S. typhimurium* strains with an *aro*A, a *pur*A, or a double mutation of *aro*A and *pur*A, showed that the *pur*A mutation resulted in a degree of attenuation that failed to result in colonization or in induction of immune responses (261). Hone and associates derived a strain of *S. typhi* (CVD 906) from Ty21 with deletion mutations in the *aro*C and *aro*D genes. It proved highly immunogenic but caused bacteremia (vaccinemia) and febrile responses in a significant number of volunteers in the phase I trial (241). Another strain of *S. typhi* made from a different parent strain, but also with mutations in *aro*C and *aro*D, and designated CVD 908 induced fewer symptoms and was highly immunogenic, but still induced silent bacteremias (241,262). Derivative strains of CVD 908 with still a third attenuating mutation in a heat shock protein have resulted in a promising vaccine strain (262). Other approaches to attenuation of Salmonella have used temperature-sensitive mutants (244,263,264), deletion of genes encoding adenylate cyclase and the cAMP receptor protein (265) and deletion of genes in the *pho*P-*pho*-Q virulence regulon (266). The latter class of organisms is of special interest because they do not multiply at all in vivo, yet are immunogenic (267). All the attenuated *Salmonella* mutants that have been made are presented in Table 6.2 (see Chapter 6). The development of an engineered strain of *S. typhi*, which does not cause bacteremia or diarrhea, but which retains immunogenicity, would appear to depend on pragmatic advances rather than on implementation of theoretical criteria. It has been difficult to predict the conditions that will result in sufficient avirulence with retention of immunogenicity.

Oral *Salmonella* vaccines are of interest not just for protection against typhoid fever, but because they have the capacity to carry and express "passenger" or "guest" antigens on their surface. The concept of making a hybrid strain of Salmonella expressing antigens of *Shigella* was introduced by Formal's group (268) and Ty21a expressing *Shigella* O antigen introduced by plasmid conjugal transfer was shown to induce serum antibody responses in rabbits and to protect mice against systemic challenge (268,269). Subsequently, Clements, El-Morshidy and colleagues constructed mutants of Ty21a and *S. enteritidis* that expressed *E. coli* heat-labile toxin (270,271). The *S. dublin* strain was capable of colonizing mice and inducing serum and mucosal antibodies to both the enterotoxin and to the *Salmonella* LPS. In addition, mucosal IgA antibody induced by the vaccine was able to neutralize the *E. coli* toxin (271). Since 1986, a variety of bacterial, parasitic, and viral antigens have been successfully cloned into attenuated *Salmonella* (see Table 6.1).

Along with testing hybrid strains for efficacy in inducing antibody to the passenger antigens, a number of theoretical questions have been addressed using the engineered strains. Among these are 1) whether cloned antigens which are not expressed at the bacterial surface of the vaccine carrier strain can induce immunity, 2) whether passenger antigens can induce cellular immune responses deemed essential for protection against some pathogens, and 3) whether repeated use of the same carrier organism, e.g., *Salmonella*, will result in less efficacy upon repeated immunizations due to preexisting immune responses to the carrier. Most of these questions have been addressed in mouse models, and the results have been encouraging. In regard to point 1, β-galactosidase expressed as an intracellular antigen in *Salmonella* was shown to induce cellular and humoral immunity when the antigen-carrying strain was given i.v. to mice (272). In regard to point 2, animals receiving this β-galactosidase-expressing strain of *Salmonella* gave positive footpad swelling to the protein antigen, indicative of DTH, and thus cellular immunity (272). Similarly, mice vaccinated with an *aro*A *aro*D mutant expressing the Tox C fragment of tetanus toxin also gave positive DTH reactions as measured by swelling of ear pinnae (273). Mice orally vaccinated with *Salmonella* expressing the circumsporozoite antigen of *Plasmodium yoelii* developed cytotoxic T cells to the malarial antigen (274), another indication of the induction of cellular immunity. Mice vaccinated with an aroA strain expressing human immunodeficiency virus (HIV) gp120 demonstrated a very weak proliferation of spleen cells presented with gp120 (275). Finally, in regard to point 3, studies by Bao and Clements (276) found that prior vaccination with a *Salmonella* carrier strain (*S. typhimurium* or *S. dublin*) did not inhibit subsequent responses to a passenger antigen (B subunit of *E. coli* heat-labile toxin) presented on that carrier; prior exposure not only did not adversely affect serum immune responses but resulted in heightened secretory immune responses. In other studies by Hormaeche, no suppression of immune responses was observed in animals primed s.c. with tetanus toxoid and subsequently immunized i.v. with an *aro*A strain of *S. typhimurium* expressing a 28-kDA antigen of *Schistosoma mansoni* or shorter peptides fused to TetC (a peptide of tetanus toxin) (277). The responses to the *Shistosoma* peptide and to tetanus toxoid were actually enhanced, and the response to the 28-kDA protein was unchanged. A similar conclusion was reached by Michalek, using an *aro*A *aro*D strain of *S. typhimurium* expressing an adhesion protein of *Streptococcus mutans* fused to cholera toxin A2/B subunits (278). Oral immunization induced serum and salivary secretory antibodies to the adhesin, cholera toxin, and *Salmonella*. A booster dose enhanced the serum response to the adhesin and cholera toxin but not *Salmonella.* By contrast, a booster did not enhance the salivary IgA response to the adhesin but did boost antibody titers to CT and *Salmonella.* In regard to the more practical aspects of the strategy of using *Salmonella* as a vector to carry passenger antigens, studies conducted by Clements are of interest. His group showed that killed *Salmonella* expressing the heat-labile toxin of *E. coli*, given orally, are as potent as live bacteria in inducing serum and secretory immune responses (279). Thus, for antibody induction, living cells are not necessary by the oral route.

A new approach to oral *Salmonella* vaccination combines use of an attenuated *Salmonella* strain with the information coding for the passenger antigen presented in the form of a transgene (280). Mice orally immunized with *Salmonella* expressing a transgene for a truncated portion of the *Listeria monocytogenes* virulence factor, listeriolysin, subsequently demonstrated cytotoxic responses against targets sensitized with the listeriolysin peptide. The transgene also induced splenic T-helper cell responses. Immunization by this method conferred protection against intravenous challenge with *Listeria* (oral challenge was not attempted). The method is postulated to work by release of the plasmid-based eukaryotic expression vectors from the dying *Salmonella* and their transcription in the cytosol of the host cell, which induces a cytotoxic T-cell response. A variation of this concept has been reported in which naked foreign phage DNA was fed to mice and found to penetrate the gastrointestinal tract and be present in gut epithelial cells, leukocytes in the Peyer's patches, in liver cells, and in B, T, and macrophages in the spleen. The DNA was linked to mouse DNA (281). The capacity of the DNA to induce immune responses was not tested.

3.3.6.6 Human Immune Responses to aroA Vaccines. The reader should recall that there were two strong rationales for pursuing the strategy of a live oral vaccine for typhoid fever. One was the perceived desirability of inducing secretory IgA, which would presumably block entry of the organisms into the Peyer's patches; the other was the superior protective efficacy of live versus killed vaccines in some mouse strains, with concomitant induction of cell-mediated immunity as evidenced by delayed-hypersensitivity reactions by live, but not killed *Salmonella.* From a theoretical point of view it is desirable to examine whether the prototype live, oral vaccines induce IgA and/or cellular immunity, or whether they simply induce protective levels of systemic antibody due to leakage of orally introduced vaccine strain organisms into the systemic compartment. Carrying out this assessment has not been an easy task. First, compared with obtaining blood samples to measure serum antibodies, collection of intestinal secretions from volunteers is more difficult, and it is more difficult to carry out the assays for sIgA levels than for serum antibody levels due to the problem of standardizing the volume of fecal fluid being tested. Second, there is no established test for the presence of cell-mediated immunity to *S. typhi* in humans, nor is there a standard skin test antigen to measure DTH, as there is for *M. tuberculosis* or *M. leprae*.

In trials using strains 541Ty and 543Ty, antibody responses to O, H, and Vi antigens were minimal in serum and intestinal fluid, the latter having been obtained by collection of jejunal fluid via a swallowed polyvinyl chloride tube (260). Cell-mediated immunity was assessed by proliferative responses of PBMC to heat-killed phenol preserved *S. typhi* and to purified LPS, and by a novel assay in which the peripheral blood mononuclear cells (PBMCs) were mixed with live, virulent *S. typhi* in heat-inactivated serum and the growth inhibition capacity of the cells was assessed (260). Most vaccinees gave proliferative responses to both antigens, and all volunteers showed positive responses in the killing assay. A puzzling aspect of the results is the meaning of the proliferative response to the O polysaccharide portion of LPS. Presumably, DTH is a response to protein, not polysaccharide antigens, but the experimental design ruled out nonspecific mitogenic effects of this polysaccharide antigen.

In a more recent study, Sztein and co-workers (282) studied responses of the peripheral blood mononuclear fraction of volunteers orally vaccinated 21 days previously with the newer *S. typhi* vaccine, CVD908 (which has mutations in *aro*C and *aro*D) and found that five of the six recipients showed marked proliferative responses to a flagellar antigen preparation. Cytokine responses of PBMCs were examined, and four of six volunteers made significant levels of IFN-γ, and only one made low levels of IL-4 in response to the flagella. The investigators interpreted the results to indicate that the vaccine induced a Th1 response. Interestingly, volunteers receiving CVD908 with a passenger malaria antigen showed even better responses to *Salmonella* flagella, with 10 of 10 showing significantly elevated proliferation. The CVD908 vaccine strain was also shown to induce cytotoxic T lymphocytes (CTLs) in an elegant experimental design in which PBMCs of volunteers were tested for their capacity to kill autologous EBV-infected lymphocytes infected with *S. typhi* (283). The effector cells were shown to be $CD8^+$ and MHC-class I restricted. This is the first demonstration in humans that CTLs can be induced that react against *Salmonella* and represents a major breakthrough in the assessment of cellular immune responses to *Salmonella*.

3.4 SUMMARY AND CONCLUSIONS

Live oral *Salmonella* vaccines have great potential as a strategy of mass vaccination that can be applied globally, regardless of the economic stratum of the country. Their capacity to carry "guest" antigens provides the opportunity to produce a vaccine that is not only easy to administer, but also might protect against several unrelated microbes with a single dose. Theoretically, a live vaccine should have an advantage over a nonviable vaccine in its capacity to induce systemic cellular immunity, and a live orally administered vaccine should also induce secretory and cellular immunity in the gastrointestinal tract. However, a point that must be continually reemphasized is that although live, oral vaccines are one effective strategy for inducing host defense to *Salmonella* infection, they are clearly not the only effective strategy. Whole killed cells, as well as a polysaccharide vaccine composed of pure Vi antigen injected s.c., both confer equal levels of protection to that of the currently licensed Ty21a oral vaccine. Thus, contrary to the prevailing notion for the last 30 years, cellular immunity is not a requirement for effective host defense to *Salmonella* infection. The conclusion that cellular immunity is required was reached using mice that are innately hypersusceptible to *Salmonella* infection. All the data support the concept that humans are more like innately resistant mice than innately susceptible mice (6), as they are well protected by nonviable vaccines.

Viable vaccines given orally may also theoretically have the undesirable effect of inducing oral tolerance, although trials in humans do not suggest that this occurs. A further consideration is that in mice, live attenuated *Salmonella* given systemically induce a subsequent window of immunosuppression to exogenous antigens that is mediated by nitric oxide. Whether a similar phenomenon could happen in humans is speculative, but it is conceivable that parenteral immunization with standard vaccines might be less effective if given after a live attenuated *Salmonella* vaccine. A further consideration is that prototype attenuated *Salmonella* have demonstrated the capacity to invade into the blood stream of human volunteers, and they may therefore pose a risk to immunosuppressed vaccinees.

Ultimately, the type of vaccine which prevails for typhoid fever will be determined empirically. The vaccine that gives acceptable levels of protection with the fewest side effects, and that is easiest and cheapest to administer, will be favored. Certainly, the studies over the last decades into the basic mechanisms underlying induction and regulation of secretory IgA responses and of the cellular arm of the immune system have inspired new and promising approaches for vaccination, not only against typhoid fever, but also against a variety of other pathogens that enter the body at mucosal surfaces.

ACKNOWLEDGMENTS

This work was supported by National Institutes of Health grants AI15613 and DA11134.

3.5 REFERENCES

1. Francis, T., Jr., R. F. Korns, R. B. Voight, M. Boisen, F. M. Hemphill, J. A. Napier, and E. Tolchinsky. 1955. An evaluation of the 1954 poliomyelitis vaccine trials: summary report. *Am. J. Public Health 45*:1.
2. Wright, A., and D. Semple. 1897. Remarks on vaccination against typhoid fever. *BMJ 1*:256.
3. Siler, J. F. 1941. *Immunization to Typhoid Fever*. Baltimore: Johns Hopkins Press.
4. Wahdan, M. H., C. Serie, Y. Cerisier, S. Sallam and R. Germanier. 1982. A controlled field trial of live *Salmonella typhi* strain Ty21a oral vaccine against typhoid: three-year results. *J. Infect. Dis. 145*:292.
5. Acharya, I. L., C. U. Lowe, R. Thapa, V. L. Gurubacharya, M. B. Shrestha, D. Bact, M. Cadoz, D. Schultz, J. Armand, D. A. Bryla, B. Trollfors, T. Cramton, R. Schneerson, and J. B. Robbins. 1987. Prevention of typhoid fever in Nepal with the Vi capsular polysaccharide of *Salmonella typhi. N. Engl. J. Med. 317*:1101.
6. Eisenstein, T. K., and B. M. Sultzer. 1983. Immunity to *Salmonella* infection. *Adv. Exp. Med. Biol. 162*:261.
7. Eisenstein, T. K., Huang, D., and Schwacha, M. G. 1996. Immunity to *Salmonella* infections. In: *Enteric Infections and Immunity*, edited by

Paradise, L. J., Bendinelli, M., and Friedman, H. New York: Plenum Press, 1996, p. 578.

8. Hsu, H. S. 1989. Pathogenesis and immunity in murine salmonellosis. *Microbiol. Rev. 53*:390.
9. Ushiba, D. 1965. Two types of immunity in experimental typhoid; "cellular immunity" and "humoral immunity." *Keio. J. Med. 14*:45.
10. Collins, F. M., G. B. Mackaness and R. V. Blanden. 1966. Infection-immunity in experimental salmonellosis. *J. Exp. Med. 124*:601.
11. Mackaness, G. B., R. V. Blanden, and F. M. Collins. 1966. Host–parasite relations in mouse typhoid. *J. Exp. Med. 124*:573.
12. Mackaness, G. B. 1964. The immunological basis of acquired cellular resistance. *J. Exp. Med. 120*:105.
13. Collins, F. M. 1978. Cellular antimicrobial immunity. *CRC. Crit. Rev. Microbiol. 7*:27.
14. Mackaness, G. B. 1971. Resistance to intracellular infection. *J. Infect. Dis. 123*:439.
15. Tomasi, T. B., Jr., and S. Zigelbaum. 1963. The selective occurrence of α_1A globulins in certain body fluids. *J. Clin. Invest. 42*:1552.
16. Heremans, J. F., M.-T. Heremans, and H. E. Schultze. 1959. Isolation and description of a few properties of the β-2A-globulin of human serum. *Clin. Chim. Acta 4*:96.
17. Hanson, L. Å. 1961. Comparative immunological studies of the immune globulins of human milk and of blood serum. *Arch. Allergy Appl. Immunol. 18*:241.
18. Tomasi, T. B., Jr., E. M. Tan, A. Solomon, and R. A. Prendergast. 1965. Characteristics of an immune system common to certain external secretions. *J. Exp. Med. 121*:101.
19. Hauptman, S. P., and T. B. Tomasi, Jr. 1975. Mechanism of immunoglobulin A polymerization. *J. Biol. Chem. 250*:3891.
20. Brandtzaeg, P. 1974. Presence of J chain in human immunocytes containing various immunoglobulin classes. *Nature 252*:418.
21. Levine, M. M., and Hone, D. M. Typhoid Fever. In: *Vaccines and Immunotherapy*, edited by Cryz, S. J. J. New York: Pergamon Press, 1991, p. 59.
22. Chodirker, W. B., and T. B. Tomasi, Jr. 1963. Gamma-globulins: quantitative relationships in human serum and nonvascular fluids. *Science 142*:1080.
23. McFarlin, D. E., W. Strober, R. D. Wochner, and T. A. Waldmann. 1965. Immunoglobulin A production in ataxia telangiectasia. *Science 150*:1175.
24. South, M. A., M. D. Cooper, F. A. Wollheim, R. Hong, and R. A. Good.

1966. The IgA system. I. Studies of the transport and immunochemistry of IgA in the saliva. *J. Exp. Med. 123*:615.

25. Ogra, P. L., and D. T. Karzon. 1969. Polio virus antibody response in serum and nasal secretions following intranasal inoculation with inactivated polio vaccine. *J. Immunol. 102*:15.
26. Ogra, P. L., and D. T. Karzon. 1969. Distribution of polio virus antibody in serum, nasopharynx and alimentary tract following segmental immunization of lower alimentary tract with polio vaccine. *J. Immunol. 102*:1423.
27. Rossen, R. D., C. Morgan, K. C. Hsu, W. T. Butler, and H. M. Rose. 1968. Localization of 11 S external secretory IgA by immunofluorescence in tissues lining the oral and respiratory passages in man. *J. Immunol. 100*:706.
28. Crabbè, P. A., D. R. Nash, H. Bazin, H. Eyssen, and J. F. Heremans. 1969. Antibodies of the IgA type in intestinal plasma cells of germ free mice after oral or parenteral immunization with ferritin. *J. Exp. Med. 130*:723.
29. Crabbè, P. A., D. R. Nash, H. Bazin, H. Eyssen, and J. F. Heremans. 1970. Immunohistochemical observations on lymphoid tissues from conventional and germ-free mice. *Lab. Invest. 22*:448.
30. Brandtzaeg, P. 1973. Structure, synthesis and external transfer of mucosal immunoglobulins. *Ann. Inst. Pasteur. 124C*:417.
31. Brandtzaeg, P. 1973. Two types of IgA immunocytes in man. *Nature New Biol. 243*:142.
32. Brandtzaeg, P. 1974. Mucosal and glandular distribution of immunoglobulin components. Differential localization of free and bound SC in secretory epithelial cells. *J. Immunol. 112*:1553.
33. Brandtzaeg, P. 1985. Role of J chain and secretory component in receptor-mediated glandular and hepatic transport of immunoglobulins in man. *Scand. J. Immunol. 22*:111.
34. Brandtzaeg, P., and H. Prydz. 1984. Direct evidence for an integrated function of J chain and secretory component in epithelial transport of immunoglobulins. *Nature 311*:71.
35. Mestecky, J., and M. W. Russell. 1986. IgA subclasses. *Allergy 19*:277.
36. Mestecky, J., and M. W. Russell. 1997. Mucosal immunoglobulins and their contribution to defense mechanisms: an overview. *Biochem. Soc. Trans. 25*:457.
37. Brandtzaeg, P., T. S. Halstensen, K. Kett, P. Krajci, D. Kvale, T. O. Rognum, H. Scott, and L. M. Sollid. 1989. Immunobiology and immunopathology of human gut mucosa: humoral immunity and intraepithelial lymphocytes. *Gastroenterology 97*:1562.
38. Conley, M. E., and D. L. Delacroix. 1987. Intravascular and mucosal

immunoglobulin A: two separate but related systems of immune defense? *Ann. Intern. Med. 106*:892.

39. Plaut, A. G., J. V. Gilbert, M. S. Artenstein, and J. D. Capra. 1975. *Neisseria gonorrhoeae* and *Neisseria meningitidis*: extracellular enzyme cleaves human immunoglobulin A. *Science 190*:1103.
40. Poulsen, K., J. Brandt, J. P. Hjorth, H. C. Thøgersen, and M. Kilian. 1989. Cloning and sequencing of the immunoglobulin A1 protease gene (*iga*) of *Haemophilus influenzae* serotype b. *Infect. Immun. 57*:3097.
41. Poulsen, K., J. Reinholdt, C. Jespersgaard, K. Boye, T. A. Brown, M. Hauge, and M. Kilian. 1998. A comprehensive genetic study of streptococcal immunoglobulin A1 proteases: evidence for recombination within and between species. *Infect. Immun. 66*:181.
42. Brandtzaeg, P. 1995. Molecular and cellular aspects of the secretory immunoglobulin system. *APMIS 103*:1.
43. Williams, R. C., and R. J. Gibbons. 1972. Inhibition of bacterial adherence by secretory immunoglobulin A: A mechanism of antigen disposal. *Science 177*:697.
44. Wold, A. E., J. Mestecky, M. Tomana, A. Kobata, H. Ohbayashi, T. Endo, and C. Svanborg-Edén. 1990. Secretory immunoglobulin A carries oligosaccharide receptors for *Escherichia coli* type 1 fimbrial lectin. *Infect. Immun. 58*:3073.
45. Mazanec, M. B., C. S. Kaetzel, M. E. Lamm, D. Fletcher, and J. G. Nedrud. 1992. Intracellular neutralization of virus by immunoglobulin A antibodies. *Proc. Natl. Acad. Sci. USA 89*:6901.
46. Burns, J. W., M. Siadat-Pajouh, A. A. Krishnaney, and H. B. Greenberg. 1996. Protective effect of rotavirus VP6-specific IgA monoclonal antibodies that lack neutralizing activity. *Science 272*:104.
47. Craig, S. W., and J. J. Cebra. 1971. Peyer's patches: an enriched source of precursors for IgA-producing immunocytes in the rabbit. *J. Exp. Med. 134*:188.
48. Williams, A. F., and J. L. Gowans. 1975. The presence of IgA on the surface of rat thoracic duct lymphocytes which contain internal IgA. *J. Exp. Med. 141*:335.
49. Parrott, D. M. V., and A. Ferguson. 1974. Selective migration of lymphocytes within the mouse small intestine. *Immunology 26*:571.
50. Guy-Grand, D., C. Griscelli, and P. Vassalli. 1974. The gut-associated lymphoid system: nature and properties of the large dividing cells. *Eur. J. Immunol. 4*:435.
51. McWilliams, M., J. M. Phillips-Quagliata, and M. E. Lamm. 1977. Mesenteric lymph node B lymphoblasts which home to the small intestine are precommitted to IgA synthesis. *J. Exp. Med. 145*:866.

52. Pierce, N. F., and J. L. Gowans. 1975. Cellular kinetics of the intestinal immune response to cholera toxoid in rats. *J. Exp. Med. 142*:1550.
53. Robertson, S. M., and J. M. Cebra. 1976. A model for local immunity. *Ric. Clin. Lab. 6*:105.
54. Holmgren, J., L. A. Hanson, B. Carlson, B. S. Lindblad, and J. Rahimtoola. 1976. Neutralizing antibodies against *Escherichia coli* and *Vibrio cholerae* enterotoxins in human milk from a developing country. *Scand. J. Immunol. 5*:867.
55. Stoliar, O. A., R. P. Pelley, E. Kaniecki-Green, M. H. Klaus, and C. C. J. Carpenter. 1976. Secretory IgA against enterotoxins in breastmilk. *Lancet 1*:1258.
56. Allardyce, R. A., D. J. C. Shearman, D. B. L. McClelland, K. Marwick, A. J. Simpson and R. B. Laidlaw. 1974. Appearance of specific colostrum antibodies after clinical infection with *Salmonella typhimurium. BMJ 3*:307.
57. Roux, M. E., M. McWilliams, J. M. Phillips-Quagliata, P. Weisz-Carrington, and M. E. Lamm. 1977. Origin of IgA-secreting plasma cells in the mammary gland. *J. Exp. Med. 146*:1311.
58. Montgomery, P. C., B. R. Rosner, and J. Cohn. 1974. The secretory antibody response. Anti-DNP antibodies induced by dinitrophenylated type III pneumococcus. *Immunol. Comm. 3*:143.
59. Goldblum, R. M., S. Ahlstedt, B. Carlsson, L. Å. Hanson, U. Jodal, G. Lidin-Janson, and A. Sohl-Åkerlund. 1975. Antibody-forming cells in human colostrum after oral immunisation. *Nature 257*:797.
60. Montgomery, P. C., I. Lemaitre-Coelho, and E. T. Lally. 1976. The effect of circulating antibodies on secretory IgA antibody induction following oral immunization with dinitrophenylated *Pneumococcus. Ric. Clin. Lab. 6(Suppl. 3)*:93.
61. Bienenstock, J., N. Johnston, and D. Y. E. Perey. 1973. Bronchial lymphoid tissue. I. Morphological characteristics. *Lab. Invest. 28*:686.
62. Bienenstock, J., N. Johnston, and D. Y. E. Perey. 1973. Bronchial lymphoid tissue. II. Functional characteristics. *Lab. Invest. 28*:693.
63. Rudzik, R., R. L. Clancy, D. Y. E. Perey, R. P. Day, and J. Bienenstock. 1975. Repopulation with IgA-containing cells of bronchial and intestinal lamina propria after transfer of homologous Peyer's patch and bronchial lymphocytes. *J. Immunol. 114*:1599.
64. Crawford, J. M., M. A. Taubman, and D. J. Smith. 1975. Minor salivary glands as a major source of secretory immunoglobulin A in the human oral cavity. *Science 190*:1206.
65. McDermott, M. R., and J. Bienenstock. 1979. Evidence for a common mucosal immunologic system. I. Migration of B immunoblasts into intestinal, respiratory, and genital tissues. *J. Immunol. 122*:1892.

66. Montgomery, P. C., A. Ayyildiz, I. M. Lemaitre-Coelho, J.-P. Vaerman, and J. H. Rockey. 1983. Induction and expression of antibodies in secretions: the ocular immune system. *Ann. NY Acad. Sci. 409*:428.

67. Kuper, C. F., P. J. Koornstra, D. M. H. Hameleers, J. Biewenga, B. J. Spit, A. M. Duijvestijn, P. J. C. van Breda Vriesman, and T. Sminia. 1992. The role of nasopharyngeal lymphoid tissue. *Immunol. Today 13*:219.

68. Berlin, C., E. L. Berg, M. J. Briskin, D. P. Andrew, P. J. Kilshaw, B. Holzmann, I. L. Weissman, A. Hamann, and E. C. Butcher. 1993. $\alpha 4\beta 7$ integrin mediates lymphocyte binding to the mucosal vascular addressin MAdCAM-1. *Cell 74*:185.

69. Streeter, P. R., E. Lakey-Berg, B. T. N. Rouse, R. F. Bargatze, and E. C. Butcher. 1988. A tissue-specific endothelial cell molecule involved in lymphocyte homing. *Nature 331*:41.

70. Orr, N., G. Robin, D. Cohen, R. Arnon, and G. H. Lowell. 1993. Immunogenicity and efficacy of oral or intranasal *Shigella flexneri* 2a and *Shigella sonnei. Infect. Immun. 61*:2390.

71. Langermanns, S., A. Palaszynski, A. Sadzlena, C. K. Stover, and S. Koenig. 1994. Systemic and mucosal immunity induced by BCG vector expressing outer-surface protein A of *Borelia burgdorferi. Nature 372*:552.

72. Gruber, W. C., R. B. Belshe, J. C. King, J. J. Treanor, P. A. Piedra, P. F. Wright, G. W. Reed, E. Anderson, and F. Newman. 1996. Evaluation of live attenuated influenza vaccines in children 6–18 months of age: safety, immunogenicity, and efficacy. *J. Infect. Dis. 173*:1313.

73. Haneberg, B., D. Kendall, H. M. Amerongen, F. M. Apter, J.-P. Kraehenbuhl, and M. R. Neutra. 1994. Induction of specific immunoglobulin A in the small intestine, colon-rectum, and vagina measured by a new method for collection of secretions from local mucosal surfaces. *Infect. Immun. 62*:15.

74. Mestecky, J., J. R. McGhee, R. R. Arnold, S. M. Michalek, S. J. Prince, and J. L. Babb. 1978. Selective induction of an immune response in human external secretions by ingestion of bacterial antigen. *J. Clin. Invest. 61*:731.

75. Alley, C. D., H. Kiyono, and J. R. McGhee. 1986. Murine bone marrow IgA responses to orally administered sheep erythrocytes. *J. Immunol. 136*:4414.

76. Mestecky, J., M. W. Russell, S. Jackson, and T. A. Brown. 1986. The human IgA system: a reassessment. *Clin. Immunol. Immunopathol. 40*:105.

77. Lycke, N., L. Lindholm, and J. Holmgren. 1985. Cholera antibody production *in vitro* by peripheral blood lymphocytes following oral immu-

nization of humans and mice. *Clin. Exp. Immunol. 62*:39.

78. Fuhrman, J. A., and J. J. Cebra. 1981. Special features of the priming process for a secretory IgA response. B cell priming with cholera toxin. *J. Exp. Med. 153*:534.
79. Komisar, J. L., J. A. Fuhrman, and J. J. Cebra. 1982. IgA-producing hybridomas are readily derived from gut-associated lymphoid tissue. *J. Immunol. 128*:2376.
80. Fubara, E. S., and R. Freter. 1972. Availability of locally synthesized and systemic antibodies in the intestine. *Infect. Immun. 6*:965.
81. Bouvet, J.-P., L. Bélec, R. Pirès, and J. Pillot. 1994. Immunoglobulin G antibodies in human vaginal secretions after parenteral injection. *Infect. Immun. 62*:3957.
82. Pier, G. B., G. Meluleni, and J. B. Goldberg. 1995. Clearance of *Pseudomonas aeruginosa* from the murine gastrointestinal tract is effectively mediated by O-antigen-specific circulating antibodies. *Infect. Immun. 63*:2818.
83. Michetti, P., M. J. Mahan, J. M. Slauch, J. J. Mekalanos, and M. R. Neutra. 1992. Monoclonal secretory immunoglobulin A protects mice against oral challenge with the invasive pathogen *Salmonella typhimurium. Infect. Immun. 60*:1786.
84. Jarvis, G. A., and J. M. Griffiss. 1991. Human IgA1 blockade of IgG-initiated lysis of *Neisseria meningitidis* is a function of antigen-binding fragment binding to the polysaccharide capsule. *J. Immunol. 147*:1962.
85. George, A. 1996. Generation of gamma interferon responses in murine Peyer's patches following oral immunization. *Infect. Immun. 64*:4606.
86. Kroese, F. G. M., E. C. Butcher, A. M. Stall, P. A. Lalor, S. Adams, and L. A. Herzenberg. 1989. Many of the IgA producing plasma cells in murine gut are derived from self-replenishing precursors in the peritoneal cavity. *Int. Immunol. 1*:75.
87. Herzenberg, L. A., A. M. Stall, P. A. Lalor, C. Sidman, W. A. Moore, and D. R. Parks. 1986. The Ly-1 B cell lineage. *Immunol. Rev. 93*:81.
88. Cantor, A. B. 1991. A new nomenclature for B cells. *Immunol. Today 12*:388.
89. Pecquet, S. S., C. Ehrat, and P. B. Ernst. 1992. Enhancement of mucosal antibody responses to *Salmonella typhimurium* and the microbial hapten phosphorylcholine in mice with X-linked immunodeficiency by B-cell precursors from the peritoneal cavity. *Infect. Immun. 60*:503.
90. Cebra, J. J., Crandall, C. A., Gearhart, P. J., Robertson, S. M., Tseng, J., and Watson, P. M. Cellular events concerned with the initiation, expression, and control of the mucosal immune response. In: *Immunology of Breast Milk*, edited by Ogra, P. L. and Dayton, D. New York: Raven Press, 1979. p. 1.

91. Guy-Grand, D., C. Griscelli, and P. Vassalli. 1975. Peyer's patches, gut IgA plasma cells and thymic function: study in nude mice bearing thymic grafts. *J. Immunol. 115*:361.
92. Elson, C. O., J. A. Heck, and W. Storber. 1979. T-cell regulation of murine IgA synthesis. *J. Exp. Med. 149*:632.
93. Coffman, R. L., D. A. Lebman, and B. Schrader. 1989. Transforming growth factor β specifically enhances IgA production by lipopolysaccharide-stimulated murine B lymphocytes. *J. Exp. Med. 170*:1039.
94. Kim, P.-H., and M. F. Kagnoff. 1990. Transforming growth factor $\beta 1$ increases IgA isotype switching at the clonal level. *J. Immunol. 145*:3773.
95. Sonoda, E., R. Matsumoto, V. Hitosni, T. Ishii, M. Sugimoto, S. Araki, A. Tominaga, and K. Takatsu. 1989. Transforming growth factor β induces IgA production and acts additively with interleukin-5 for IgA production. *J. Exp. Med. 170*:1415.
96. Lebman, D. A., F. D. Lee, and R. L. Coffman. 1990. Mechanism for transforming growth factor β and IL-2 enhancement of IgA expression in lipopolysaccharide-stimulated B cell cultures. *J. Immunol. 144*:952.
97. van Vlasselaer, P., J. Punnonen, and J. E. de Vries. 1992. Transforming growth factor-β directs IgA switching in human B cells. *J. Immunol. 148*:2062.
98. Defrance, T., B. Vanbervliet, F. Brière, I. Durand, F. Rousset, and J. Banchereau. 1992. Interleukin 10 and transforming growth factor β cooperate to induce anti-CD40-activated naive human B cells to secrete immunoglobulin A. *J. Exp. Med. 175*:671.
99. McIntyre, T. M., M. R. Kehry, and C. M. Snapper. 1995. Novel in vitro model for high-rate IgA class switching. *J. Immunol. 154*:3156.
100. Stavnezer, J. 1995. Regulation of antibody production and class switching by TGF-β. *J. Immunol. 155*:1647.
101. Coffman, R. L., B. Shrader, J. Carty, T. R. Mosmann, and M. W. Bond. 1987. A mouse T cell product that preferentially enhances IgA production. I. Biologic characterization. *J. Immunol. 139*:3685.
102. Beagley, K. W., J. H. Eldridge, F. Lee, H. Kiyono, M. P. Everson, W. J. Koopman, T. Hirano, T. Kishimoto, and J. R. McGhee. 1989. Interleukins and IgA synthesis. Human and murine interleukin 6 induce high rate IgA secretion in IgA-committed B cells. *J. Exp. Med. 169*:2133.
103. Taguchi, T., J. R. McGhee, R. L. Coffman, K. W. Beagley, J. H. Eldridge, K. Takatsu, and H. Kiyono. 1990. Analysis of Th1 and Th2 cells in murine gut-associated tissues: frequencies of $CD4^+$ and $CD8^+$ T cells that secrete IFN-γ and IL-5. *J. Immunol. 145*:68.

104. Wilson, A. D., M. Bailey, N. A. Williams, and C. R. Stokes. 1991. The *in vitro* production of cytokines by mucosal lymphocytes immunized by oral administration of keyhole limpet hemocyanin using cholera toxin as an adjuvant. *Eur. J. Immunol. 21*:2333.

105. Xu-Amano, J., H. Kiyono, R. J. Jackson, H. F. Staats, K. Fujihashi, P. D. Burrows, C. O. Elson, S. Pillai, and J. R. McGhee. 1993. Helper T cell subsets for immunoglobulin A responses: oral immunization with tetanus toxoid and cholera toxin as adjuvant selectively induces Th2 cells in mucosa associated tissues. *J. Exp. Med. 178*:1309.

106. Klimpel, G. R., M. Asuncion, J. Haithcoat, and D. W. Niesel. 1995. Cholera toxin and *Salmonella typhimurium* induce different cytokine profiles in the gastrointestinal tract. *Infect. Immun. 63*:1134.

107. VanCott, J. L., H. F. Staats, D. W. Pascual, M. Roberts, S. N. Chatfield, M. Yamamoto, M. Coste, P. B. Carter, H. Kiyono, and J. R. McGhee. 1996. Regulation of mucosal and systemic antibody responses by T helper cell subsets, macrophages, and derived cytokines following oral immunization with live recombinant *Salmonella. J. Immunol. 156*:1504.

108. Hörnquist, C. E., L. Ekman, K. D. Grdic, K. Schön, and N. Y. Lycke. 1995. Paradoxical IgA immunity in CD4-deficient mice: lack of cholera toxin-specific protective immunity despite normal gut mucosal IgA differentiation. *J. Immunol. 155*:2877.

109. Okahashi, N., M. Yamamoto, J. L. VanCott, S. N. Chatfield, M. Roberts, H. Bluethmann, T. Hiroi, H. Kiyono, and J. R. McGhee. 1996. Oral immunization of interleukin-4 (IL-4) knockout mice with a recombinant *Salmonella* strain or cholera toxin reveals that $CD4^+$ Th2 cells producing IL-6 and IL-10 are associated with mucosal immunoglobulin A responses. *Infect. Immun. 64*:1516.

110. Owens, W. E., and R. D. Berg. 1980. Bacterial translocation from the gastrointestinal tract of athymic (*nu*/*nu*) mice. *Infect. Immun. 27*:461.

111. Owens, W. E., and R. D. Berg. 1982. Bacterial translocation from the gastrointestinal tract of thymectomized mice. *Curr. Microbiol. 7*:169.

112. Gautreaux, M. D., E. A. Deitch, and R. D. Berg. 1994. T lymphocytes in the host defense against bacterial translocation from the gastrointestinal tract. *Infect. Immun. 62*:2874.

113. Guy-Grand, D., N. Cerf-Bensussan, B. Malissen, M. Malassis-Seris, C. Briottet, and P. Vassalli. 1991. Two gut intraepithelial $CD8^+$ lymphocyte populations with different T cell receptors: a role for the gut epithelium in T cell differentiation. *J. Exp. Med. 173*:471.

114. Balk, S. P., E. C. Ebert, and R. L. Blumenthal. 1991. Oligoclonal expansion and CD1 recognition by human intestinal intraepithelial lymphocytes. *Science 253*:1411.

115. Dogan, A., D. K. Dunn-Walters, T. T. MacDonald, and J. Spencer. 1996. Demonstration of local clonality of mucosal T cells in human colon using DNA obtained by microdissection of immunohistochemically stained tissue sections. *Eur. J. Immunol. 26*:1240.

116. Goodman, T. and L. Lefrançois. 1988. Expression of the $\gamma\delta$ T cell receptor on intestinal $CD8^+$ intraepithelial lymphocytes. *Nature 333*:855.

117. Takagaki, Y., A. DeCloux, M. Bonneville, and S. Tonegawa. 1989. Diversity of $\gamma\delta$ T-cell receptors of murine intestinal intraepithelial lymphocytes. *Nature 339*:712.

118. Itohara, S., A. G. Farr, J. J. Lafaille, M. Bonneville, Y. Takagaki, W. Haas, and S. Tonegawa. 1990. Homing of $\gamma\delta$ thymocyte subset with homogeneous T-cell receptors to mucosal epithelia. *Nature 343*:754.

119. Fujihashi, K., J. R. McGhee, M.-N. Kweon, M. D. Cooper, S. Tonegawa, I. Takahashi, T. Hiroi, J. Mestecky, and H. Kiyono. 1996. γ/δ T cell-deficient mice have impaired mucosal immunoglobulin A responses. *J. Exp. Med. 183*:1929.

120. Lefrançois, L., R. LeCorre, J. Mayo, J. A. Bluestone, and T. Goodman. 1990. Extrathymic selection of TCR-$\gamma\delta^+$ T cells by class II major histocompatibility molecules. *Cell 63*:333.

121. Bandeira, A., S. Itohara, M. Bonneville, O. Burlen-Defranoux, T. Mota-Santos, A. Coutinho, and S. Tonegawa. 1990. Extrathymic origin of intestinal intraepithelial lymphocytes bearing T-cell antigen receptor $\gamma\delta$. *Proc. Natl. Acad. Sci. USA 88*:43.

122. Emoto, M., Y. Emoto, and S. H. E. Kaufmann. 1996. Development of CD8 α/β^+ TCR $\alpha\beta$ intestinal intraepithelial lymphocytes in athymic *nu/nu* mice and participation in regional immune responses. *Immunology 88*:531.

123. Guy-Grand, D., B. Cuenod-Jabri, M. Malassis-Seris, F. Selz, and P. Vassalli. 1996. Complexity of the mouse gut T cell immune system: identification of two distinct natural killer T cell intraepithelial lineages. *Eur. J. Immunol. 26*:2248.

124. Buzoni-Gatel, D., A. C. Lepage, I. H. Dimier-Poisson, D. T. Bout, and L. H. Kasper. 1997. Adoptive transfer of gut intraepithelial lymphocytes protects against murine infection with *Toxoplasma gondii. J. Immunol. 158*:5883.

125. Weiner, H. L., A. Friedman, A. Miller, S. J. Khoury, A. Al-Sabbagh, L. Santos, M. Sayegh, R. B. Nussenblatt, D. E. Trentham, and D. A. Hafler. 1994. Oral tolerance: Immunologic mechanisms and treatment of animal and human organ-specific autoimmune diseases by oral administration of autoantigens. *Annu. Rev. Immunol. 12*:809.

126. Pierce, N. F. 1984. Induction of optimal mucosal antibody responses:

effects of age, immunization route(s), and dosing schedule in rats. *Infect. Immun. 43*:341.

127. Wells, H. G., and T. B. Osborne. 1911. The biological properties of the vegetable proteins. I. Anaphylaxis. *J. Infect. Dis. 8*:66.
128. Weiner, H. L. 1997. Oral tolerance: immune mechanisms and treatment of autoimmune diseases. *Immunol. Today 18*:335.
129. Chase, M. W. 1946. Inhibition of experimental drug allergy by prior feeding of sensitizing agent. *Proc. Soc. Exp. Biol. Med. 61*:257.
130. Asherton, G. L., M. Zembala, M. A. C. C. Perera, B. Mayhew, and W. R. Thomas. 1977. Production of immunity and unresponsiveness in the mouse by feeding contact sensitizing agents and the role of suppressor cells in the Peyer's patches, mesenteric lymph nodes and other lymphoid tissues. *Cell. Immunol. 33*:145.
131. Freidman, A., and H. L. Weiner. 1994. Induction of anergy or active suppression following oral tolerance is determined by antigen dosage. *Proc. Natl. Acad. Sci. USA 91*:6688.
132. Takahashi, I., I. Nakagawa, H. Kiyono, J. R. McGhee, J. D. Clements, and S. Hamada. 1995. Mucosal T cells induce systemic anergy for oral tolerance. *Biochem. Biophys. Res. Commun. 206*:414.
133. Chen, Y., V. K. Kuchroo, J. Inobe, D. A. Hafler, and H. L. Weiner. 1994. Regulatory T-cell clones induced by oral tolerance: suppression of autoimmune encephalitis. *Science 265*:1237.
134. Miller, A., O. Lider, A. B. Roberts, M. B. Sporn, and H. L. Weiner. 1992. Suppressor T cells generated by oral tolerization to myelin basic protein suppress both *in vitro* and *in vivo* immune responses by the release of transforming growth factor β after antigen-specific triggering. *Proc. Natl. Acad. Sci. USA 89*:421.
135. Bergerot, I., C. Ploix, J. Petersen, V. Moulin, C. Rask, N. Fabien, M. Lindblad, A. Mayer, C. Czerkinsky, J. Holmgren, and C. Thivolet. 1997. A cholera toxoid-insulin conjugate as an oral vaccine against spontaneous autoimmune diabetes. *Proc. Natl. Acad. Sci. USA 94*:4610.
136. Trentham, D. E., R. A. Dynesius-Trentham, E. J. Orav, D. Combitchi, C. Lorenzo, K. L. Sewell, D. A. Hafler, and H. L. Weiner. 1993. Effects of oral administration of type II collagen on rheumatoid arthritis. *Science 261*:1727.
137. Bitar, D., and C. C. Whitacre. 1988. Suppression of experimental autoimmune encephalomyelitis by the oral administration of myelin basic protein. *Cell. Immunol. 112*:364.
138. Weiner, H. L., G. A. Mackin, M. Matsui, E. J. Orav, S. J. Khoury, D. M. Dawson, and D. A. Hafler. 1993. Double-blind pilot trial of oral tolerization with myelin antigens in multiple sclerosis. *Science 259*:1321.
139. Blanas, E., F. R. Carbone, J. Allison, J. F. A. P. Miller, and W. R.

Heath. 1996. Induction of autoimmune diabetes by oral administration of autoantigen. *Science 274*:1707.

140. Kauffmann, F. *Enterobacteriaceae*. Copenhagen: Ejnar Munksgaard, 1951.

141. Pegues, D. A., Hohmann, E. L., and Miller, S. I. *Salmonella* including *S. typhi*. In: *Infections of the gastrointestinal tract*, edited by Blaser, M. J., Smith, P. D., Ravdin, J. I.,; Greenberg, H. B., and Guerrant, R. L. New York: Raven Press, 1995, p. 785.

142. Edelman, R., and M. M. Levine. 1986. Summary of an international workshop on typhoid fever. *Rev. Infect. Dis. 8*:329.

143. Woodward, T. E., J. E. Smadel, H. L. Ley, R. Green, and D. S. Mankikar. 1948. Preliminary report on the beneficial effect of chloromycetin in the treatment of typhoid fever. *Ann. Intern. Med. 29*:131.

144. Heyns, K., G. Kiessling, H. Paulsen, and M. E. Webster. 1959. D-galaktosaminvornsaure (2-amino-2-desoxy-D-galakturonsaure) als baustein des Vi-antigens. *Chem. Ber. 92*:2435.

145. Hone, D. M., S. R. Attridge, B. Forrest, R. Morona, D. Daniels, J. T. LaBrooy, D. J. Shearman, and J. Hackett. 1988. A *galE via* (Vi antigen-negative) mutant of *Salmonella typhi* Ty2 retains virulence in humans. *Infect. Immun. 56*:1326.

146. Eisenstein, T. K., Deakins, L. W., and Sultzer, B. W. The C3HeB/FeJ mouse, a strain in the C3H lineage which separates *Salmonella* susceptibility and immunizability from mitogenic responsiveness to lipopolysaccharide. In: *Proceedings of an International Symposium on Genetic Control of Natural Resistance to Infection and Malignancy*, edited by Skamene, E., Kongshaven, P. A. L., and Landy, M. New York: Academic Press, 1980, p. 115.

147. Eisenstein, T. K., L. W. Deakins, L. Killar, P. H. Saluk, and B. M. Sultzer. 1982. Dissociation of innate susceptibility to *Salmonella* infection and endotoxin responsiveness in C3HeB/FeJ mice and other strains in the C3H lineage. *Infect. Immun. 36*:696.

148. Eisenstein, T. K., L. M. Killar, and B. M. Sultzer. 1984. Immunity to infection with *Salmonella typhimurium*: mouse-strain differences in vaccine- and serum-mediated protection. *J. Infect. Dis. 150*:425.

149. Plant, J., and A. A. Glynn. 1974. Natural resistance to *Salmonella* infection, delayed hypersensitivity and Ir genes in different strains of mice. *Science 248*:345.

150. O'Brien, A. D., I. Scher, G. H. Campbell, R. P. MacDermott, and S. B. Formal. 1979. Susceptibility of CBA/N mice to infection with *Salmonella typhimurium*: influence of the X-linked gene controlling B lymphocyte function. *J. Immunol. 123*:720.

151. O'Brien, A. D., D. L. Rosenstreich, I. Scher, G. H. Campbell, R. P.

MacDermott, and S. B. Formal. 1980. Genetic control of susceptibility to *Salmonella typhimurium* in mice: role of the lps gene. *J. Immunol. 124*:20.

152. Vidal, S. M., D. Malo, K. Vogan, E. Skamene, and P. Gros. 1993. Natural resistance to infection with intracellular parasites: isolation of a candidate for *Bcg. Cell 73*:469.
153. Klugman, K., I. T. Gilberson, H. J. Koornhof, J. B. Robbins, R. Schneerson, D. Schulz, M. Cadoz, and J. Armand. 1987. Vaccination advisory committee: protective activity of Vi capsular polysaccharide vaccine against typhoid fever. *Lancet* 2:1165.
154. Collins, F. M. 1972. Salmonellosis in orally infected specific pathogen-free C57B1 mice. *Infect. Immun. 5*:191.
155. Collins, F. M. 1970. Immunity to enteric infection in mice. *Infect. Immun. 1*:243.
156. Gaines, S., H. Sprinz, J. G. Tully, and W. D. Tigertt. 1968. Studies on infection and immunity in experimental typhoid fever. VII. The distribution of *Salmonella typhi* in chimpanzee tissue following oral challenge, and the relationship between the numbers of bacilli and morphologic lesions. *J. Infect. Dis. 118*:293.
157. Carter, P. B., and F. M. Collins. 1974. The route of enteric infection in normal mice. *J. Exp. Med. 139*:1189.
158. Collins, F. M., and P. B. Carter. 1972. Comparative immunogenicity of heat-killed and living oral *Salmonella* vaccines. *Infect. Immun. 6*:451.
159. Collins, F. M., and P. B. Carter. 1978. Growth of salmonellae in orally infected germ free mice. *Infect. Immun. 21*:41.
160. Hohmann, A. W., G. Schmidt, and D. Rowley. 1978. Intestinal colonization and virulence of *Salmonella* in mice. *Infect. Immun. 22*:763.
161. Kohbata, S., H. Yokoyama, and E. Yabuuchi. 1986. Cytopathogenic effect of *Salmonella typhi* GIFU 10007 on M cells of murine ileal Peyer's patches in ligated ileal loops: an ultrastructural study. *Microbiol. Immunol. 30*:1225.
162. Jones, B. D., N. Ghori, and S. Falkow. 1994. *Salmonella typhimurium* initiates murine infection by penetrating and destroying the specialized epithelial M cells of the Peyer's patches. *J. Exp. Med. 180*:15.
163. Clark, M. A., M. A. Jepson, N. L. Simmons, and B. H. Hirst. 1994. Preferential interaction of *Salmonella typhimurium* with mouse Peyer's patch M cells. *Res. Microbiol. 145*:543.
164. Neutra, M. R., P. J. Giannasca, K. T. Giannasca, and J.-P. Kraehenbuhl, M cells and microbial pathogens. In: *Infections of the Gastrointestinal Tract*, edited by M. J. Blaser, P. D. Smith, J. I. Ravdin, H. B. Greenberg, and R. L. Guerrant, New York: Raven Press, 1995, p. 163.
165. Takeuchi, A. 1967. Electron microscopic studies of experimental

Salmonella infection. 1. Penetration into the intestinal epithelium by *Salmonella typhimurium. Am. J. Pathol. 50*:109.

166. Tannock, G. W., R. V. H. Blumershine, and D. C. Savage. 1975. Association of *Salmonella typhimurium* with, and its invasion of, the ileal mucosa in mice. *Infect. Immun. 11*:365.
167. Ginocchio, C., J. Pace, and J. E. Galan. 1992. Identification and molecular characterization of a *Salmonella typhimurium* gene involved in triggering the internalization of salmonellae into cultured epithelial cells. *Proc. Natl. Acad. Sci. USA 89*:5976.
168. Jones, B. D., H. F. Paterson, A. Hall, and S. Falkow. 1993. *Salmonella typhimurium* induces membrane ruffling by a growth factor-receptor-independent mechanism. *Proc. Natl. Acad. Sci. USA 90*:10390.
169. Francis, C. L., T. A. Ryan, B. D. Jones, S. J. Smith, and S. Falkow. 1993. Ruffles induced by *Salmonella* and other stimuli direct macropinocytosis of bacteria. *Nature 364*:639.
170. Francis, C. L., M. N. Starnbach, and S. Falkow. 1992. Morphological and cytoskeletal changes in epithelial cells occur immediately upon interaction with *Salmonella typhimurium* grown under low-oxygen conditions. *Mol. Microbiol. 6*:3077.
171. Finlay, B. B. and S. Falkow. 1998. Comparison of the invasion strategies used by *Salmonella cholerae-suis, Shigella flexneri*, and *Yersinia enterocolitica* to enter cultured animal cells: endosome acidification is not required for bacterial invasion or intracellular replication. *Biochemistry 70*:1089.
172. Bukholm, G., B. V. Johansen, E. Namork, and J. Lassen. 1982. Bacterial adhesiveness and invasiveness in cell culture monolayer. *Acta Pathol. Microbiol. Immunol. Scand. Sect. B 90*:403.
173. Finlay, B. B., and S. Falkow. 1990. *Salmonella* interactions with polarized human intestinal Caco-2 epithelial cells. *J. Infect. Dis. 162*:1096.
174. Finlay, B. B., B. Gumbiner, and S. Falkow. 1988. Penetration of *Salmonella* through a polarized Madin-Darby canine kidney epithelial cell monolayer. *J. Cell Biol. 107*:221.
175. McCormick, B. A., S. P. Colgan, C. Delp-Archer, S. I. Miller, and J. L. Madara. 1993. *Salmonella typhimurium* attachment to human intestinal epithelial monolayers: transcellular signaling to subepithelial neutrophils. *J. Cell Biol. 123*:895.
176. Rubin, F. A., P. D. McWhirter, D. Burr, N. H. Punjabi, E. Lane, S. Kumala, P. Sudarmono, S. P. Pulungsih, M. Lesmana, and P. Tjaniadi. 1990. Rapid diagnosis of typhoid fever through identification of *Salmonella typhi* within 18 hours of specimen acquisition by culture of the mononuclear cell-platelet fraction of blood. *J. Clin. Microbiol. 28*:825.

177. Joo, I. Bacterial diseases: The problem, and control by vaccines. Present status and perspectives of vaccination against typhoid fever. In: *International Conference on the Application of Vaccines Against Viral, Rickettsial, and Bacterial Diseases of Man. Scientific Publication No. 226*, edited by Pan-American World Health Organization, Washington, DC: Pan American World Health Organization, 1971, p. 329.

178. Ashcroft, M. T., J. M. Ritchie, and C. C. Nicholson. 1964. Controlled field trial in British Guiana school children of heat-killed phenolized and acetone-killed lyophilized typhoid vaccines. *Am. J. Hyg. 79*:196.

179. Yugoslav Typhoid Commission, 1962. A controlled field trial of the effectiveness of phenol and alcohol typhoid vaccines. *Bull. WHO 26*:357.

180. Hejfec, L. B. 1965. Results of the study of typhoid vaccines in four controlled field trials in the U.S.S.R. *Bull. WHO 32*:1.

181. Goodlow, R. J., S. C. Rittenberg, and J. H. Silliker. 1949. Coproantibody response in humans following T.A.B. infection. *Proc. Soc. Exp. Biol. Med. 10*:543.

182. Hobson, D. 1957. Resistance to reinfection in experimental mouse typhoid. *J. Hyg. 55*:334.

183. Ushiba, D., K. Saito, T. Akiyama, M. Nakano, T. Sugiyama, and S. Shirono. 1959. Studies on experimental typhoid: bacterial multiplication and host cell response after infection with *Salmonella enteritidis* in mice immunized with live and killed vaccines. *Jpn. J. Microb. 3*:231.

184. Collins, F. M. 1969. Effect of specific immune mouse serum on the growth of *Salmonella enteritidis* in mice preimmunized with living or ethyl alcohol-killed vaccines. *J. Bacteriol. 97*:676.

185. Collins, F. M. 1969. Effect of specific immune mouse serum on the growth of *Salmonella enteritidis* in nonvaccinated mice challenged by various routes. *J. Bacteriol. 97*:667.

186. Ushiba, D., M. Yoshioka, R. Iwahata, and S. Yamagata. 1953. Studies on the immunity of experimental typhoid. II. Effects of the immunization with killed vaccines on *Salmonella enteritidis* infection of mice. *Keio. J. Med. 2*:75.

187. Blanden, R. V., G. B. Mackaness, and F. M. Collins. 1966. Mechanisms of acquired resistance in mouse typhoid. *J. Exp. Med. 124*:585.

188. Collins, F. M., and G. B. Mackaness. 1968. Delayed hypersensitivity and Arthus reactivity in relation to host resistance in *Salmonella*-infected mice. *J. Immunol. 101*:830.

189. Mosmann, T. R., H. Cherwinski, M. W. Bond, M. A. Giedlin, and R. L. Coffman. 1986. Two types of murine helper T cell clone. 1. Definition according to profiles of lymphokine activities and secreted proteins. *J. Immunol. 136*:2348.

190. Ornellas, E. P., R. J. Roantree, and J. P. Steward. 1970. The specificity and importance of humoral antibody in the protection of mice against intraperitoneal challenge with complement-sensitive and complement-resistant *Salmonella. J. Infect. Dis. 121*:113.

191. Angerman, C. R., and T. K. Eisenstein. 1978. Comparative efficacy and toxicity of a ribosomal vaccine, acetone-killed cells, lipopolysaccharide, and a live cell vaccine prepared from *Salmonella typhimurium. Infect. Immun. 19*:575.

192. Jenkin, C. R., and D. Rowley. 1965. Partial purification of the "protective" antigen of *Salmonella typhimurium* and its distribution amongst various strains of bacteria. *Aust. J. Exp. Biol. Med. Sci. 43*:65.

193. Herzberg, M., P. Nash, and S. Hino. 1972. Degree of immunity induced by killed vaccines to experimental salmonellosis in mice. *Infect. Immun. 5*:83.

194. Svenson, S. B., M. Nurminen, and A. A. Lindberg. 1979. Artificial *Salmonella* vaccines: O-antigenic oligosaccharide-protein conjugates induce protection against infection with *Salmonella typhimurium. Infect. Immun. 25*:863.

195. Jenkin, C. R., D. Rowley, and I. Auzins. 1965. The basis for immunity to mouse typhoid. I. The carrier state. *Aust. J. Exp. Biol. Med. Sci. 42*:215.

196. Lindberg, A. A., L. T. Rosenberg, A. Ljunggren, P. J. Garegg, S. Svensson, and Wallin, N. H. 1974. Effect of synthetic disaccharide-protein conjugate as an immunogen in *Salmonella* infection in mice. *Infect. Immun. 10*:541.

197. Svenson, S. B., and A. A. Lindberg. 1978. Immunochemistry of *Salmonella* O-antigens: preparation of an octasaccharide-bovine serum albumin immunogen representative of *Salmonella* serogroup B O-antigen and characterization of the antibody response. *J. Immunol. 120*:1750.

198. Hochadel, J. F., and K. F. Keller. 1977. Protective effects of passively transferred immune T- or B-lymphocytes in mice infected with Salmonella typhimurium. *J. Infect. Dis. 135*:813.

199. Morris, J. A., C. Wray, and W. J. Sojka. 1976. The effect of T and B lymphocyte depletion on the protection of mice vaccinated with a *Gal E* mutant of *Salmonella typhimurium. Br. J. Exp. Pathol. 57*:354.

200. Nauciel, C. 1990. Role of $CD4^{+}$ T cells and T-independent mechanisms in acquired resistance to *Salmonella typhimurium* infection. *J. Immunol. 145*:1265.

201. Davies, R., and I. Kotlarski. 1976. The role of thymus-derived cells in immunity to salmonella infection. *Aust. J. Exp. Biol. Med. Sci. 54*:221.

202. Chander, R., K. B. Sainis, and N. F. Lewis. 1995. Role of thymus-

derived lymphocytes in acquired immunity to salmonellosis in mice. *Microbiol. Immunol. 30*:1299.

203. Guilloteau, L., D. Buzoni-Gatel, F. Bernard, I. Lantier, and F. Lantier. 1993. *Salmonella abortus ovis* infection in susceptible BALB/cby mice: importance of Lyt-2^+ and L3T4^+ T cells in acquired immunity and granuloma formation. *Microb. Pathog. 14*:45.
204. Hougen, H. P., B. Klausen, and E. T. Jensen. 1989. Are $CD4^+$ cells responsible for protection against salmonellosis? Remarks from studies on athymic and thymus-grafted rats. *Thymus 13*:213.
205. Killar, L. M., and T. K. Eisenstein. 1984. Differences in delayed-type hypersensitivity responses in various mouse strains in the C3H lineage infected with *Salmonella typhimurium*, strain SL3235. *J. Immunol. 133*:1190.
206. Killar, L. M., and T. K. Eisenstein. 1986. Delayed-type hypersensitivity and immunity to *Salmonella typhimurium. Infect. Immun. 52*:504.
207. Killar, L. M., and T. K. Eisenstein. 1985. Immunity to *Salmonella typhimurium* infection in C3H/HeJ and C3H/HeNCrlBR mice: studies with an aromatic-dependent live *S. typhimurium* strain as a vaccine. *Infect. Immun. 47*:605.
208. Kotlarski, I., M. Pope, K. Doherty, and S. R. Attridge. 1989. The in vitro proliferative response of lymphoid cells of mice infected with *Salmonella enteriditis* 11RX. *Immunol. Cell Biol. 67*:19.
209. Cookson, B. T., and M. J. Bevan. 1997. Identification of a natural T cell epitope presented by *Salmonella*-infected macrophages and recognized by T cells from orally immunized mice. *J. Immunol. 158*:4310.
210. Hess, J., C. Ladel, D. Miko, and S. H. E. Kaufmann. 1996. *Salmonella typhimurium aroA*$^-$ infection in gene-targeted immunodeficient mice. Major role of $CD4^+$ TCR-$\alpha\beta$ cells and IFN-γ in bacterial clearance independent of intracellular location. *J. Immunol. 156*:3321.
211. De Libero, G., and S. H. Kaufmann. 1986. Antigen-specific Lyt-2^+ cytolytic T lymphocytes from mice infected with the intracellular bacterium *Listeria monocytogenes. J. Immunol. 137*:2688.
212. Mastroeni, P., B. Villarreal-Ramos, and C. E. Hormaeche. 1993. Adoptive transfer of immunity to oral challenge with virulent salmonellae in innately susceptible BALB/c mice requires both immune serum and T cells. *Infect. Immun. 61*:3981.
213. Mastroeni, P., B. Villarreal-Ramos, and C. E. Hormaeche. 1992. Role of T cells, TNF alpha and IFN gamma in recall of immunity to oral challenge with virulent salmonellae in mice vaccinated with live attenuated aro$^-$ *Salmonella* vaccines. *Microb. Pathog. 13*:477.
214. Hormaeche, C. E. 1979. Genetics of natural resistance to salmonellae in mice. *Immunology 37*:319.

215. O'Brien, A. D., and E. S. Metcalf. 1982. Control of early *Salmonella typhimurium* growth in innately *Salmonella*-resistant mice does not require functional T lymphocytes. *J. Immunol. 129*:1349.
216. Schafer, R., and T. K. Eisenstein. 1992. Natural killer cells mediate protection induced by a *Salmonella aroA* mutant. *Infect. Immun. 60:*791.
217. Hof, H., P. Emmerling, J. Hacker, and C. Hughes. 1982. The role of macrophages in primary and secondary infection of mice with *Salmonella typhimurium. Ann. Immunol.* (*Inst. Pasteur*) *133*:21.
218. O'Brien, A. D., I. Scher, and S. B. Formal. 1979. Effect of silica on the innate resistance of inbred mice to *Salmonella typhimurium* infection. *Infect. Immun. 25*:513.
219. Van Dissel, J. T., J. J. Stikkelbroeck, B. C. Michel, P. C. Leijh, and R. van Furth. 1987. *Salmonella typhimurium*-specific difference in rate of intracellular killing by resident peritoneal macrophages from salmonella-resistant CBA and salmonella-susceptible C57BL/10 mice. *J. Immunol. 138*:4428.
220. Lissner, C. R., D. L. Weinstein, and A. D. O'Brien. 1985. Mouse chromosome 1 Ity locus regulates microbicidal activity of isolated peritoneal macrophages against a diverse group of intracellular and extracellular bacteria. *J. Immunol. 135*:544.
221. Trinchieri, G. 1995. Interleukin-12: a proinflammatory cytokine with immunoregulatory functions that bridge innate resistance and antigen specific adaptive immunity. *Annu. Rev. Immunol. 13*:251.
222. Matsumura, H., K. Onozuka, Y. Terada, Y. Nakano, and M. Nakano. 1990. Effect of murine recombinant interferon-γ in the protection of mice against *Salmonella. Int. J. Immunopharmacol. 12*:49.
223. Nauciel, C., and F. Espinasse-Maes. 1992. Role of gamma infection and tumor necrosis factor alpha in resistance to *Salmonella typhimurium* infection. *Infect. Immun. 60*:450.
224. Ramarathinam, L., D. W. Niesel, and G. R. Klimpel. 1993. Ity influences the production of IFN-gamma by murine splenocytes stimulated in vitro with *Salmonella typhimurium. J. Immunol. 150*:3965.
225. Mastroeni, P., J. A. Harrison, J. A. Chabalgoity, and C. E. Hormaeche. 1996. Effect of interleukin 12 neutralization on host resistance and gamma interferon production in mouse typhoid. *Infect. Immun. 64*:189.
226. Nakano, Y., K. Onozuka, Y. Terada, H. Shinomiya, and M. Nakano. 1990. Protective effect of recombinant tumor necrosis factor-α in murine salmonellosis. *J. Immunol. 144*:1935.
227. Morrissey, P. J., and K. Charrier. 1994. Treatment of mice with IL-1 before infection increases resistance to a lethal challenge with *Salmonella typhimurium*. The effect correlates with the resistance allele at the Ity locus. *J. Immunol. 153*:212.

228. Eckmann, L., J. Fierer, and M. F. Kagnoff. 1996. Genetically resistant (*Ity*^{r}) and susceptible (*Ity*^{s}) congenic mouse strains show similar cytokine responses following infection with *Salmonella dublin. J. Immunol. 156*:2894.

229. Lee, J. C., C. W. Gibson, and T. K. Eisenstein. 1985. Macrophage-mediated mitogenic suppression induced in mice of the C3H lineage by a vaccine strain of *Salmonella typhimurium. Cell. Immunol. 91*:75.

230. Eisenstein, T. K., L. M. Killar, B. A. Stocker, and B. M. Sultzer. 1984. Cellular immunity induced by avirulent *Salmonella* in LPS-defective C3H/HeJ mice. *J. Immunol. 133*:958.

231. Deschenes, M., E. Guenounou, F. Ronco, F. Vacheron, and C. Nauciel. 1986. Impairment of lymphocyte proliferative responses and interleukin-2 production in susceptible (C57BL/6) mice infected with *Salmonella typhimurium. Immunology 58*:225.

232. Al-Ramadi, B. K., M. A. Brodkin, D. M. Mosser, and T. K. Eisenstein. 1991. Immunosuppression induced by attenuated *Salmonella*. Evidence for mediation by macrophage precursors. *J. Immunol. 146*:2737.

233. Al-Ramadi, B. K., J. M. Greene, J. J. Meissler, Jr., and T. K. Eisenstein. 1992. Immunosuppression induced by attenuated *Salmonella*: effect of LPS responsiveness on development of suppression. *Microb. Pathog. 12*:267.

234. Al-Ramadi, B. K., J. J. Meissler, Jr., D. Huang, and T. K. Eisenstein. 1992. Immunosuppression induced by nitric oxide and its inhibition by interleukin-4. *Eur. J. Immunol. 22*:2249.

235. Huang, D., M. G. Schwacha, and T. K. Eisenstein. 1996. Attenuated salmonella vaccine induced suppression of murine spleen cell mitogen responses is mediated by macrophage nitric oxide: quantitative aspects. *Infect. Immun. 64*:3786.

236. Eisenstein, T. K., J. J. Meissler, B. A. D. Stocker, and S. I. Miller. 1998. Immunosuppression and nitric oxide induced by attenuated *Salmonella* vaccines do not correlate with protective capacity: a *phoP* mutant does not suppress but does protect. *Vaccine 16*:24.

237. Schwacha, M. G., and T. K. Eisenstein. 1997. Interleukin-12 is critical for induction of nitric oxide-mediated immunosuppression following vaccination of mice with attenuated *Salmonella typhimurium. Infect. Immun. 65*:4897.

238. Saito, S., K. Onozuka, H. Shinomiya, and M. Nakano. 1991. Sensitivity of bacteria to $NaNO_2$ and to L-arginine-dependent system in murine macrophages. *Microbiol. Immunol. 354*:325.

239. De Groote, M. A., D. Granger, Y. Xu, G. Campbell, R. Prince, and F. C. Fang. 1995. Genetic and redox determinants of nitric oxide cyto-

toxicity in a *Salmonella typhimurium* model. *Proc. Natl. Acad. Sci. USA 92*:6399.

240. Eisenstein, T. K., D. Huang, J. J. Meissler, Jr., and B. al-Ramadi. 1994. Macrophage nitric oxide mediates immunosuppression in infectious inflammation. *Immunobiology 191*:493.
241. Hone, D. M., C. O. Tacket, A. M. Harris, B. Kay, G. Losonsky, and M. M. Levine. 1992. Evaluation in volunteers of a candidate live oral attenuated *Salmonella typhi* vector vaccine. *J. Clin. Invest. 90*:412.
242. MacMicking, J., Q.-W. Xie, and C. Nathan. 1997. Nitric oxide and macrophage function. *Annu. Rev. Immunol. 15*:323.
243. Archer, G. T. L., and J. L. Whitby. 1957. Protection of mice by living Vi and O vaccines against death caused by *Salmonella paratyphi C. J. Hyg. 55*:513.
244. Fahey, K. J., and G. N. Cooper. 1970. Oral immunization against experimental Salmonellosis. *Infect. Immun. 1*:263.
245. DuPont, H. L., R. B. Hornick, M. J. Snyder, A. T. Dawkins, G. G. Heiner, and T. E. Woodward. 1971. Studies of immunity in typhoid fever. Protection induced by killed oral antigens or by primary infection. *Bull. WHO 44*:667.
246. Phalipon, A., M. Kaufmann, P. Michetti, J.-M. Cavaillon, M. Huerre, P. Sansonetti, and J.-P. Kraehenbuhl. 1995. Monoclonal immunoglobulin A antibody directed against serotype-specific epitope of *Shigella flexneri* lipopolysaccharide protects against murine experimental shigellosis. *J. Exp. Med. 182*:769.
247. Michetti, P., N. Porta, M. J. Mahan, J. M. Slauch, J. J. Mekalanos, A. L. Blum, J.-P. Kraehenbuhl, and M. R. Neutra. 1994. Monoclonal immunoglobulin A prevents adherence and invasion of polarized epithelial cell monolayers by *Salmonella typhimurium. Gastroenterol. 107*:915.
248. Ramarathinam, L., R. A. Shaban, D. W. Niesel, and G. R. Klimpel. 1991. Interferon gamma (IFN-γ) production by gut-associated lymphoid tissue and spleen following oral *Salmonella typhimurium* challenge. *Microb. Patho. 11*:347.
249. Kincy-Cain, T., J. D. Clements, and K. L. Bost. 1996. Endogenous and exogenous interleukin-12 augment the protective immune response in mice orally challenged with *Salmonella dublin. Infect. Immun. 64*:1437.
250. Harrison, J. A., B. Villarreal-Ramos, P. Mastroeni, R. Demarco de Hormaeche, and C. E. Hormaeche. 1997. Correlates of protection induced by live aro$^-$ *Salmonella typhimurium* vaccines in the murine typhoid model. *Immunology 90*:618.
251. Mixter, P. F., V. Camerini, B. J. Stone, V. L. Miller, and M. Kronenberg. 1994. Mouse T lymphocytes that express a gamma delta T-cell antigen

receptor contribute to resistance to *Salmonella* infection in vivo. *Infect. Immun. 62*:4618.

252. Germanier, R., and E. Fürer. 1975. Isolation and characterization of *Gal*E mutant Ty 21a of *Salmonella typhi*: a candidate strain for a live, oral typhoid vaccine. *J. Infect. Dis. 131*:553.
253. Germanier, R. 1970. Immunity in experimental salmonellosis. I. Protection induced by rough mutants of *Salmonella typhimurium. Infect. Immun. 2*:309.
254. Gilman, R. H., R. B. Hornick, W. E. Woodward, H. L. DuPont, M. J. Snyder, M. M. Levine, and J. P. Libonati. 1977. Evaluation of a UDP-glucose-4-epimeraseless mutant of *Salmonella typhi* as a live oral vaccine. *J. Infect. Dis. 136*:717.
255. Levine, M. M., C. Ferreccio, R. E. Black, R. Germanier, and Chilean Typhoid Committee. 1987. Large-scale field trial of Ty21a live oral typhoid vaccine in enteric-coated capsule formulation. *Lancet 1*:1049.
256. Ferreccio, C., M. M. Levine, H. Rodriguez, R. Contreras, and Chilean Typhoid Committee. 1989. Comparative efficacy of two, three or four doses of Ty21a live oral typhoid vaccine in enteric-coated capsules. A field trial in an endemic area. *J. Infect. Dis. 159*:766.
257. Hirschel, B., R. Wuthrich, B. Somaini, and R. Steffen. 1985. Inefficacy of the commercial live oral Ty 21a vaccine in the prevention of typhoid fever. *Eur. J. Clin. Microbiol. 4*:295.
258. Silva, B. A., C. Gonzales, G. C. Mora, and F. Cabello. 1987. Genetic characteristics of the *Salmonella typhi* strain Ty21a vaccine. *J. Infect. Dis. 155*:1077.
259. Hoiseth, S. K., and B. A. D. Stocker. 1981. Aromatic-dependent *Salmonella typhimurium* are non-virulent and effective as live vaccines. *Nature 291*:238.
260. Levine, M. M., D. Herrington, J. R. Murphy, J. G. Morris, G. Losonsky, B. Tall, A. A. Lindberg, S. Svenson, S. Baqar, M. F. Edwards, and B. Stocker. 1987. Safety, infectivity, immunogenicity, and in vivo stability of two attenuated auxotrophic mutant strains of *Salmonella typhi*, 541Ty and 543Ty, as live oral vaccines in man. *J. Clin. Invest. 79*:888.
261. Sigwart, D. F., B. A. Stocker, and J. D. Clements. 1989. Effect of a purA mutation on efficacy of *Salmonella* live-vaccine vectors. *Infect. Immun. 57*:1858.
262. Tacket, C. O., M. B. Sztein, G. A. Losonsky, S. S. Wasserman, J. P. Nataro, R. Edelman, D. Pickard, G. Dougan, S. N. Chatfield, and M. M. Levine. 1997. Safety of live oral *Salmonella typhi* vaccine strains with deletions in *htrA* and *aroC aroD* and immune response in humans. *Infect. Immun. 65*:452.
263. Hooke, A. M., Z. Wang, M. C. Cerquetti, and J. A. Bellanti. 1991.

Immunization with temperature-sensitive mutants of *Salmonella typhi* induces protection in mice. *Vaccine 9*:238.

264. Gherardi, M. M., V. E. García, V. Brizzio, D. O. Sordelli, and M. C. Cerquetti. 1993. Differential persistence, immunogenicity and protective capacity of temperature-sensitive mutants of *Salmonella enteritidis* after oral or intragastric administration to mice. *FEMS. Immunol. Med. Microb. 7*;161.
265. Curtiss, R., and S. M. Kelly. 1987. *Salmonella typhimurium* deletion mutants lacking adenylate cyclase and cyclic AMP receptor protein are avirulent and immunogenic. *Infect. Immun. 55*:3035.
266. Miller, S. I., and J. J. Mekalanos. 1990. Constitutive expression of the phoP regulon attenuates *Salmonella* virulence and survival within macrophages. *J. Bacteriol. 172*:2485.
267. Hohmann, E. L., C. A. Oletta, K. P. Killeen, and S. I. Miller. 1996. *phop/phoQ*-deleted *Salmonella typhi* (Ty800) is a safe and immunogenic single-dose typhoid fever vaccine in volunteers. *J. Infect. Dis. 173*:1408.
268. Formal, S. B., L. S. Baron, D. J. Kopecko, O. Washington, C. Powell, and C. A. Life. 1981. Construction of a potential bivalent vaccine strain: introduction of *Shigella sonnei* Form I antigen genes into the *galE Salmonella typhi* Ty21a typhoid vaccine strain. *Infect. Immun. 34*:746.
269. Keren, D. F., H. H. Collins, L. S. Baron, D. J. Kopecko, and S. B. Formal. 1982. Intestinal immunoglobulin A response in rabbits to a *Salmonella typhi* strain harboring a *Shigella sonnei* plasmid. *Infect. Immun. 37*:387.
270. Clements, J. D., and S. El-Morshidy. 1984. Construction of a potential live oral bivalent vaccine for typhoid fever and cholera-*Escherichia coli*-related diarrheas. *Infect. Immun. 46*:564.
271. Clements, J. D., F. L. Lyon, K. L. Lowe, A. L. Farand, and S. El-Morshidy. 1986. Oral immunization of mice with attenuated *Salmonella enteritidis* containing a recombinant plasmid which codes for production of the B subunit of heat-labile *Escherichia coli* enterotoxin. *Infect. Immun. 53*:685.
272. Brown, A., C. E. Hormaeche, R. Demarco de Hormaeche, M. Winther, G. Dougan, and B. A. Stocker. 1987. An attenuated aroA *Salmonella typhimurium* vaccine elicits humoral and cellular immunity to cloned beta-galactosidase in mice. *J. Infect. Dis. 155*:86.
273. Karem, K. L., S. Chatfield, N. Kuklin, and B. Rouse. 1995. Differential induction of carrier antigen-specific immunity by *Salmonella typhimurium* live-vaccine strains after single mucosal or intravenous immunization of BALB/c mice. *Infect. Immun. 63*:4557.

274. Sadoff, J. C., W. R. Ballou, L. S. Baron, W. R. Majarian, R. N. Brey, W. T. Hockmeyer, S. J. Cryz, J. Ou, G. H. Lowell, et al. 1988. Oral *Salmonella typhimurium* vaccine expressing circumsporozoite protein protects against malaria. *Science 240*:336.

275. Berggren, R. E., A. Wunderlich, E. Ziegler, M. Schleicher, R. C. Duke, D. Looney, and F. C. Fang. 1995. HIV gp120-specific cell-mediated immune responses in mice after oral immunization with recombinant *Salmonella. J. AIDS Hum. Retrovirus 10*:489.

276. Bao, J. X., and J. D. Clements. 1991. Prior immunologic experience potentiates the subsequent antibody response when *Salmonella* strains are used as vaccine carriers. *Infect. Immun. 59*:3841.

277. Chabalgoity, J. A., B. Villareal-Ramos, C. M. Anjam Khan, S. N. Chatfield, R. Demarco de Hormaeche, and C. E. Hormaeche. 1995. Influence of preimmunization with tetanus toxoid on immune responses to tetanus toxin fragment C-guest antigen fusions in a *Salmonella* vaccine carrier. *Infect. Immun. 63*:2564.

278. Harokopakis, E., G. Hajishengallis, T. E. Greenway, M. W. Russell, and S. M. Michalek. 1997. Mucosal immunogenicity of a recombinant *Salmonella typhimurium*-cloned heterologous antigen in the absence or presence of coexpressed cholera toxin A2 or B subunits. *Infect. Immun. 65*:1445.

279. Cardenas, L., U. Dasgupta, and J. D. Clements. 1994. Influence of strain viability and antigen dose on the use of attenuated mutants of *Salmonella* as vaccine carriers. *Vaccine 12*:833.

280. Darji, A., C. A. Guzman, B. Gerstel, J. Wachholz, K. N. Timmis, J. Wehland, T. Chakraborty, and S. Weiss. 1997. Oral somatic transgene vaccination using attenuated *S. typhimurium. Cell 91*:765.

281. Schubbert, R., D. Renz, B. Schmitz, and W. Doerfler. 1997. Foreign (M13) DNA ingested by mice reaches peripheral leukocytes, spleen, and liver via the intestinal wall mucosa and can be covalently linked to mouse DNA. *Proc. Natl. Acad. Sci. USA 94*:961.

282. Sztein, M. B., S. S. Wasserman, C. O. Tacket, R. Edelman, D. Hone, A. A. Lindberg, and M. M. Levine. 1994. Cytokine production patterns and lymphoproliferative responses in volunteers orally immunized with attenuated vaccine strains of *Salmonella typhi. J. Infect. Dis. 170*:1508.

283. Sztein, M. B., M. K. Tanner, Y. Polotsky, J. M. Orenstein, and M. M. Levine. 1995. Cytotoxic T lymphocytes after oral immunization with attenuated vaccine strains of *Salmonella typhi* in humans. *J. Immunol. 155*:3987.

CHAPTER 4

CELL BIOLOGY AND IMMUNE RESPONSE TO *Listeria monocytogenes*, AN INTRACELLULAR PATHOGEN

SUJATA VIJH and ERIC G. PAMER

4.1 INTRODUCTION

Listeria monocytogenes was first identified as a pathogenic organism in the early part of the twentieth century. In one early report, a fatal disease of wild gerbils in South Africa was attributed to a previously undescribed gram-positive bacillus. In honor of Lord Joseph Lister and because the bacterium caused severe infection of the liver, it was named *Listerella hepatolytica* (1). At about the same time, a fatal disease of laboratory rabbits in England was found to result from infection by a gram-positive bacillus (2) as well. Because the infection was associated with a pronounced monocytosis, the bacterium was named *Bacterium monocytogenes*. Not long after these two descriptions of animal infection by this bacterium came the first case report of human infection (3). This bacterium, eventually renamed *Listeria*

Abbreviations: APC, antigen-presenting cell; β2-M, β2-microglobulin; CTL, cytotoxic T lymphocyte; ELISA, enzyme-linked immunosorbent assay; HIV, human immunodeficiency virus; hly, hemolysin; HPLC, high performance liquid chromatography; inl, internalin; IFN, interferon; IL, interleukin; LLO, listeriolysin O; LPS, lipopolysaccharide; MHC, major histocompatibility antigen; MPL, metalloprotease; NK, natural killer; NO, nitric oxide; PI-PLC, phosphatidylinositol-specific phospholipase C; PC-PLC, phosphatidylcholine-specific phospholipase C; RAG, recombination activating gene; SCID, severe combined immunodeficiency; TAP, transporters associated with antigen processing; TCR, T-cell receptor; Th, T helper; TNF, tumor necrosis factor.

Intracellular Bacterial Vaccine Vectors, Edited by Yvonne Paterson.
ISBN 0-471-17278-2

monocytogenes, has since been recognized as an important cause of severe, often fatal, infections of immunocompromised human beings.

4.2 INFECTIONS CAUSED BY *Listeria monocytogenes*

Human infection with *Listeria monocytogenes* typically occurs in individuals with an underlying immunodeficiency (4). In immunocompetent people, infection with *Listeria monocytogenes* may be accompanied by flu-like symptoms, and spontaneous resolution is usual (4). In patients with illnesses that compromise the immune system, such as cancer, chronic liver disease, and renal failure, or in patients who are pharmacologically immunosuppressed, such as transplant recipients or patients treated with chemotherapy for cancer or autoimmunity, *Listeria monocytogenes* can cause severe, frequently fatal, infections. In these patients, *L. monocytogenes* causes bacteremia or meningitis, or both. Another important syndrome caused by *L. monocytogenes* is septic abortion, which typically occurs during the third trimester of pregnancy. Although mothers usually recover uneventfully, fetal infection, which in its most severe form is called granulomatosis infantisepticum, is frequently fatal. Neonates can also be infected after birth, in which case *Listeria monocytogenes* causes either meningitis or bacteremia, or both. Finally, the immunosuppression that results from human immunodeficiency virus (HIV) infection also increases the risk of symptomatic *L. monocytogenes* infection (5).

Although strains of *Listeria monocytogenes* containing plasmids that confer antibiotic resistance have been isolated from patients, it is fortunate that this is an unusual event (6). Infections with *L. monocytogenes* are generally treated with ampicillin, however the mortality remains as high as 50%, perhaps because clinically apparent infection occurs in a more vulnerable patient population (4).

4.3 EPIDEMIOLOGY OF *Listeria monocytogenes* INFECTIONS

Listeria monocytogenes is an environmental organism cultivated from water, silage, and soil. *L. monocytogenes* can infect a remarkable range of vertebrate animals, including cattle, sheep, chickens, wild fowl, and even fish (7). The ability of a single strain of *L. monocytogenes* to infect such a diverse group of animals suggests that its virulence factors must foil defense mechanisms that are common to its different hosts.

An important consequence of *L. monocytogenes*' prevalence in the environment is that human exposure to this pathogen is common. One study showed that most healthy individuals have serum antibodies that recognize *L. monocytogenes* antigens (8). It is unclear, however, whether exposed individuals have protective immunity to *L. monocytogenes*. The most important route for human exposure to *L. monocytogenes* is the oral ingestion of contaminated food (9). That *L. monocytogenes* is a food-borne pathogen was first demonstrated during the 1980s, after an outbreak of listeriosis in the Canadian Maritime provinces (10). In this epidemic, coleslaw made with cabbage that had been fertilized with manure from *L. monocytogenes*-infected sheep was the likely cause of more than 40 clustered cases of listeriosis. Subsequent outbreaks of listeriosis have been attributed to contaminated cheeses or other dairy products (11). Although epidemics of listeriosis occur periodically, most clinical cases are isolated and sporadic. In sporadic listeriosis, a variety of food sources, including undercooked chicken, uncooked sausages, and deli food have been implicated (12). The current U.S. Department of Agriculture (USDA) policy does not tolerate any contamination of ready-to-eat food products with *L. monocytogenes*. However, foods that should be cooked prior to ingestion, such as meat products, can be, and very frequently are, contaminated with *L. monocytogenes* (13).

4.4 *Listeria monocytogenes* MICROBIOLOGY

Listeria monocytogenes is a gram-positive bacterium that is rod shaped. It is motile in liquid culture and can grow well as 37°C, but it also multiplies at temperatures as low as 4°C. *L. monocytogenes* is very easy to cultivate in the laboratory. In rich media such as trypticase soy broth or brain/heart infusion, bacteria divide approximately every 30–35 minutes, nearly as fast as *Escherichia coli*. There are now numerous genetic tools, such as transposons (14,15), conjugatable plasmids (16), and temperature-sensitive plasmids (17,18), that can be used to manipulate *L. monocytogenes*. Temperature-sensitive plasmids that undergo site-specific integration at nonpermissive temperatures have been used to generate attenuated strains of *L. monocytogenes* that lack virulence factors or to generate strains of *L. monocytogenes* that produce heterologous antigens (17,21,22).

4.5 PATHOGENESIS AND CELL BIOLOGY OF *Listeria monocytogenes* INFECTIONS

Although *L. monocytogenes* is an important cause of infection in humans, our understanding of the pathogenesis and immunology of human listeriosis is incomplete. By contrast, the pathogenesis and immunology of listeriosis in mice is understood to a far greater extent. In this chapter, unless stated otherwise, the pathogenesis of *L. monocytogenes* infection and the subsequent immune response have been deduced from either in vitro infection of cell lines or in vivo infection of mice. It is widely assumed that these findings are relevant to human infection with *L. monocytogenes*.

Listeria monocytogenes causes natural infection by invading intestinal epithelial cells following ingestion of contaminated food. Since epithelial cells are not actively phagocytic, *L. monocytogenes* must enter these cells by an invasive process that requires the association of a bacterial surface protein with a receptor on the surface of the host cell. A surface protein of *L. monocytogenes*, internalin, was discovered to play an essential role in the invasion of epithelial cells (23). Internalin contains repeat regions that are similar to previously described streptococcal and staphylococcal surface proteins. There are two different internalin molecules, internalin A (InlA) and internalin B (InlB), which are structurally similar (23). Strains of *L. monocytogenes* that lack both forms of internalin are less virulent and cause markedly diminished infection of the liver (24). Both forms of internalin appear to play important but different roles in *L. monocytogenes* invasion of epithelial cells (24–26). While InlA is essential for internalization by intestinal epithelial cells, InlB appears to be important for internalization by hepatocytes. In order for *L. monocytogenes* to be fully virulent, both forms of internalin must be expressed. Recently, the ligand for internalin on the surface of epithelial cells was found to be E-cadherin (27).

After cellular entry, intracellular *L. monocytogenes* escape the vacuole by secreting a protein called listeriolysin-O (LLO), which lyses the vacuolar membrane (28). LLO is an essential virulence factor and *L. monocytogenes* that lack LLO are avirulent in mice (14,15,29). While LLO is the major virulence factor implicated in escape from the vacuole, it does not act alone. Three other proteins, phosphatidylinositol-specific phospholipase C (PI-PLC), a broad-range phospholipase C (PC-PLC), and the secreted metalloprotease (MPL), also participate in escape from the vacuole. In fact, in some epithelial cell lines, LLO is not essential for escape from the vacuole (20). PC-PLC is a secreted protein activated by MPL (30). Thus, LLO independent escape from the vacuole requires both PC-PLC and the metalloprotease (20). Although *L. monocytogenes* that express LLO but lack PC-PLC escape primary vacuoles normally, they are less virulent in mice and defective in cell to cell spread. Studies with strains of *L. monocytogenes* that lack both Pl-PLC and PC-PLC suggest that these secreted proteins have overlapping functions in pathogenesis (31). It has been proposed that PC-PLC plays a major role in escape from double-membraned vacuoles as *L. monocytogenes* spreads from one cell to another (20).

In the cytosol *L. monocytogenes* multiplies rapidly and spreads to adjacent cells. Intracellular and intercellular movement of *L. monocytogenes* results from the asymmetric polymerization of actin on one pole of the bacterium (32), which pushes the bacterium through the host cells cytosol (33). Through this process, intracellular bacteria can be pushed into neighboring cells without re-entering the extracellular space. ActA is a surface protein of *L. monocytogenes* that is essential for actin polymerization and motility in the host cell cytosol (34,35). Strains of *L. monocytogenes* that lack ActA are markedly less virulent in mice, indicating that movement in the cytosol of infected cells in vivo, and cell to cell spread by this mechanism are essential for pathogenesis. Expression of *L. monocytogenes* ActA in the mitochondria of eukaryotic cells demonstrated that it functions independently as a nucleator of the actin cytoskeleton (36).

Thus, infection of host cells by *L. monocytogenes* and spread to neighboring cells require expression of these multiple virulence factors. The genes encoding these factors are clustered in the virulence region of the *L. monocytogenes* chromosome and are regulated by the prfA regulator (37). Although the virulence genes are regulated by the same factor, and in the absence of this factor expression of the virulence factors is downregulated, the virulence factors appear not to be expressed in concert (38,39). Since some of the *L. monocytogenes* virulence factors, in particular LLO, can be toxic to the host cell, it is clear that their expression must be regulated. It appears that the genes for the different virulence factors have different sensitivities to prfA, allowing ActA to be highly expressed in the host cell cytosol (18), while LLO expression is very low (39). Thus, the important task of expressing the appropriate virulence factor in the appropriate subcellular location may be accomplished by graded responsiveness of virulence genes to prfA levels. Different environmental stimuli may affect the level of prfA expression. The role of the different *L. monocytogenes* virulence factors during cellular infection is tabulated in Table 7.2 and presented schematically in Figure 4.1.

While *L. monocytogenes* multiplies in the host cell cytosol the host cells metabolic machinery remains remarkably unaffected. Thus, host cell protein synthesis and protein trafficking occur with near normal kinetics in *L. monocytogenes* infected cells. However, studies of the glycosylation of host cell glycoproteins have shown that *L. monocytogenes* infection reduces the sialic acid content of lysosomal and cell surface glycoproteins (40). The downmodulation of cell surface sialic acid may serve as a signal to the innate immune system of cellular

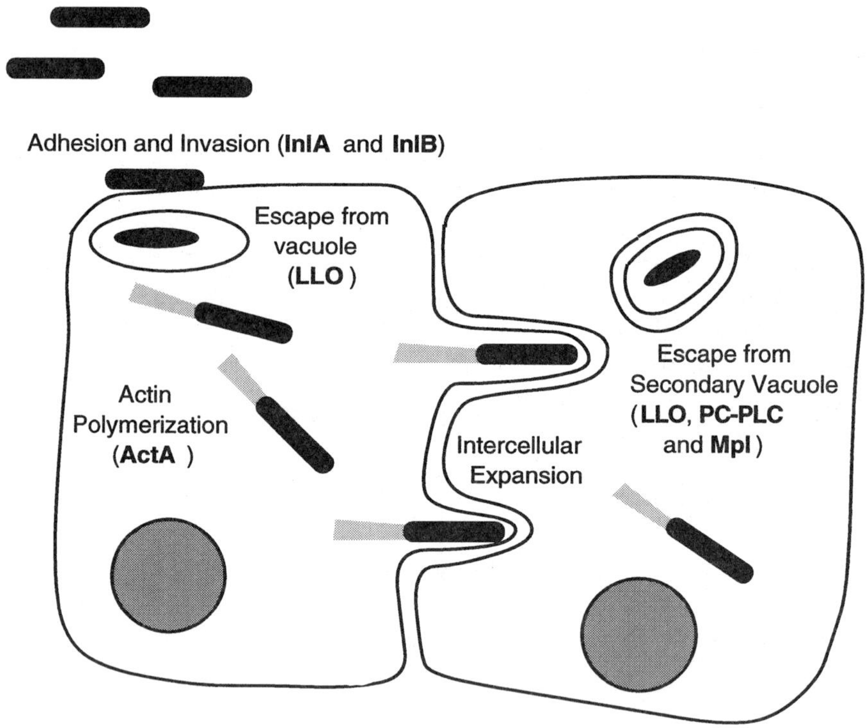

Figure 4.1 Interaction of *Listeria monocytogenes* with eukaryotic host cells. There are four major steps in cellular infection by *L. monocytogenes:* 1, adhesion and invasion, mediated by InlA and InlB; 2, escape from the phagosomal vacuole, mediated by LLO; 3, motility within the host cell cytosol, mediated by ActA, which nucleates actin at one pole of the bacterium; and 4, cell-to-cell spread, which requires LLO, PC-PLC, and the metalloprotease for escape from the secondary vacuole.

infection. In contrast to macrophage infection, infection of hepatocytes with *L. monocytogenes* appears to induce host cell apoptosis (41). This is reminiscent of the effect of another pathogenic bacterium that enters the host cell cytosol, *Shigella flexneri* (42).

4.6 THE IMMUNE RESPONSE TO *Listeria monocytogenes* INFECTION

L. monocytogenes infection of mice has been one of the most useful models for investigating cell mediated immunity. Over the past 40 years, many aspects of the mammalian immune system have been investigated with this model. Mice can be infected with *L. monocytogenes* intravenously, subcutaneously, intraperitoneally, or orally. The lethal dose of intravenous *L. monocytogenes* varies with the mouse strain being infected and with the strain of *L. monocytogenes* used for infection but is usually around 1,000–10,000 bacilli per animal. After intravenous infection with a sublethal dose of *L. monocytogenes*, mice clear the infection and develop long term immunity to infection with much higher doses (43). This model is simple and highly reproducible. As a result, the murine response to *L. monocytogenes* is perhaps the best understood immune response to any pathogenic organism.

4.7 EARLY RESPONSES TO *Listeria monocytogenes* INFECTION

The immune response to pathogenic organisms can be divided into the innate responses, which occur early and are not antigen specific, and the specific immune responses, which occur later. The importance of innate immunity to *L. monocytogenes* infection became apparent from work with athymic mice (44,45) and mice with severe combined immunodeficiency (SCID) (45). Surprisingly, infection of mice with absent cell-mediated and humoral immune responses resulted in chronic but, reasonably well-controlled, infections. Therefore, the nonspecific innate immune system limits the growth of *L. monocytogenes* in the mammalian host. In the last decade much has been learned about the innate response to murine infection with *L. monocytogenes*.

Ingestion and killing by neutrophils is one of the major defenses against many extracellular bacteria. It has now become apparent that neutrophils also play a very important role in the defense against infection by intracellular pathogens such as *L. monocytogenes*. Initial investigation of liver and spleen histology after *L. monocytogenes* infection showed many neutrophils during the first few days after infection. Although it remained unclear whether neutrophils reduce the number of viable bacilli in vivo, the fact that immune-mediated resistance to *L. monocytogenes* infection correlated with enhanced accumulation of neutrophils at sites of infection suggested that neutrophils play a role in defense against infection (46). More compelling evidence for a protective role of neutrophils in the defense against *L. monocytogenes* infection came from experiments in which antibodies that prevent the migration of neutrophils and monocytes were administered to mice. Blocking neutrophil migration greatly exacerbated *L. monocytogenes* infection in the liver (47), suggesting that neutrophils lyse infected hepatocytes and kill *L. monocytogenes* to curtail infection (48). Recently, studies with more specific monoclonal antibodies that deplete neutrophils in infected mice demonstrate that neutrophils play a more important role in containing *L. monocytogenes* infection in the liver than in the spleen (49). Studies in SCID mice showed that the major defensive role of neutrophils occurs in the first few days after infection (50). Neutrophil depletion does not impair the development of T-lymphocyte-mediated immunity, since splenocytes from *L. monocytogenes*-infected, but neutrophil-depleted, mice can confer specific immunity upon transfer to naive mice (51). While specific immunity can develop in the absence of neutrophils, immune T cells appear to require neutrophils to abolish *L. monocytogenes* infection, as transfer of immune splenocytes to neutrophil-depleted recipient mice does not result in protection. This finding suggests an important role for neutrophils in completing the work of lymphocytes (52).

Natural killer (NK) cells represent another branch of the nonspecific, innate immune system and they also participate in the early defense against *L. monocytogenes* infection. Depletion of NK cells from mice with specific antibodies results in exacerbation of *L. monocytogenes* infection (53). After tissue infection with *L. monocytogenes*, draining lymph nodes contain large numbers of interferon-γ (IFN-γ) secreting cells that are predominantly NK cells (54,55). These findings suggest that NK cells play a major role in the early defense against *L. monocytogenes* infection, although the stimulus that results in NK cell migration to sites of *L. monocytogenes* infection is unknown. It has been shown that heat-killed *L. monocytogenes* can induce IFN-γ secretion by NK cells in the presence of tumor necrosis factor (55).

Although lysis of infected cells by NK cells may be important in antilisterial defense, it is likely that IFN-γ production by NK cells is of greater importance. The role of IFN-γ in the defense against *L. monocytogenes* infection was demonstrated in mice lacking the receptor for IFN-γ or the gene for IFN-γ. Both mutations result in mice that are much more susceptible to infection with *L. monocytogenes* (56,57). Subsequent studies have shown that MHC class I restricted CTL do not have to express IFN-γ to be protective (56,58). These findings, taken together, suggest that IFN-γ produced by NK cells is critical for early defense against *L. monocytogenes* infection.

Lymphocytes bearing the $\gamma\delta$ T-cell receptor (TCR) also contribute to the early defense against *L. monocytogenes* infection. *L. monocytogenes* infection of the mouse peritoneum results in the early influx of $\gamma\delta$ T cells, followed by the appearance of $\alpha\beta$ T cells (59). The severity of *L. monocytogenes* infection influences the kinetics of the $\gamma\delta$ T-cell response (60). Depletion of $\gamma\delta$ T cells from infected mice with specific antibodies exacerbates *L. monocytogenes* infection, resulting in roughly 100-fold more bacteria in the spleens of mice 5 days postinfection (61). However, $\gamma\delta$ T-cell-depleted mice eventually clear the infection, in contrast to mice depleted of $\alpha\beta$ T cells (61). Studies in mice that lack $\alpha\beta$ T cells, $\gamma\delta$ T cells, or both $\alpha\beta$ and $\gamma\delta$ T cells (62) demonstrate that early *L. monocytogenes* infection is controlled to a much greater extent by $\gamma\delta$ T cells than by $\alpha\beta$ T cells. In the case of $\alpha\beta$ and $\gamma\delta$ T-cell knockout mice, however, sublethal doses of *L. monocytogenes* are eventually cleared (62). As might be expected from previous studies with nude mice, if *L. monocytogenes*-infected mice lack both $\gamma\delta$ and $\alpha\beta$ T cells, a chronic infection develops (62). The antigen specificity of the $\gamma\delta$ T-cell response to *L. monocytogenes* infection is unknown. It is possible that $\gamma\delta$ T cells may not be expanding in response to bacterial antigens, as there is evidence that the cytokines IL-1 and IL-12, which are produced by *L. monocytogenes*-infected macrophages, can drive expansion of this T-cell subset (63).

The early defense against *L. monocytogenes* infection is mediated by macrophages, neutrophils, natural killer cells and $\gamma\delta$ T lymphocytes. Neutrophils appear to attack infected cells and ingest and kill bacteria in the liver and spleen. This battle, which occurs during the first 24–48 hours after infection, is a major defense against *L. monocytogenes*. Neutrophil mediated defenses are complemented by macrophages, which are activated to become more bacteriocidal by IFN-γ, which is produced by NK and $\gamma\delta$ T cells. These defenses, which are not antigen specific and which are activated quickly in response to *L. monocytogenes* infection, control a potentially lethal infection. Indeed, early innate immune responses may eliminate a greater number of bacteria than the subsequent adaptive immune response.

4.8 T-LYMPHOCYTE RESPONSES TO *Listeria monocytogenes*

Although the innate immune system limits the early stages of *L. monocytogenes* infection, clearance of the infection and development of long term immunity require specific immunity. In contrast to infections by extracellular bacteria, infections caused by intracellular bacteria generally do not induce protective humoral immunity. This is also the case after infection by *L. monocytogenes*. Thus, although mice that have recovered from *L. monocytogenes* have serum antibodies that recognize a number of different bacterial antigens, transfer of immune serum to naive mice does not confer protection. Early studies of protective immunity after *L. monocytogenes* infection demonstrated that immunity could only be transferred to naive mice with cells (64). In the past 15 years it has become clear that T lymphocytes bearing the $\alpha\beta$ T-cell receptor (TCR) clear *L. monocytogenes* infection and provide long-term immunity (62).

T lymphocytes can be divided into subsets that express $CD4^+$ or $CD8^+$ on their cell surface. $CD4^+$ T cells generally interact with MHC class II molecules presenting peptides derived from exogenous or vacuolar antigens. By contrast, $CD8^+$ T cells recognize peptides that are generally of cytosolic origin which are presented by MHC class I molecules (65). The role of $CD8^+$ and $CD4^+$ T cells in the defense against *L. monocytogenes* infection was first investigated by transferring these T-cell subsets from *L. monocytogenes*-immunized mice to naive recipients. These adoptive transfer experiments demonstrated that *L. monocytogenes* specific $CD8^+$ cytolytic T lymphocytes can protect naive mice from lethal infection (66). More recently, mice lacking $CD4^+$ or $CD8^+$ T cells were used to determine the relative importance of these T-cell subsets in protection from *L. monocytogenes* infection (67). To determine the role of $CD8^+$ T cells, mice in which the gene for β2-microglobulin (β2-M) was disrupted were used. Because β2-M is essential for MHC class I surface expression, positive selection of $CD8^+$ T cells does not occur in these knockout mice and they therefore have greatly reduced numbers of $CD8^+$ T lymphocytes. To determine the role of $CD4^+$ T cells, mice in which the gene for the I-A β chain was disrupted were used. Disrupting the I-A β chain in C57BL/6 mice, which lack I-E MHC class II molecules, results in mice that do not express any cell surface MHC class II molecules and thus have greatly reduced numbers of $CD4^+$ T lymphocytes. These knockout mice were infected with *L. monocytogenes* and the course of their infection was determined (67). It was found that mice that lack $CD4^+$ T cells have a slightly prolonged course of *L. monocytogenes* infection as compared with control mice, but the infection resolves. In mice lacking $CD8^+$ T cells, however, *L. monocytogenes* infection was significantly prolonged. Although mice lacking $CD8^+$ T cells also recovered from infection, recovered mice appeared to have a lower level of immunity than that of immune mice lacking $CD4^+$ T cells. These studies demonstrated that neither $CD4^+$ nor $CD8^+$ T cells are absolutely essential for clearance of infection or immunity. However, both $CD4^+$ and $CD8^+$ cells contribute to the protective immune response to *L. monocytogenes* infection. Experiments with adoptive transfer of T-cell subsets or with the T-cell subset knockout mice indicate that $CD8^+$ T cells play a greater role in the generation of protective immunity than $CD4^+$ T cells.

$CD8^+$ cytolytic T lymphocytes were believed to mediate resistance to *L. monocytogenes* infection by lysing infected cells and secreting IFN-γ in the infected microenvironment, which would activate local macrophages. The importance of cell lysis by CTL was demonstrated in mice in which the gene for perforin was disrupted (68). These perforin knockout mice have diminished resistance to primary infection and reduced levels of immunity after sublethal infection. Furthermore, adoptive transfer of perforin-deficient immune splenocytes conferred approximately 100-fold less protection than control immune splenocytes (68). Thus, lysis of *L. monocytogenes* infected cells appears to play a significant role in the ability of CTL to confer protection. Studies using bone marrow chimeric mice indicate that CTL-mediated lysis of bone marrow derived and non-bone marrow-derived cells, perhaps hepatocytes, is essential for optimal bacterial clearance (69).

4.9 CYTOKINES AND SOLUBLE MEDIATORS OF HOST DEFENSE

While lysis of *L. monocytogenes*-infected cells requires direct contact between the effector and the target cell, many intercellular interactions during the course of infection occur by means of cytokine secretion. The following sections summarize the role of the major cytokines in combating infection with *L. monocytogenes*.

4.9.1 Interferon-γ

Interferon-γ (IFN-γ) is an important cytokine in the host defense against many infections. Its major activity is to activate macrophages to become more effective microbial killers and to increase the capacity of many different cell types to process and present antigens to T lymphocytes. Administration of specific antibodies that neutralize IFN-γ to mice infected with *L. monocytogenes* demonstrated that IFN-γ plays a key role in controlling infection (70). This finding was confirmed with mice in which the receptor for IFN-γ or the gene for IFN-γ were disrupted. Both knockout mouse strains were found to be much more sensitive to *L. monocytogenes* infection (56,57). Macrophages lacking the receptor for IFN-γ are more permissive for *L. monocytogenes* infection (71). Although the major effector functions of $CD8^+$ T cells are lysis of infected cells and secretion of IFN-γ, $CD8^+$ T cells are not the only source of IFN-γ. Since NK cells, $\gamma\delta$ T lymphocytes and $CD4^+$ T lymphocytes also produce IFN-γ, it was not clear which source of IFN-γ is important and which might be dispensable. *L. monocytogenes*-specific $CD8^+$ T cells can protect naive mice from infection upon adoptive transfer. To determine whether secretion of IFN-γ is an important effector function of adoptively transferred CTL, $CD8^+$ T cells were transferred with and without IFN-γ neutralizing antibody. It was found that protection conferred by the adoptive transfer of *L. monocytogenes*-specific CTL was not diminished by the co-administration of anti IFN-γ antibodies (58). When *L. monocytogenes*-specific $CD4^+$ T lymphocytes were adoptively transferred, however, protection was diminished by the administration of IFN-γ specific antibodies. This study suggested that IFN-γ is not an essential effector mechanism for CTL mediated protection.

This issue was addressed more rigorously in subsequent studies using mice in which the IFN-γ gene was disrupted. Because IFN-γ deficient mice are highly susceptible to wild type *L. monocytogenes* infection, knockout mice were immunized with a strain of *L. monocytogenes* that was attenuated by deleting a portion of the ActA gene (18,56). This strain of *L. monocytogenes*, which cannot induce the polymerization of cytosolic actin and thus cannot spread from cell to cell, has a similar LD_{50} in IFN-γ knockout and wild-type mice.

Infection of IFN-γ knock-out mice with a sublethal dose of ActA-deficient *L. monocytogenes* induces partial immunity to infection with wild-type bacteria. This finding indicates that at least a portion of protective immunity is independent of IFN-γ (56). When $CD8^+$ T cells were obtained from immunized IFN-γ-deficient mice and transferred to naive mice, it was found that they were able to confer protection. This study proved that CTL can confer protection by a mechanism other than IFN-γ production. This suggests that lysis of infected cells is the major effector mechanism $CD8^+$ T cells use to control infection by *L. monocytogenes*.

4.9.2 Tumor Necrosis Factor-α

Tumor necrosis factor-α (TNF-α) is best known for its role during septic shock after infections with gram-negative bacteria. Many of the systemic symptoms associated with gram-negative septic shock can be replicated by administering TNF-α to animals. Furthermore, administering antibodies that bind to TNF-α can prevent death in animals infused with lipopolysaccharide (LPS) from gram-negative bacteria. In marked contrast to infection by certain gram-negative bacteria, TNF-α appears to play a protective role in the defense against *L. monocytogenes* infection. A potential role for TNF-α in the defense against *L. monocytogenes* infection was first found when TNF-α-specific antibodies were administered to infected mice (72). These studies demonstrated that blocking TNF-α markedly increased the lethality of *L. monocytogenes* infection. In other studies it was found that TNF-α plays a role in the activation of macrophages of SCID mice (73). These studies were extended with mice in which the gene encoding the 55-kD receptor for TNF-α was disrupted (74,75). Although these mice were resistant to endotoxin, they were much more susceptible to *L. monocytogenes* infection. Taken together, these studies indicate that TNF-α is a critical factor in the defense against *L. monocytogenes*. Studies with *Salmonella typhimurium*-infected mice also demonstrate that TNF-α plays a protective role (76,77). Thus, TNF-α may be most important in the defense against intracellular bacterial infection.

4.9.3 Interleukin-1

Interleukin-1 (IL-1), like TNF-α, is a cytokine that mediates many of the systemic symptoms associated with severe infection. In *L.*

monocytogenes-infected mice IL-1 is expressed in the livers and spleens as early as 1 day after infection. The amount of IL-1 found correlates with the severity of infection (78). When antibodies specific for the type I IL-1 receptor were administered to infected mice, it resulted in 100- to 1,000-fold higher numbers of *L. monocytogenes* in liver and spleen 5 days after infection than in untreated mice (78). This study was confirmed when antibodies specific for IL-1α, IL-1β, and the type I IL-1 receptor were administered to SCID mice. These mice developed more severe infections with *L. monocytogenes* than occurred in control SCID mice and suffered higher mortality rates (79). Several mechanisms for the IL-1-mediated protection have been suggested. Interestingly, blocking IL-1 inhibited the characteristic influx of neutrophils into the peritoneal cavity following infection, suggesting that IL-1 plays a role in neutrophil recruitment. IL-1 blockade also diminished macrophage sensitivity to IFN-γ and the expression of MHC class II molecules by macrophages after infection by *L. monocytogenes* (80). These experiments suggest that IL-1 may mediate its protective effect by facilitating the activation of macrophages. This activity of IL-1 may not be limited to macrophages since IL-1 in combination with IL-12 has been shown to enhance $\gamma\delta$ T-cell proliferation and expression of IFN-γ (63). Recently, mice in which the gene for IL-1β was disrupted were shown to have similar resistance to *L. monocytogenes* infection as that exhibited by wild-type mice (81). Thus, it is possible that IL-1α and IL-1β may have overlapping roles in the defense against *L. monocytogenes* infection.

4.9.4 Interleukin-12

IL-12 has been shown to enhance NK cell proliferation and $CD8^+$ T-cell expansion and to enhance the differentiation of $CD4^+$ T cells into Th1 (IFN-γ and IL-2), rather than Th2 (IL-4 and IL-10) cells (82). Macrophages exposed to heat-killed *L. monocytogenes* secrete IL-12. Thus, heat-killed *L. monocytogenes* have been used to sway the $CD4^+$ T-cell response in the direction of the Th1 instead of the Th2 phenotype (83). A protective role for IL-12 in the response to *L. monocytogenes* infection was shown by administering IL-12 to mice. IL-12 was found to enhance their resistance to *L. monocytogenes* infection (84). By contrast, blocking IL-12 with specific antibody exacerbated *L. monocytogenes* infection and resulted in 100- to 1,000-fold more bacteria in spleen and liver than in control animals (84). In SCID mice, IL-12-blocking antibodies also worsened *L. monocytogenes* infection.

The deleterious effect of anti-IL-12 antibody could be reversed by concomitant administration of IFN-γ (85). This finding suggests that IL-12 production after *L. monocytogenes* infection is critical for generating early, IFN-γ mediated responses.

It is possible that IL-12 may play a role in the development of *L. monocytogenes* specific immunity. A recent study in which mice were immunized with heat-killed *L. monocytogenes* and IL-12 showed that they developed protective immunity (86). Immunization of mice with dead *L. monocytogenes* generally does not prime a protective immune response, although a recent study found protective immunity after multiple injections of high doses of heat-killed *L. monocytogenes* (87). Other investigators have shown that heat-killed *L. monocytogenes* can be processed by macrophages and that epitopes can be presented by MHC class I molecules to $CD8^+$ T lymphocytes (88). It is possible that IL-12, either induced by heat-killed listeria or administered exogenously, may induce a protective $CD4^+$ Th1 response in this setting (86).

4.9.5 Interleukin-6

IL-6, which like IL-1 is a cytokine that mediates the acute inflammatory response, has also been shown to play a positive role in the immune response to *L. monocytogenes* infection. The levels of IL-6 found in mice during *L. monocytogenes* infection are directly correlated with the severity of infection (89). The protective role of IL-6 in *L. monocytogenes* infections was demonstrated by administering IL-6 shortly before infection. Mice that received IL-6 had 10-fold fewer bacteria in the spleen and liver at 2 and 4 days after infection. The protective effect of IL-6 administration was demonstrated in recombination activating gene (RAG) knockout mice, which lack B and T lymphocytes, to require the presence of neutrophils (90). Disruption of the gene encoding IL-6 renders mice more susceptible to *L. monocytogenes* infection (90,91). These knockout mice had greater liver infection and fewer circulating neutrophils than control mice (90). Taken together, these studies suggest that neutrophils mediate protective effects of IL-6.

4.9.6 Interleukin-4, Interleukin-10, and Interleukin-13

Cytokines associated with enhanced inflammation or swaying of the immune response in the direction of cell-mediated immunity (Th1 type

$CD4^+$ T-cell responses) play a positive role in the defense against *L. monocytogenes* infection. By contrast, cytokines associated with Th2 type $CD4^+$ T-cell responses appear to exacerbate *L. monocytogenes* infections. For examples, in mice injected with antibodies specific for IL-4, the number of *L. monocytogenes* in the liver and spleen is reduced by a factor of up to 100 after infection (92). Interestingly, while IL-4 is generally undetectable in normal mice during *L. monocytogenes* infection, in infected mice lacking the receptor for IFN-γ, IL-4 is readily detected (93). Even in normal mice, however, IL-4-producing cells can be found in the liver during very early infection; this IL-4 production has been proposed to play a role in the production of monocyte chemoattractant protein-1 (94). Studies of the role of IL-10 during *L. monocytogenes* infection have also been performed. In these studies, SCID mice were injected with immune complexes, which promote IL-10 secretion by macrophages. Mice treated with immune complexes were found to be more susceptible to *L. monocytogenes* infection. When infected SCID mice were treated with immune complexes and IL-10-specific antibodies, however, exacerbation of infection was prevented (95). More recently, it has been shown that mice with a disrupted gene for IL-10 have greater resistance to *L. monocytogenes* infection, with enhanced clearance of bacteria early after infection and increased production of proinflammatory cytokines (96). These experiments indicate that both IL-4 and IL-10 expression are detrimental to T lymphocyte independent clearance of *L. monocytogenes*. Recently, the role of the Th2-like IL-13 was investigated in *L. monocytogenes*-infected mice (97). Surprisingly, administration of IL-13 to mice enhanced their resistance to infection. Determining the mechanisms by which these cytokines influence the clearance of bacteria will require further investigation.

4.9.7 NF-κB and NF-IL6 Transcription Factors

The regulation of gene expression after infection is complex, but certain transcription factors appear to play central roles in the activation of gene expression for multiple cytokines. One such factor is NF-κB, which is a transcription factor that regulates the expression of interleukin-1β, IL-2, IL-6, IFN-β, and tumor necrosis factor-α (TNF-α). The gene for the p50 subunit of NF-κB has been disrupted in mice. The knockout mice are developmentally normal but, not surprisingly, more susceptible to *L. monocytogenes* infection (98). Another transcription factor, NF-IL6, regulates the expression of IL-6,

IL-1α, IL-8, TNF-α, granulocyte colony-stimulating factor (G-CSF) and nitric oxide synthase. Mice in which NF-IL6 has been knocked out are also more susceptible to *L. monocytogenes* infection (99). Interestingly, macrophages deficient in NF-IL6 have a decreased ability to kill vacuolar *L. monocytogenes;* thus, a greater proportion of bacteria escape into the cytosol. These studies are beginning to address one of the most fundamental questions of host parasite interaction: How are the genes involved in host defense activated?

4.9.8 Nitric Oxide

The importance of nitric oxide in defense against microbial pathogens has recently received much attention. Nitric oxide (NO) can be directly bacteriocidal; it can also react with hydrogen peroxide to form peroxynitrite, to enhance killing by the oxidative burst (100). NO production has been shown to participate in macrophage-mediated killing of *L. monocytogenes*. Aminoguanidine, a competitive inhibitor of nitric oxide synthase, decreases the ability of macrophages to kill intracellular *L. monocytogenes* (101). If aminoguanidine is administered to mice it dramatically increases the mortality of normal and SCID mice to infection with *L. monocytogenes* (101). Thus, although other microbicidal mechanisms are, surely, also involved, nitric oxide appears to play a critical role in macrophage mediated clearance of *L. monocytogenes* in infected mice.

4.9.9 Summary of Innate Responses to *L. monocytogenes*

The murine immune response to *L. monocytogenes* is complex, with distinct cell types and cytokines performing sequential, in some cases complementary and in others overlapping, functions. Figure 4.2 summarizes the immune response to *L. monocytogenes* infection. All the immune activities appear to circle around the infected macrophage, which is at center stage. Early in infection, inflammatory and immune cells are recruited by the secretion of IL-1, IL-6, IL-12, and TNF-α. The rapid, nonspecific elimination of *L. monocytogenes* at sites of infection requires neutrophil recruitment, which is mediated, at least in part, by IL-1 and IL-6. It is likely that macrophage produced IL-12 stimulates NK cells and $\gamma\delta$ T cells during the first few days of murine infection. In turn, these cells become activated and secrete IFN-γ, which activates infected and uninfected macrophages. Activated macrophages are far more effective at killing *L. monocyto-*

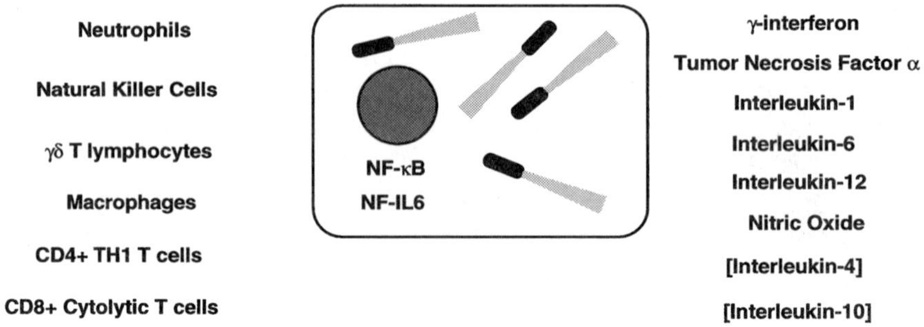

Figure 4.2 Immune defenses against *Listeria monocytogenes* infection. The cellular response to *L. monocytogenes* infection can be divided into two major components: 1, the innate cellular responses mediated by neutrophils, natural killer (NK) cells, $\gamma\delta$ T cells, and macrophages; and 2, the specific immune responses mediated by $CD4^+$ and $CD8^+$ T lymphocytes. The nuclear transcription factors NF-κB and NF-IL6 play a major role in the activation of inflammatory cytokine gene transcription. The cytokines that play a protective role in the response to *L. monocytogenes* infection are indicated on the right. Cytokines that worsen *L. monocytogenes* infections are shown in brackets.

genes, in part by NO production. The early, nonspecific responses are followed by specific T-cell responses to *L. monocytogenes* antigens presented by infected macrophages. The nature of the T-cell response is very likely influenced by the cytokines produced in the preceding inflammatory response. Thus, the expansion and phenotype of T cells is also driven by IL-12 produced by infected macrophages. Clearance of infection and long term immunity are mediated principally by $CD4^+$ T cells, which secrete IL-2 and IFN-γ, and $CD8^+$ T cells, which lyse *L. monocytogenes*-infected cells. Although the murine defense against *L. monocytogenes* infection contains some redundancies, optimal clearance of infection requires each step to be intact.

4.10 ANTIGEN SPECIFICITY OF T LYMPHOCYTES

4.10.1 MHC Class II-Restricted T Cells

The importance of $CD4^+$ and $CD8^+$ T lymphocytes in the clearance of *L. monocytogenes* after infection and the establishment of protective immunity was outlined earlier in this chapter. T lymphocytes that respond to intracellular infection recognize peptide fragments that are either in the groove of MHC class I or MHC class II molecules (102). $CD4^+$ T cells recognize peptide fragments that are generated in the endosomal compartment of antigen-presenting cells (APCs) from proteins that have either been engulfed from the cell surroundings or transported there from the other cellular compartments (103). Since *L. monocytogenes* traverses the endosomal compartment on its way to becoming an intracellular pathogen, and since the majority of macrophage ingested bacteria are killed and degraded (104), MHC class II molecules present *L. monocytogenes*-derived peptides to $CD4^+$ T cells.

One of the first *L. monocytogenes* antigens shown to be detected by T lymphocytes was listeriolysin (LLO), the essential virulence factor required for bacterial escape into the cytosol (105). Subsequent analysis with peptide fragments of LLO showed that this antigen contains several epitopes that are presented by MHC class II molecules to $CD4^+$ lymphocytes (106). The MHC class II-restricted T-cell response is not limited to LLO, since another epitope derived from a previously unknown *L. monocytogenes* antigen was identified by expression cloning (107). The complexity of the $CD4^+$ T lymphocyte response was analyzed by separation of *L. monocytogenes* proteins by two-dimensional electrophoresis, and assessment of T-cell reactivity with the separated proteins. These experiments demonstrated that many different *L. monocytogenes* proteins are recognized by T cells (108). Thus, it appears that many different proteins feed into the MHC class II antigen processing pathway during the course of *L. monocytogenes* infection. Because of the relatively small number of antigens that have been identified, it is too early to say whether any particular subset of bacterial proteins (i.e., secreted, cell wall associated or intrabacterial) form the major targets of *L. monocytogenes*-specific $CD4^+$ T lymphocytes.

4.10.2 MHC Class Ia-Restricted CTL

In contrast to the MHC class II antigen processing pathway, the peptides presented by MHC class I molecules principally derive from proteins that are degraded in the cytosol of the antigen presenting cell (65). Most cytosolic peptides are generated by proteasomes, which are multicatalytic, multicomponent protease complexes that are prevalent in the cytosol and nucleus of eukaryotic cells. The cytosolic peptides are transported into the lumen of the endoplasmic reticulum by the heterodimeric transporters associated with antigen processing (TAP) proteins. MHC class I molecules that have been newly synthesized associate with β2-M and bind antigenic peptides in the endoplasmic reticulum. The MHC class I/β2-M/peptide trimer trafficks to the cell surface, where the complex is detected by the T-cell receptor (TCR) of $CD8^+$ T lymphocytes (65). The MHC class I antigen-processing pathway is present in most nucleated cells and is believed to function primarily in the defense against viral infection. *L. monocytogenes*, however, feeds into the MHC class I antigen processing pathway because it enters the cytosol of infected cells (110). Thus, $CD8^+$ T lymphocytes, in contrast to many other intracellular bacterial infections, are recruited to fight this infection.

Early studies with T-cell lines and clones derived from immunized mice demonstrated that specific $CD8^+$ T cells could lyse *L. monocytogenes*-infected macrophages (66). Subsequent studies found that an H2-K^d-restricted CTL clone could lyse a syngeneic tumor cell line transfected with the gene for LLO, the major virulence factor of *L. monocytogenes*. The precise epitope recognized by this clone was found to be residues 91–99 of LLO (111). The antigenicity of LLO was confirmed when target cells infected with *Bacillus subtilis* expressing LLO were recognized by *L. monocytogenes*-specific CTL (112). Some CTL clones derived from $H2^d$ mice and also restricted by H2-K^d were found not to be specific for LLO 91–99. The antigen specificity of one of these clones was determined by affinity-purifying H2-K^d from *L. monocytogenes*-infected cells, isolating and high-performance liquid chromatography (HPLC) purifying the bound peptides. The fraction recognized by the CTL clone was subjected to amino acid sequence analysis, which identified the epitope as residues 217–225 of the secreted *L. monocytogenes* murein hydrolase, p60 (113). Subsequently, it was found that amino acids 449–457 of p60 are also presented to CTL by the H-2K^d MHC class I molecule (114). The antigenicity of p60 was demonstrated in previous studies that showed that immunization of mice with *Salmonella* expressing *L. monocytogenes* p60 could protect them from subsequent *L. monocytogenes* infection (8). The important role of CTL specific for the LLO and p60 epitopes in protective immunity was demonstrated by adoptive transfer of CTL specific for either LLO 91–99 or p60 to naive mice. Recipients of specific CTL were significantly protected from *L. monocytogenes* infection (115,116). A fourth H2-K^d-restricted CTL epitope derived from the *L. monocytogenes* metalloprotease has also been identified (117).

It is remarkable that all the H2-K^d-restricted epitopes described above derive from proteins that are secreted by *L. monocytogenes*. This finding suggests that secreted proteins have the greatest access to the MHC class I antigen processing pathway. Presentation of the *L. monocytogenes* epitopes requires active bacterial protein synthesis, since tetracycline, an inhibitor of bacterial protein synthesis, rapidly abrogates the production of LLO 91–99 or p60 217–225 (118,119). Once secreted by *L. monocytogenes* into the host cell cytosol, the bacterial proteins are rapidly degraded. Using two inhibitors of cytosolic proteases, it was demonstrated that proteasomes degrade the majority of proteins secreted by *L. monocytogenes* into the host cell cytosol (39,120). Taken together, these studies make a strong case for the notion that proteins secreted by intracellular bacteria are the most likely to be antigenic at the T-cell level. An important implication of this finding is that secretion of antigenic proteins by bacteria functioning as "vaccine vehicles" may be essential for their success. Several recent studies have directly addressed the role of bacterial antigen secretion in the priming of CTL responses. While studies with *Salmonella typhimurium* demonstrated that protein secretion is essential for the generation of protective immunity (123), another group determined that even proteins that are not secreted by *L. monocytogenes* can induce CTL responses and protective immunity (123). Because these studies have used different antigens and bacteria to address this question, and have obtained different, but not conflicting results, it is fair to say that the role of antigen secretion by bacteria in protective immunity warrants further investigation (124).

4.10.3 Efficiency of MHC Class I Antigen Processing

Although the major *L. monocytogenes*-derived CTL epitopes are all presented on the cell surface by H2-K^d, they are present in different amounts. These quantitative differences are partially a function of the intracellular expression levels of LLO and p60. LLO is very toxic to eukaryotic cells, and its expression is highly regulated. Under stressful conditions, such as might be found in the phagolysosome, its expression is upregulated, while in complete media its level of expression is very low (37). By contrast, p60, which is not toxic to eukaryotic cells, is expressed constitutively (125). Two-dimensional gel electrophoresis of metabolically labeled bacterial proteins demonstrated that following cellular infection p60 is one of the most highly expressed secreted proteins (118). Pulse-chase analysis demonstrated that p60 is degraded in the cytosol with a half-life of 90 minutes. Quantitation of p60 secretion by enzyme-linked immunosorbent assay (ELISA) demonstrated that, on average, individual *L. monocytogenes* bacteria secrete roughly 60 molecules of p60 per minute. With this information it was possible to estimate that roughly 35 p60 molecules are degraded for every p60 217–225 epitope generated (118). Because p60 449–457 is generated from p60 with roughly 10-fold greater efficiency, only three to four molecules of p60 have to be degraded to generate one p60 449–457 epitope (114).

In contrast to p60, the expression of LLO in the cytosol of infected cells is almost undetectable (39). Intracellular metabolic labeling of *L. monocytogenes* proteins shows that the rate of LLO secretion is approximately 2% the level of p60 secretion. It is remarkable, therefore, that LLO is one of the major antigens detected by CTL. The remarkable antigenicity of LLO may result from its very rapid rate of degradation in the host cell cytosol and the great efficiency of LLO 91–99 generation from whole LLO. Based on the efficiency of p60 processing, it is estimated that only 5–10 LLO molecules must be degraded for every LLO 91–99 epitope generated in the host cell (39). Thus, the likelihood that an antigen will be detected by CTL is influenced not only by the absolute amount of antigen secreted into the cytosol, but by the rate of its degradation and the efficiency with which nonamer epitopes can be generated by the host cell as well. An important unresolved issue concerns the mechanism of host cell recognition of bacterial proteins in the cytosol. Along these lines, a recent study demonstrated that the identity of the N-terminal amino acid of p60 can dramatically influence its rate of degradation in the host cell cytosol (126), indicating that degradation of this bacterial antigen adheres to the eukaryotic host cells' N-end rule for protein degradation (127).

Studies of the CTL antigens of *L. monocytogenes* have provided important information for vaccine development. First, there is a tight linkage between the rate of protein degradation and the number of epitopes that are ultimately presented on the cell surface. Second, if protein degradation is rapid, it may not be essential to have high levels of intracellular secretion of the antigen. Third, MHC class I antigen processing of bacterial proteins is actually very efficient, especially if one considers the hurdles that an epitope must surmount in order to be presented on the cell surface. Given this efficiency, it may not be necessary for antigens to be expressed at high levels to be of immunologic significance.

4.10.4 Magnitude and Kinetics of MHC Class Ia-Restricted CTL Responses

The magnitude of the T-cell response to the four H2-K^d-restricted *L. monocytogenes* epitopes was determined by ELISPOT, and demonstrated that LLO 91–99 elicits the largest T-cell response, p60 217–225 an intermediate response and mpl 84–92 and p60 449–457 elicit only minor T-cell responses (128,129). This result was surprising because the magnitude of the T-cell response did not correlate with the number of respective epitopes that are presented by *L. monocytogenes*-infected macrophages. Further studies performed with strains of *L. monocytogenes* that secrete mutant forms of p60 that are processed into p60 217–225 with a range of different efficiencies demonstrated that once a threshold amount of epitope is produced, increasing the amount of epitope that is presented does not significantly effect the magnitude of the T-cell response (130). Analysis of the TCR repertoire of CTL specific for each of the four H2-K^d-restricted epitopes showed that the dominant epitopes elicit a broad range of receptors, while the subdominant epitopes elicit a restricted range of receptors (128). Further studies investigating the expansion of CTL following *L. monocytogenes* infection were performed with H2-K^d tetramers complexed with each of the epitopes (131). Surprisingly, CTL specific for these different peptides expand and contract synchronously in response to infection, suggesting that they are coordinately regulated (131). Direct analysis of TCR diversity during expansion demonstrates that expansion rates vary for different clones, resulting in the focusing of T-cell responses after repeated infections (132).

4.10.5 MHC Class Ib-Restricted CTL

Early investigations of *L. monocytogenes*-specific CTL demonstrated that some CTL clones could recognize *L. monocytogenes*-infected macrophages derived from strains of mice that differed in the MHC (133–135). Although these CTL were initially considered to be MHC unrestricted, the solution to their mysterious specificity was ultimately found in the MHC. In addition to the classical MHC class I molecules (H-2K, D, and L), mice also have many MHC class Ib molecules. These molecules, which are also referred to as nonclassical class I molecules, are structurally similar to classical MHC class I molecules, in that they contain three major domains and associate with β2-M. One feature of MHC class Ib molecules is their conservation between mouse strains. Thus, mouse strains as diverse as BALB/c ($H2^d$), C57BL/6 ($H2^b$), SJL ($H2^s$), and C3H ($H2^k$) share common MHC class Ib molecules, while their MHC class Ia molecules are distinct (136). There are more than 20 MHC class Ib genes in the mouse, however, with respect to the immune response to bacterial infection one molecule, H2-M3, stands out. H2-M3 was first identified to present peptides derived from mitochondria to alloreactive CTL (137). Subsequently it was determined that H2-M3 presents almost exclusively peptides that contain N-formyl methionine at the N-terminus (138). The prediction that H2-M3 may play an important role in presentation of bacterial antigens was fulfilled when the specificity of "unrestricted," *L. monocytogenes*-specific CTL was determined (139,140). These studies demonstrated that H-2M3 presented *L. monocytogenes* peptides, and possibly other bacterial products, to CTL. Recently, the exact peptide specificity of three H2-M3 restricted CTL clones was determined (141–143). All three are short, formyl-methionine peptides. One peptide derives from an *L. monocytogenes* integral membrane protein of unknown function (141), while the most recently identified peptide derives from a short open reading frame that may play a regulatory role in the expression of some nearby genes (142). An interesting aspect of peptide presentation by H2-M3 is the finding that macrophages can present both formyl-methionine peptides if they are fed heat-killed *L. monocytogenes* (144). The implication of this finding is that H2-M3 can bind peptides that originate in an endosomal compartment, rather than in the cytosol. Alternate MHC class I antigen processing pathways have been described previously for bacterial antigens and particulate antigens (145,146). Thus, H2-M3 may participate in such an alternate MHC class I antigen processing pathway. An interesting recent finding suggests that CTL clones restricted by H2-M3 may recognize multiple *L. monocytogenes*-derived peptides (147). The molecular basis for this cross-reactivity remains undefined. The antigen specificity of MHC class I restricted CTL is summarized in Fig. 4.3.

An exciting aspect of antigen presentation by MHC class Ib molecules is their conservation, with the practical implication that the same peptide antigen can be presented to T cells in individuals with disparate MHC haplotypes. In the case of the murine immune response to *L. monocytogenes*, H2-M3-restricted CTL have been shown to confer protection against infection. Mice with disparate MHC haplotypes all respond to the same H2-M3-presented peptide (143). In the face of the difficulties presented by MHC polymorphism in outbred ani-

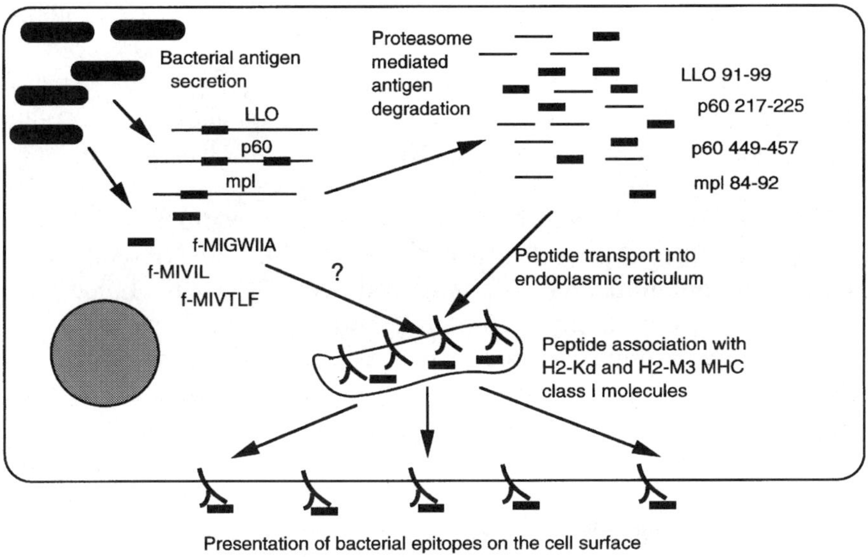

Figure 4.3 Antigen specificity of CTL after infection with *Listeria monocytogenes*. There are seven *L. monocytogenes* peptides recognized by CTL derived from BALB/c ($H2^d$) mice after infection. Three of these peptides, f-MIVIL, f-MIVTLF, and f-MIGWIIA, are presented to CTL by the H2-M3 MHC class Ib molecules. Four other peptides—LLO 91–99, p60 217–225, p60 449–457, and mpl 84–92—result from the cytosolic degradation of bacterially secreted LLO, p60, and mpl. Peptides are transported into the lumen of the endoplasmic reticulum, where they are bound by newly synthesized $H2\text{-}K^d$ MHC class I molecules. After transport to the cell surface, *L. monocytogenes* peptide epitopes are presented to $CD8^+$ cytolytic T lymphocytes.

mals, peptide-based vaccines may be better directed to MHC class Ib molecules.

4.11 CONCLUSION

Listeria monocytogenes is a remarkable and well-characterized pathogenic bacterium. It can survive and grow in the environment, and it can infect a broad range of vertebrate hosts. To be pathogenic, *L. monocytogenes* must express virulence factors that (i) allow it to adhere to and invade epithelial cells, (ii) escape from the phagocytic vacuole, (iii) move within cells by polymerizing actin, and (iv) move from cell to cell and lyse double membrane vacuoles. To be fully virulent, *L. monocytogenes* must express a series of virulence proteins. Strains of *L. monocytogenes* lacking one or more of the virulence proteins are attenuated. While the degree of attenuation varies depending on which virulence factor is defective, as long as bacteria gain access to the host cell cytosol, a potent, MHC class I-restricted T-cell response is elicited.

By means of mechanisms that are not yet fully elucidated, *L. monocytogenes* infection provokes a brisk neutrophil and NK cell mediated innate inflammatory response, followed by a Th1 helper and $CD8^+$ CTL-specific immune response. Understanding the mechanisms that move this complex response in the direction of protective, cell-mediated immunity will be essential for the development of vaccines against pathogens that evade the specific immune system.

4.12 REFERENCES

1. Pirie, J. H. 1927. A new disease of veld rodents. Tiger River Disease. *Publ. S. Afr. Inst. Med. Res. 3*:163.
2. Murray, E. G. D., R. A. Webb, and M. B. R. Swann. 1926. A disease of rabbits characterised by a large mononuclear leucocytosis, caused by a hitherto undescribed bacillus *Bacterium monocytogenes. J. Pathol. Biol. 29*:407.
3. Nyfeldt, A. 1929. Etiologie de la mononucleose infectieuse. *Soc. Biol. 101*:590.
4. Gellin, B. G., and C. V. Broome. 1989. Listeriosis. *JAMA 261*:1313.
5. Gellin, B. G., C. V. Broome, W. F. Bibb, R. E. Weaver, S. Gaventa, and L. Mascola. 1991. The epidemiology of listeriosis in the United States—1986. *Am. J. Epidemiol. 133*:392.
6. Poyart-Salmeron, C., C. Carlier, P. Trieu-Cuot, A. L. Courtieu, and P. Courvalin. 1990. Transferable plasmid-mediated antibiotic resistance in *Listeria monocytogenes. Lancet 335*:1422.
7. Farber, J. M., and P. I. Peterkin. 1991. *Listeria monocytogenes*, a food-borne pathogen. *Microbiol. Rev. 55*:476.
8. Gentschev, I., Z. Sokolovic, S. Kohler, G. F. Krohne, H. Hof, J. Wagner, and W. Goebel. 1992. Identification of p60 antibodies in human sera and presentation of this listerial antigen on the surface of attenuated Salmonellae by the HlyB-HlyD secretion system. *Infect. Immun. 60*:5091.
9. Jones, D. 1990. Listeriosis. *Lancet 336*:1171.
10. Schlech, W. F., P. M. Lavigne, R. A. Bortolussi, A. C. Allen, E. V.

Haldane, A. J. Wort, A. W. Hightower, S. E. Johnson, S. H. King, E. S. Nicholls, and C. V. Broome. 1983. Epidemic listeriosis—evidence for transmission by food. *N. Engl. J. Med. 308*:203.

11. Linnan, M. J., L. Mascola, X. D. Lou, V. Goulet, S. May, C. Salminen, D. W. Hird, M. L. Yonekura, P. Hayes, R. Weaver, A. Audurier, B. D. Plikaytis, S. L. Fannin, A. Kleks, and C. V. Broome. 1988. Epidemic listeriosis associated with Mexican-style cheese. *N. Engl. J. Med. 319*:823.
12. Schuchat, A., K. A. Deaver, J. D. Wenger, P. D. Plikaytis, L. Mascola, R. W. Pinner, A. L. Reingold, and C. V. Broome. 1992. Role of foods in sporadic listeriosis. I. Case-control study of dietary risk factors. *JAMA 267*:2041.
13. Pinner, R. W., A. Schuchat, B. Swaminathan, P. S. Hayes, K. A. Deaver, R. E. Weaver, P. D. Plikaytis, M. Reeves, C. V. Broome, and J. D. Wenger. 1992. Role of foods in sporadic listeriosis. II. Microbiologic and epidemiologic investigation. *JAMA 267*:2046.
14. Gaillard, J. L., P. Berche, and P. Sansonetti. 1986. Transposon mutagenesis as a tool to study the role of hemolysin in the virulence of *Listeria monocytogenes. Infect. Immun. 52*:50.
15. Kathariou, S., P. Metz, H. Hof, and W. Goebel. 1987. Tn916-induced mutations in the hemolysin determinant affecting virulence of *Listeria monocytogenes. J. Bacteriol. 169*:1291.
16. Trieu-Cuot, P., C. Carlier, P. Martin, and P. Courvalin. 1987. Plasmid transfer by conjugation from *Escherichia coli* to Gram-positive bacteria. *FEMS Microbiol. Lett. 48*:289.
17. Shen, H., M. K. Slifka, M. Matloubian, E. R. Jensen, R. Ahmed, and J. F. Miller. 1995. Recombinant Listeria monocytogenes as a live vaccine vehicle for the induction of protective anti-viral cell-mediated immunity. *Proc. Natl. Acad. Sci. USA 92*:3987.
18. Brundage, R. A., G. A. Smith, A. Camilli, J. A. Theriot, and D. A. Portnoy. 1993. Expression and phosphorylation of the *Listeria monocytogenes* ActA protein in mammalian cells. *Proc. Natl. Acad. Sci. USA 90*:11890.
19. Camilli, A., L. G. Tilney, and D. A. Portnoy. 1993. Dual roles of plcA in *Listeria monocytogenes* pathogenesis. *Mol. Microbiol. 8*:143.
20. Marquis, H., V. Doshi, and D. A. Portnoy. 1995. The broad-range phospholipase C and a metalloprotease mediate listeriolysin O-independent escape of *Listeria monocytogenes* from a primary vacuole in human epithelial cells. *Infect. Immun. 63*:4531.
21. Frankel, F. R., S. Hedge, J. Lieberman, and Y. Patterson. 1995. Induction of cell-mediated immune responses to human immunodeficiency

virus type 1 Gag protein by using Listeria monocytogenes as a live vaccine vector. *J. Immunol. 155*:4775.

22. Jensen, E. R., R. Selvakumar, H. Shen, R. Ahmed, F. O. Wettstein, and J. F. Miller. 1998. Recombinant *Listeria monocytogenes* vaccination eliminates papillomavirus-induced tumors and prevents papilloma formation from viral DNA. *J. Virol. 71*:8467.
23. Gaillard, J. L., P. Berche, C. Frehel, E. Gouin, and P. Cossart. 1991. Entry of *L. monocytogenes* into cells is mediated by internalin, a repeat protein reminiscent of surface antigens from Gram-positive cocci. *Cell 65*:1127.
24. Gaillard, J. L., F. Jaubert, and P. Berche. 1996. The inlAB locus mediates the entry of *Listeria monocytogenes* into hepatocytes in vivo. *J. Exp. Med. 183*:359.
25. Dramsi, S., C. Kocks, C. Forestier, and P. Cossart. 1993. Internalin-mediated invasion of epithelial cells by *Listeria monocytogenes* is regulated by the bacterial growth state, temperature and the pleiotropic activator prfA. *Mol. Microbiol. 9*:931.
26. Dramsi, S., I. Biswas, E. Maguin, L. Braun, P. Mastroeni, and P. Cossart. 1995. Entry of *Listeria monocytogenes* into hepatocytes requires expression of inlB, a surface protein of the internalin multigene family. *Mol. Microbiol. 16*:251.
27. Mengaud, J., H. Ohayon, P. Gounon, R. M. Mege, and P. Cossart. 1996. E-cadherin is the receptor for internalin, a surface protein required for entry of *L. monocytogenes* into epithelial cells. *Cell 84*:923.
28. Bielecki, J., P. Youngman, P. Connelly, and D. A. Portnoy. 1990. Bacillus subtilis expressing a haemolysin gene from *Listeria monocytogenes* can grow in mammalian cells. *Nature 345*:175.
29. Portnoy, D. A., P. S. Jacks, and D. J. Hinrichs. 1988. Role of hemolysin for the intracellular growth of *Listeria monocytogenes. J. Exp. Med. 167*:1459.
30. Poyart, C., E. Abachin, I. Razafimanantsoa, and P. Berche. 1993. The zinc metalloprotease of *Listeria monocytogenes* is required for maturation of phosphatidylcholine phospholipase C: direct evidence obtained by gene complementation. *Infect. Immun. 61*:1576.
31. Smith, G. A., H. Marquis, S. Jones, N. C. Johnston, D. A. Portnoy, and H. Goldfine. 1995. The two distinct phospholipases C of *Listeria monocytogenes* have overlapping roles in escape from a vacuole and cell-to-cell spread. *Infect. Immun. 63*:4231.
32. Tilney, L. G., and D. A. Portnoy. 1989. Actin filaments and the growth, movement, and spread of the intracellular parasite, *Listeria monocytogenes. J. Cell Biol. 109*:1597.
33. Theriot, J. A., T. J. Mitchison, L. G. Tilney, and D. A. Portnoy. 1992.

The rate of actin-based motility of intracellular *Listeria monocytogenes* equals the rate of actin polymerization. *Nature 357*:257.

34. Kocks, C., E. Gouin, M. Tabouret, P. Berche, H. Ohayon, and P. Cossart. 1992. L. monocytogenes-induced actin assembly requires the actA gene product, a surface protein. *Cell 68*:521.
35. Domann, E., J. Wehland, M. Rohde, S. Pistor, M. Hartl, W. Goebel, M. Leimeister-Wachter, and T. Chakraborty. 1992. A novel bacterial virulence gene in *Listeria monocytogenes* required for host cell microfilament interaction with homology to the proline-rich region of vinculin. *EMBO J. 11*:1981.
36. Pistor, S., T. Chakraborty, K. Niebuhr, E. Domann, and J. Wehland. 1994. The ActA protein of *Listeria monocytogenes* acts as a nucleator inducing reorganization of the actin cytoskeleton. *EMBO J. 13*:758.
37. Leimeister-Wachter, M., C. Haffner, E. Domann, W. Goebel, and T. Chakraborty. 1990. Identification of a gene that positively regulates expression of listeriolysin, the major virulence factor of *Listeria monocytogenes. Proc. Natl. Acad. Sci. USA 87*:8336.
38. Sheehan, B., A. Klarsfeld, T. Msadek, and P. Cossart. 1995. Differential activation of virulence gene expression by PrfA, the *Listeria monocytogenes* virulence regulator. *J. Bacteriol. 177*:6469.
39. Villanueva, M. S., A. J. A. M. Sijts, and E. G. Pamer. 1995. Listeriolysin is processed efficiently into an MHC class I-associated epitope in *Listeria monocytogenes*-infected cells. *J. Immunol. 155*:5227.
40. Villanueva, M. S., C. J. M. Beckers, and E. G. Pamer. 1994. Infection with *Listeria monocytogenes* impairs sialic acid addition to host cell glycoproteins. *J. Exp. Med. 62*:1881.
41. Rogers, H. W., M. P. Callery, B. Deck, and E. R. Unanue. 1996. *Listeria monocytogenes* induces apoptosis of infected hepatocytes. *J. Immunol. 156*:679.
42. Zychlinsky, A., M. C. Prevost, and P. J. Sansonetti. 1992. *Shigella flexneri* induces apoptosis in infected macrophages. *Nature 358*:167–169.
43. Mackaness, G. B. 1962. Cellular resistance to infection. *J. Exp. Med. 116*:381.
44. Emmerling, P., H. Finger, and H. Hof. 1977. Cell mediated resistance to infection with *Listeria monocytogenes* in nude mice. *Infect. Immun. 15*:382.
45. Bancroft, G. J., R. D. Schreiber, and E. R. Ununue. 1991. Natural immunity: a T-cell-independent pathway of macrophage activation defined in the SCID mouse. *Immunol. Rev. 124*:5.
46. Czuprynski, C. J., P. M. Henson, and P. A. Campbell. 1985. Enhanced accumulation of inflammatory neutrophils and macrophages mediated

by transfer of T cells from mice immunized with *Listeria monocytogenes. J. Immunol. 134*:3449.

47. Rosen, H., S. Gordon, and R. J. North. 1989. Exacerbation of murine listeriosis by a monoclonal antibody specific for the type 3 complement receptor of myelomonocytic cells. *J. Exp. Med. 170*:27.
48. Conlan, J. W., and R. J. North. 1991. Neutrophil-mediated dissolution of infected host cells as a defense strategy against a facultative intracellular bacterium. *J. Exp. Med. 174*:741.
49. Conlan, J. W., and R. J. North. 1994. Neutrophils are essential for early anti-*Listeria* defense in the liver, but not in the spleen or peritoneal cavity, as revealed by a granulocyte-depleting monoclonal antibody. *J. Exp. Med. 179*:259.
50. Rogers, H. W., and E. R. Unanue. 1993. Neutrophils are involved in acute, nonspecific resistance to *Listeria monocytogenes* in mice. *Infect. Immun. 91*:5090.
51. Czuprynski, C. J., J. F. Brown, N. Maroushek, R. D. Wagner, and H. Steinberg. 1994. Administration of anti-granulocyte mAb RB6-8C5 impairs the resistance of mice to *Listeria monocytogenes* infection. *J. Immunol. 152*:1836.
52. Appelberg, R., A. G. Castro, and M. T. Silva. 1994. Neutrophils as effector cells of T-cell-mediated, acquired immunity in murine Listeriosis. *Immunology 83*:302.
53. Dunn, P. L., and R. J. North. 1991. Early gamma interferon production by natural killer cells is important in defense against murine Listeriosis. *Infect. Immun. 59*:2892.
54. Teixeira, H. C., and S. H. E. Kaufmann. 1994. Role of $NK1.1^+$ cells in experimental Listeriosis. *J. Immunol. 152*:1873.
55. Wherry, J. C., R. D. Schreiber, and E. R. Unanue. 1991. Regulation of IFN-production by natural killer cells in SCID mice: role of TNF and bacterial stimuli. *Infect. Immun. 59*:1709.
56. Harty, J. T., and M. J. Bevan. 1995. Specific immunity to *Listeria monocytogenes* in the absence of INF gamma. *Immunity 3*:109.
57. Huang, S., W. Hendriks, A. Althage, S. Hemmi, H. Bluethmann, R. Kamijo, J. Vilcek, R. M. Zinkernagel, and M. Aguet. 1993. Immune response in mice that lack the interferon-γ receptor. *Science 259*:1742.
58. Harty, J. T., R. D. Schreiber, and M. J. Bevan. 1992. CD8 T cells can protect against an intracellular bacterium in an interferon gamma-independent fashion. *Proc. Natl. Acad. Sci. USA 89*:11612.
59. Ohga, S., Y. Yoshikai, Y. Takeda, K. Hiromatsu, and K. Nomoto. 1990. Sequential appearance of gamma/delta- and alpha/beta-bearing T cells in the peritoneal cavity during an i.p. infection with *Listeria monocytogenes. Eur. J. Immunol. 20*:533.

60. Belles, C., A. K. Kuhl, A. J. Donoghue, Y. Sano, R. L. O'Brien, W. Born, K. Bottomly, and S. R. Carding. 1996. Bias in the gamma delta T cell response to *Listeria monocytogenes*. V delta 6.3$^+$ cells are a major component of the gamma delta T cell response to *Listeria monocytogenes*. *J. Immunol.* *156*:4280.

61. Hiromatsu, K., Y. Yoshikai, G. Matsuzaki, S. Ohga, K. Muramori, K. Matsumoto, J. A. Bluestone, and K. Nomoto. 1992. A protective role of γ/δ T cells in primary infection with *Listeria monocytogenes* in mice. *J. Exp. Med.* *175*:49.

62. Mombaerts, P., J. Arnoldi, F. Russ, S. Tonegawa, and S. H. Kaufmann. 1993. Different roles of alpha beta and gamma delta T cells in immunity against an intracellular bacterial pathogen. *Nature* *365*:53.

63. Skeen, M. J., and H. K. Ziegler. 1995. Activation of $\gamma\delta$ T cells for production of IFN-γ is mediated by bacteria via macrophage-derived cytokines IL-1 and IL-12. *J. Immunol.* *154*:5832.

64. Miki, K., and G. B. Mackaness. 1964. The passive transfer of acquired resistance to *Listeria monocytogenes*. *J. Exp. Med.* *120*:93.

65. Pamer, E. G., and P. Cresswell. 1998. Mechanisms of MHC class I-restricted antigen processing. *Annu. Rev. Immunol.* *16*:323.

66. Kaufmann, S. H. E., E. Hug, and G. DeLibero. 1986. *Listeria monocytogenes* reactive T lymphocyte clones with cytolytic activity against infected target cells. *J. Exp. Med.* *164*:363.

67. Ladel, C. H., I. E. F. Flesch, J. Arnoldi, and S. H. E. Kaufmann. 1994. Studies with MHC deficient knock out mice reveal impact of both MHC I- and MHC II-dependent T cell responses on *Listeria monocytogenes* infection. *J. Immunol.* *153*:3116.

68. Kagi, D., B. Ledermann, K. Burki, H. Hengartner, and R. F. Zinkernagel. 1994. CD8 T cell-mediated protection against an intracellular bacterium by perforin-dependent cytotoxicity. *Eur. J. Immunol.* *24*:3068.

69. Harty, J. T., and M. J. Bevan. 1996. CD8 T cell recognition of macrophages and hepatocytes results in immunity to *Listeria monocytogenes*. *Infect. Immun.* *64*:3632.

70. Buchmeier, N. A., and R. D. Schreiber. 1985. Requirement of endogenous interferon-γ production for resolution of *Listeria monocytogenes* infection. *Proc. Natl. Acad. Sci. USA* *82*:7404.

71. Dai, W. J., W. Bartens, G. Kohler, M. Hufnagel, M. Kopf, and F. Brombacher. 1997. Impaired macrophage listericidal and cytokine activities are responsible for the rapid death of *Listeria monocytogenes*-infected IFN-gamma receptor-deficient mice. *J. Immunol.* *158*:5297.

72. Havell, E. 1989. Evidence that tumor necrosis factor has an important role in antibacterial resistance. *J. Immunol.* *143*:2894.

73. Bancroft, G. J., K. C. Sheehan, R. D. Schreiber, and E. R. Unanue. 1989. Tumor necrosis factor is involved in the T cell-independent pathway of macrophage activation in SCID mice. *J. Immunol. 143*:127.
74. Pfeifer, K., T. Matsuyama, T. M. Kundig, A. Wakeham, K. Kenjihara, A. Shahinian, K. Wiegmann, P. S. Ohashi, M. Kronke, and T. W. Mak. 1993. Mice deficient for the 55 kd tumor necrosis factor receptor are resistant to endotoxic shock, yet succumb to *L. monocytogenes* infection. *Cell 73*:457.
75. Rothe, J., W. Lesslauer, H. Lotscher, Y. Lang, P. Koebel, F. Kontgen, A. Althage, R. Zinkernagel, M. Steinmetz, and H. Bluethmann. 1993. Mice lacking the tumour necrosis factor receptor 1 are resistant to TNF-mediated toxicity but highly susceptible to infection by *Listeria monocytogenes. Nature 364*:798.
76. Mastroeni, P., B. Villareal-Ramos, and C. Hormaeche. 1992. Role of T cells, TNF alpha and IFN gamma in recall of immunity to oral challenge with virulent salmonellae in mice vaccinated with live attenuated aro^- salmonella vaccines. *Microb. Pathog. 13*:477.
77. Nauciel, C., and F. Espinasse-Maes. 1992. Role of gamma interferon and tumor necrosis factor alpha in resistance to *Salmonella typhimurium* infection. *Infect. Immun. 60*:450.
78. Havell, E. A., L. L. Moldawer, D. Helfgott, P. L. Kilian, and P. G. Sehgal. 1992. Type I IL-1 receptor blockade exacerbates murine Listeriosis. *J. Immunol. 148*:1486.
79. Rogers, H. W., K. C. F. Sheehan, L. M. Brunt, S. K. Dower, E. R. Unanue, and R. D. Schreiber. 1992. Interleukin 1 participates in the development of anti-Listeria responses in normal and SCID mice. *Proc. Natl. Acad. Sci. USA 89*:1011.
80. Rogers, H. W., C. S. Tripp, R. D. Schreiber, and E. R. Unanue. 1994. Endogenous IL-1 is required for neutrophil recruitment and macrophage activation during murine Listeriosis. *J. Immunol. 153*:2093.
81. Zheng, H., D. Fletcher, W. Kozak, M. Jiang, K. J. Hofmann, C. A. Conn, D. Soszynski, C. Grabiec, M. E. Trumbauer, A. Shaw, M. J. Kostura, K. Stevens, H. Rosen, R. J. North, H. Y. Chen, M. J. Tocci, M. J. Kluger, and L. H. T. V. d. Ploeg. 1995. Resistance to fever induction and impaired acute-phase response in interleukin-1β-deficient mice. *Immunity 3*:9.
82. Biron, C. A., and R. T. Gazzinelli. 1995. Effects of IL-12 on immune responses to microbial infections: a key mediator in regulating disease outcome. *Curr. Opin. Immunol. 7*:485.
83. Hsieh, C. S., S. E. Macatonia, C. S. Tripp, S. F. Wolf, A. O'Garra, and K. M. Murphy. 1993. Development of TH1 $CD4^+$ T cells through IL-12 produced by *Listeria*-induced macrophages. *Science 260*:547.

84. Wagner, R. D., H. Steinberg, J. F. Brown, and C. J. Czuprynski. 1994. Recombinant interleukin-12 enhances resistance of mice to *Listeria monocytogenes* infection. *Microb. Pathog. 17*:175.

85. Tripp, C. S., M. K. Gately, J. Hakimi, P. Ling, and E. R. Unanue. 1994. Neutralization of IL-12 decreases resistance to Listeria in SCID and C.B-17 mice. Reversal by IFN-gamma. *J. Immunol. 152*:1883.

86. Miller, M. A., M. J. Skeen, and H. K. Ziegler. 1995. Nonviable bacterial antigens administered with IL-12 generate antigen-specific T cell responses and protective immunity against *Listeria monocytogenes. J. Immunol. 155*:4817.

87. Szalay, G., C. H. Ladel, and S. H. Kaufmann. 1995. Stimulation of protective $CD8^+$ T lymphocytes by vaccination with nonliving bacteria. *Proc. Natl. Acad. Sci. USA 92*:12389.

88. Zwickey, H. L., and T. A. Potter. 1996. Peptide epitopes from noncytosolic Listeria monocytogenes can be presented by major histocompatibility complex class I molecules. *Infect. Immun. 64*:1870.

89. Liu, Z., R. J. Simpson, and C. Cheers. 1992. Recombinant interleukin-6 protects mice against experimental infection. *Infect. Immun. 60*:4402.

90. Dalrymple, S. A., L. A. Lucian, R. Slattery, T. McNeil, D. M. Aud, S. Fuchino, F. Lee, and R. Murray. 1995. Interleukin-6-deficient mice are highly susceptible to *Listeria monocytogenes* infection: correlation with inefficient neutrophilia. *Infect. Immun. 63*:2262.

91. Kopf, M., H. Baumann, G. Freer, M. Freudenberg, M. Lamers, T. Kishimoto, R. Zinkernagel, H. Bluethmann, and G. Kohler. 1994. Impaired immune and acute-phase responses in interleukin-6-deficient mice. *Nature 368*:339.

92. Haak Frendscho, M., J. F. Brown, Y. Iizawa, R. D. Wagner, and C. J. Czuprynski. 1992. Administration of anti-IL-4 monoclonal antibody 11B11 increases the resistance of mice to *Listeria monocytogenes* infection. *J. Immunol. 148*:3978.

93. Szalay, G., C. H. Ladel, C. Blum, and S. H. Kaufmann. 1996. IL-4 neutralization or TNF-alpha treatment ameliorate disease by an intracellular pathogen in IFN-gamma receptor-deficient mice. *J. Immunol. 157*:4746.

94. Flesch, I. E., A. Wandersee, and S. H. Kaufmann. 1997. IL-4 secretion by $CD4^+$ $NK1^+$ T cells induces monocyte chemoattractant protein-1 in early listeriosis. *J. Immunol. 159*:7.

95. Tripp, C. S., K. P. Beckerman, and E. R. Unanue. 1995. Immune complexes inhibit antimicrobial responses through interleukin-10 production. *J. Clin. Invest. 95*:1628.

96. Dai, W. J., G. Kohler, and F. Brombacher. 1997. Both innate and ac-

quired immunity to *Listeria monocytogenes* infection are increased in IL-10 deficient mice. *J. Immunol. 158*:2259.
97. Flesch, I. E., A. Wandersee, and S. H. Kaufmann. 1997. Effects of IL-13 on murine listeriosis. *Int. Immunol. 9*:467.
98. Sha, W. C., H. C. Liou, E. I. Tuomanen, and D. Baltimore. 1995. Targeted disruption of the p50 subunit of NF-κB leads to multifocal defects in immune responses. *Cell 80*:321.
99. Tanaka, T., S. Akira, K. Yoshida, M. Umemoto, Y. Yoneda, N. Shirafuji, H. Fujiwara, S. Suematsu, N. Yoshida, and T. Kishimoto. 1995. Targeted disruption of the NF-IL6 gene discloses its essential role in bacteria killing and tumor cytotoxicity by macrophages. *Cell 80*:353.
100. Pryor, W. A., and G. L. Squadrito. 1995. The chemistry of peroxynitrite: a product from the reaction of nitric oxide with superoxide. *Am. J. Physiol. 268*: L699.
101. Beckerman, K. P., H. W. Rogers, J. A. Corbett, R. D. Schreiber, M. L. McDaniel, and E. R. Unanue. 1993. Release of nitric oxide during the T cell-independent pathway of macrophage activation. *J. Immunol. 150*:888.
102. Germain, R. N. 1994. MHC-dependent antigen processing and peptide presentation: providing ligands for T lymphocyte activation. *Cell 76*:287.
103. Cresswell, P. 1994. Assembly, transport and function of MHC class II molecules. *Annu. Rev. Immunol. 12*:259.
104. Portnoy, D. A., R. D. Schreiber, P. Connelly, and L. G. Tilney. 1989. Gamma interferon limits access of *Listeria monocytogenes* to the macrophage cytoplasm. *J. Exp. Med. 170*:2141.
105. Berche, P., J. L. Gaillard, C. Geoffroy, and J. E. Alouf. 1987. T cell recognition of listeriolysin O is induced during infection with *Listeria monocytogenes. J. Immunol. 139*:3813.
106. Safley, S. A., C. W. Cluff, N. E. Marshall, and H. K. Ziegler. 1991. Role of listeriolysin-O (LLO) in the T lymphocyte response to infection with *Listeria monocytogenes*. Identification of T cell epitopes of LLO. *J. Immunol. 146*:3604.
107. Sanderson, S., D. J. Campbell, and N. Shastri. 1995. Identification of a $CD4^+$ T cell-stimulating antigen of pathogenic bacteria by expression cloning. *J. Exp. Med. 182*:1751.
108. Daugelat, S., C. H. Ladel, B. Schoel, and S. H. E. Kaufmann. 1994. Antigen-specific T-cell responses during primary and secondary *Listeria monocytogenes* infection. *Infect. Immun. 62*:1881.
109. Cresswell, P., M. J. Androlewicz, and B. Ortmann. 1994. Assembly and transport of class I MHC–peptide complexes. *Ciba Found. Symp. 187*:150.

110. Brunt, L. M., D. A. Portnoy, and E. R. Unanue. 1990. Presentation of *Listeria monocytogenes* to CD8$^+$ T cells requires secretion of hemolysin and intracellular bacterial growth. *J. Immunol. 145*:3540.

111. Pamer, E. G., J. T. Harty, and M. J. Bevan. 1991. Precise prediction of a dominant class I MHC-restricted epitope of *Listeria monocytogenes. Nature 353*:852.

112. Bouwer, H. G., C. S. Nelson, B. L. Gibbins, D. A. Portnoy, and D. J. Hinrichs. 1992. Listeriolysin O is a target of the immune response to *Listeria monocytogenes. J. Exp. Med. 175*:1467.

113. Pamer, E. G. 1994. Direct sequence identification and kinetic analysis of an MHC class I-restricted *Listeria monocytogenes* CTL epitope. *J. Immunol. 152*:686.

114. Sijts, A. J. A. M., A. Neisig, J. Neefjes, and E. G. Pamer. 1996. Two Listeria monocytogenes CTL epitopes are processed from the same antigen with different efficiencies. *J. Immunol. 156*:685.

115. Harty, J. T., and M. J. Bevan. 1992. CD8 T cells specific for a single nonamer epitope of *Listeria monocytogenes* are protective in vivo. *J. Exp. Med. 175*:1531.

116. Harty, J. T., and E. G. Pamer. 1995. CD8 T lymphocytes specific to the secreted p60 antigen protect against *Listeria monocytogenes* infection. *J. Immunol. 154*:4642.

117. Busch, D. H., A. G. A. Bouwer, D. Hinrichs, and E. G. Pamer. 1997. A nonamer peptide derived from *Listeria monocytogenes* metalloprotease is presented to cytolytic T lymphocytes. *Infect. Immun. 65*:5326.

118. Villanueva, M. S., P. Fischer, K. Feen, and E. G. Pamer. 1994. Efficiency of antigen processing: a quantitative analysis. *Immunity 1*:479.

119. Sijts, A. J. A., and E. G. Pamer. 1997. Enhanced intracellular dissociation of Major Histocompatibility Complex Class I-associated peptides: a mechanism for optimizing the spectrum of cell surface-presented cytotoxic T lymphocyte epitopes. *J. Exp. Med. 185*:1403.

120. Sijts, A. J. A. M., M. S. Villanueva, and E. G. Pamer. 1996. CTL epitope generation is tightly linked to cellular proteolysis of a *Listeria monocytogenes* antigen. *J. Immunol. 156*:1497.

121. Hess, J., I. Gentschev, D. Miko, M. Welzel, C. Ladel, W. Goebel, and S. H. E. Kaufmann. 1996. Superior efficacy of secreted over somatic antigen display in recombinant *Salmonella* vaccine induced protection against listeriosis. *Proc. Natl. Acad. Sci. USA 93*:1458.

122. Hess, J., G. Dietrich, I. Gentschev, D. Miko, W. Goebel, and S. H. E. Kaufmann. 1997. Protection against murine listeriosis by an attenuated recombinant *Salmonella typhimurium* vaccine strain that secretes the naturally somatic antigen superoxide dismutase. *Infect. Immun. 65*:1286.

123. Shen, H., J. F. Miller, X. Fan, D. Kolwyck, R. Ahmed, and J. T. Harty. 1998. Compartmentalization of bacterial antigens: differential effects on priming of CD8 T cells and protective immunity. *Cell 92*:535.
124. Pamer, E. G. 1998. Cell mediated immunity: the role of bacterial protein secretion. *Curr. Biol. 8*:457.
125. Wuenscher, M. D., S. Kohler, A. Bubert, U. Gerike, and W. Goebel. 1993. The *iap* gene of *Listeria monocytogenes* is essential for cell viability, and its gene product, p60, has bacteriolytic activity. *J. Bacteriol. 175*:3491.
126. Sijts, A. J. A. M., I. Pilip, and E. G. Pamer. 1997. The *Listeria monocytogenes* p60 protein is an N-end rule substrate in the cytosol of infected cells: implications for MHC class I antigen processing of bacterial proteins. *J. Biol. Chem. 272*:19261.
127. Varshavsky, A. 1992. The N-end rule. *Cell 69*:725.
128. Busch, D. H., and E. G. Pamer. 1998. MHC class I/peptide stability: implications for immunodominance, in vitro proliferation and diversity of responding CTL. *J. Immunol. 160*:4441.
129. Vijh, S., and E. G. Pamer. 1997. Immunodominant and subdominant CTL responses to *Listeria monocytogenes* infection. *J. Immunol. 158*:3366.
130. Vijh, S., I. M. Pilip, and E. G. Pamer. 1998. Effect of antigen processing efficiency on in vivo T cell response magnitudes. *J. Immunol. 160*:3971.
131. Busch, D. H., I. M. Pilip, S. Vijh, and E. G. Pamer. 1998. Coordinate regulation of complex T cell populations responding to bacterial infection. *Immunity 8*:353.
132. Busch, D. H., I. Pilip, and E. G. Pamer. 1998. Evolution of a complex T cell receptor repertoire during primary and recall bacterial infection. *J. Exp. Med. 188*:61.
133. Kaufmann, S. H. E., H. R. Rodewald, E. Hug, and G. D. Libero. 1988. Cloned Listeria monocytogenes specific non-MHC-restricted Lyt-2^+ T cells with cytolytic and protective activity. *J. Immunol. 140*:3173.
134. Lukacs, K., and R. J. Kurlander. 1989. MHC-unrestricted transfer of antilisterial immunity by freshly isolated immune CD8 spleen cells. *J. Immunol. 143*:3731.
135. Brown, M. L., P. E. Fields, and R. J. Kurlander. 1992. Metabolic requirements for macrophage presentation of *Listeria monocytogenes* to immune CD8 cells. *J. Immunol. 148*:555.
136. Pamer, E. G., M. J. Bevan, and K. F. Lindahl. 1993. Do nonclassical, class Ib MHC molecules present bacterial antigens to T cells? *Trends Microbiol. 1*:35.
137. Loveland, B. E., C. R. Wang, H. Yonekawa, E. Hermel, and K. F.

Lindahl. 1990. Maternally transmitted histocompatibility antigen of mice: a hydrophobic peptide of a mitochondrially encoded protein. *Cell 60*:971.

138. Shawar, S. M., R. G. Cook, J. R. Rodgers, and R. R. Rich. 1990. Specialized functions of MHC class I molecules. I. An N-formyl peptide receptor is required for construction of the class I antigen Mta. *J. Exp. Med. 171*:897.
139. Pamer, E. G., C. R. Wang, L. Flaherty, K. F. Lindahl, and M. J. Bevan. 1992. H2-M3 presents a *Listeria monocytogenes* peptide to cytotoxic T lymphocytes. *Cell 70*:215.
140. Kurlander, R. J., S. M. Shawar, M. L. Brown, and R. R. Rich. 1992. Specialized role for a murine class I-b MHC molecule in prokaryotic host defenses. *Science 257*:678.
141. Lenz, L. L., B. Dere, and M. J. Bevan. 1996. Identification of an H2-M3-restricted *Listeria* epitope: implications for antigen presentation by M3. *Immunity 5*:63.
142. Princiotta, M. F., L. L. Lenz, M. J. Bevan, and U. D. Staerz. 1998. H2-M3 restricted presentation of a *Listeria*-derived leader peptide. *J. Exp. Med. 187*:1711.
143. Gulden, P. H., P. Fischer, N. E. Sherman, W. Wang, V. H. Engelhard, J. Shabanowitz, D. H. Hunt, and E. G. Pamer. 1996. A *Listeria monocytogenes* pentapeptide is presented to cytolytic T lymphocytes by the H2-M3 MHC class Ib molecule. *Immunity 5*:73.
144. Lenz, L. L., and M. J. Bevan. 1996. H2-M3 restricted presentation of *Listeria monocytogenes* antigens. *Immunol. Rev. 151*:107.
145. Kovacsovics-Bankowski, M., and K. L. Rock. 1995. A phagosome-to-cytosol pathway for exogenous antigens presented on MHC class I molecules. *Science 267*:243.
146. Pfeifer, J. D., M. J. Wick, R. L. Roberts, K. Findlay, S. J. Normark, and C. V. Harding. 1993. Phagocytic processing of bacterial antigens for class I MHC presentation to T cells. *Nature 361*:359.
147. Nataraj, C., G. R. Huffman, and R. J. Kurlander. 1998. H2M3wt-restricted, *Listeria monocytogenes*-immune CD8 T cells respond to multiple formylated peptides and to a variety of gram-positive and gram-negative bacteria. *Int. Immunol. 10*:7.

PART II

VACCINE STRATEGIES USING LIVE RECOMBINANT INTRACELLULAR BACTERIA

CHAPTER 5

RECOMBINANT BCG VACCINES

ANNA ALDOVINI and RICHARD YOUNG

5.1 INTRODUCTION AND OVERVIEW OF RECOMBINANT BCG AS A VACCINE VEHICLE

A new generation of vaccines against a broad spectrum of infectious diseases is being developed, using viral and bacterial live recombinant vaccine vehicles. A live recombinant vehicle vaccine is composed of a viable but harmless organism that can produce various pathogen proteins and deliver them to the immune system. In principle, this type of vaccine can be engineered to stimulatc immunity to a broad spectrum of different pathogens through a single vaccination. The ideal live recombinant vehicle vaccine would be safe, inexpensive, and stable during storage and transport (1).

The human tuberculosis vaccine *Mycobacterium bovis* bacillus Calmette-Guérin (BCG) is a strain of *M. bovis* that has been attenu-

Abbreviations: *aph*, aminoglycoside phosphotransferase gene; attP, phage attachment site P; BCG: bacillus Calmette-Guérin; GM-CSF, granulocyte-macrophage colony-stimulating factor; HIV, human immunodeficiency virus; hsp, heat shock protein; IFN-γ, interferon-γ; IL, interleukin; *leuD*, leucine biosynthetic gene D; MIp, mycobacterial integrating protein; MRP, mycobacterial replicating plasmid; OMP-DCase, orotidine-5-monophosphate decarboxylase gene; OspA, outer surface protein A; PBMC, peripheral blood mononuclear cells; PPD, purified protein derivative; PspA, pneumococcal surface protein A; *pyrF*, pyrimidine synthesis gene F (alternate names: uracil phosphoribosyltransferase or orotidine-5-monophosphate decarboxylase gene); rBCG, recombinant BCG; recA, recombinase A (gene or protein); rpsL, ribosomal protein S12; SCID, severe combined immunodeficiency; SIV, simian immunodeficiency virus; STORE, selection technique of recombination events; UMP, uracil-monophosphate; uraA, orotidine-5-monophosphate decarboxylase; ureA, urease A (gene or protein, part of urease operon); ureB, urease B (gene or protein, part of urease operon); ureC urease C (gene or protein, part of urease operon).

Intracellular Bacterial Vaccine Vectors, Edited by Yvonne Paterson.
ISBN 0-471-17278-2

ated by 230 serial passages in vitro (2). BCG has features that make it a particularly attractive live recombinant vaccine vehicle. With nearly 2 billion immunizations, BCG has a long record of safe use in humans (3–6). It can be given at birth and engenders long-lived immune responses with only a single dose; there is a worldwide distribution network with experience in BCG vaccination.

Improved understanding of mycobacterial biology and the development of powerful molecular genetic tools provide additional impetus and rationale to use mycobacteria as live vaccine vehicles for a variety of clinical purposes. The antigens that are targets of the immune response to infection by mycobacteria have been studied extensively, and the immune response to mycobacteria is well understood (7–15). We have an improved understanding of the molecular mechanisms involved in resistance to antimycobacterial antibiotics (16,17). Genome mapping and sequencing projects are providing valuable information about the *M. tuberculosis* and *M. leprae* genomes that will facilitate further study of the biology of these pathogens (14,18). A wide variety of molecular genetic tools have been developed that permit molecular genetic manipulation of mycobacteria and allow the construction of recombinant BCG vaccine vehicles (18–30). As the size of its genome allows the introduction of more than one gene, BCG has the potential to become a multivalent vaccine (21).

5.2 *Mycobacteria* AS HOSTS FOR MOLECULAR GENETICS

5.2.1 DNA Vectors and Transformation

To construct a BCG recombinant vehicle, investigators have developed a variety of molecular genetic tools and methods for use in *Mycobacteria*. Three items were essential: a transformation method, plasmid or phage vectors that can be manipulated in vitro, and selectable genetic markers. This section describes the transformation methods that are favored for introducing DNA into mycobacteria, replicating and integrating vectors that have been developed for mycobacteria, and the drug-resistance and nutritional markers that are available for monitoring plasmid DNA introduced into mycobacteria.

5.2.1.1 Transformation. Three different methods have been used for mycobacterial transformation. *Mycobacteria* are autocompetent and can be transformed at a low frequency without special treatments.

To obtain greater transformation frequencies, spheroplasts can be produced after transient growth in glycine-containing medium, and these can be transformed in the presence of polyethylene glycol (PEG) (23). The best transformation frequencies in both slow- and fast-growing *Mycobacteria* are obtained by electroporation; this technique is currently the method of choice (8,29,30).

5.2.1.2 Plasmid and Phage Vectors. The two types of plasmid vectors that are useful for introducing foreign genes into mycobacteria are autonomously replicating plasmids (19,29) and integrating plasmids (22). We refer to them here as mycobacterial replicating plasmids (MRp plasmids) and mycobacterial integrating plasmids (MIp plasmids). The MRp and the MIp plasmids are shuttle plasmids; they have been constructed to permit plasmid maintenance in *Escherichia coli*, using origins of replication that allow autonomous replication at high copy number in *E. coli*. The MRp plasmids also contain an origin of replication from a *Mycobacterium fortuitum* plasmid (29). These plasmids are maintained at approximately 25 copies per cell in BCG. The MIp plasmids lack the ability to replicate autonomously in mycobacteria but carry an *E. coli* origin of replication that allows easy manipulation of these plasmids in *E. coli*. It must integrate into the mycobacterial genome to be maintained. This integration takes place through recombination with mycobacterial sequences carried by the MIp vector (22).

Bacteriophages can also be useful tools to construct recombinant *Mycobacteria* that carry a gene of interest stably integrated in the bacterial genome. A temperate phage, L5, that allows integration of foreign genes at a specific site in the mycobacterial chromosome has been extensively characterized (20,25). Plasmid vectors carrying segments of L5 DNA including the attP site, the integrase gene and a selectable antibiotic marker have been constructed. These vectors cannot replicate autonomously in mycobacteria, yet they transform both fast- and slow-growing mycobacteria with the same efficiency as extrachromosomal plasmids. The transformants obtained with these vectors are much more stable than transformants obtained with extrachromosomal plasmids when they are grown in absence of antibiotic selection. This type of vector has been used for the expression of genes such as human immunodeficiency virus (HIV) gp120.

5.2.1.3 Selectable Genetic Markers. The two types of selectable genetic markers that have been used for molecular genetic manipulation of *Mycobacteria* are genes that lead to drug resistance and prototrophy. *Mycobacteria* are sensitive to kanamycin and the aminoglycoside phosphotransferase gene (*aph*) confers resistance to kanamycin in mycobacteria (22,28,29). *M. smegmatis* and *M. bovis* BCG are sensitive to 10 mg/ml kanamycin in plates and in liquid medium, and the *aph* gene from Tn903 (28) confers resistance to kanamycin at levels of >100 mg/ml. *Mycobacteria* are also sensitive to hygromycin (31).

Nutritional markers have several advantages as selectable markers, and mycobacterial genes responsible for pyrimidere (*pyrF*), urease (*ureC*) and leucine (*leuD*) have been isolated and used as selectable markers (22,32–34). Genes that encode essential metabolic enzymes can provide a more powerful genetic selection than can drug-resistance genes. When metabolic genes are deleted, the mutant cells cannot revert to their wild-type state, unless the appropriate gene is reintroduced into the cell. By contrast, spontaneous drug resistance is acquired through a variety of mechanisms (alterations in cell wall permeability, changes in susceptible enzymes), sometimes making the frequency of spontaneous revertants a problem for investigators. There may also be concerns with the use of drug resistance genes in bacteria that are destined for human use; there are no such concerns with nutritional markers. Both positive and negative selections can be employed in manipulating some genes that encode essential metabolic enzymes.

Genes encoding orotidine monophosphate decarboxylase (OMP-DCase) are widely used as genetic markers in diverse fungi, in slime molds, and in prokaryotes (35–37). These genes are useful because they are nutritional markers and can permit the development of genetic systems that do not rely on drug-resistance markers. Such systems may be advantageous when drug resistance is a concern. Genes encoding OMP-DCase are also useful as genetic markers because they allow the development of both positive and negative selection schemes (35). For example, a functional *pyrF* gene, which encodes OMP-DCase, allows cells to grow in medium lacking uracil, yet is lethal to cells grown in the presence of 5-fluoro-orotic acid (22,35). The fact that all organisms display the same basic uracil-monophosphate (UMP) biosynthesis pathway, that all organisms examined to date have a single OMP-DCase gene, and that this gene can be readily cloned by complementation of *E. coli pyrF* mutants has also contributed to interest in the BCG OMP-DCase gene.

The *M. smegmatis* and *M. bovis* BCG *pyrF* genes have been isolated and used to investigate the value of *pyrF* in the manipulation of genes in *M. smegmatis* (22,32). Mutations in the *pyrF* gene have been introduced into the *M. smegmatis* genome, using 5-fluoro-orotic acid to select for the mutant cells, creating uracil auxotrophs. The mutant gene in these uracil auxotrophs can be replaced by homologous recombination with the wild-type *pyrF* gene upon transformation and selection for uracil prototrophy.

The *leuD* and *ureABC* genes of *Mycobacterium tuberculosis* have been cloned and used as selectable markers (33,34). A suicide vector containing a *ureC* gene disrupted by a kanamycin marker (*aph*) was used to construct a urease-negative BCG mutant by allelic exchange involving replacement of the *ureC* gene with the *aph* : : *ureC* construct (34). Similarly, a recombination substrate containing a *leuD* allele disrupted with a kanamycin-resistance gene has been used to generate leucine auxotrophs by homologous recombination in the Erdman and H37Rv strains of *M. tuberculosis* (33).

5.2.2 Genome Manipulation in *Mycobacteria*

The ability to achieve homologous recombination in slow-growing mycobacteria provides an important approach to understanding the pathogenesis of tuberculosis and should permit construction of attenuated strains of *M. tuberculosis* for vaccine purposes. Investigators have struggled to obtain homologous recombination in slow-growing mycobacteria such as *M. tuberculosis* and *M. bovis* BCG by classical suicide vectors (24,32), despite being able to accomplish this fairly easily in the fast-growing *Mycobacterium smegmatis* (22). Among the reasons that have been proposed to be responsible for the difficulty in obtaining efficient homologous recombination in slow-growing mycobacteria are poor transformation efficiency, limited activity of the machinery involved in homologous recombination, the relatively high level of illegitimate recombination, and the singular biology of the *recA* gene in slow-growing mycobacteria (27).

Homologous recombination and consequent gene replacement has also been obtained using the nutritional markers *ureC* (32) and *leuD* (33) disrupted by a kanamicin resistance gene. Similarly, replacement of the mycocerosic acid synthetase gene by a hygromycin-resistance gene led to bacteria incapable of synthesizing mycocerosic acids and mycosides, fatty acids present only in slow-growing mycobacteria and thought to be important for pathogenesis (31).

A combined positive/negative selection system has been developed for gene replacement in mycobacteria (38). This one-step double selection procedure provides a means to distinguish strictly between gene replacement by double crossover versus homologous recombination by single crossover events. In this system, the host cell is first made streptomycin sensitive. The vector insert DNA contains a kanamycin-resistance gene within the region destined for genome insertion, allowing selection for the presence of these sequences. A wild-type *rpsL* gene, which codes for ribosomal protein S12 and confers a dominant streptomycin-sensitivity phenotype, is placed in the vector outside of sequences that are destined for homologous integration. By placing the gene for positive selection within, and that used for negative selection outside, the target gene of interest, and by selecting for kanomycin and streptomycin resistance simultaneously, gene replacement at the homologous locus is obtained.

A technique called selection technique of recombination events (STORE) has been developed to facilitate identification of cells in which homologous recombination has taken place (39). It is based on the use of replicative plasmids that facilitate the detection of rare recombination events, because the proportion of recombined molecules increases over time. The technique may be useful for organisms for which homologous recombination is difficult to achieve.

The genomes of *M. bovis* and *M. tuberculosis* are very similar and *M. bovis* is capable of producing a pulmonary disease indistinguishable from that caused by *M. tuberculosis*. Thus, markers used successfully in *M. bovis* BCG should prove to be a useful tool for genetic manipulation of *M. tuberculosis*. Similarly, the methods used to obtain targeted integration in the *M. bovis* BCG genome should be useful in achieving targeted integration in *M. tuberculosis*.

5.3 EXPRESSION OF FOREIGN PROTEINS IN *Mycobacteria*

5.3.1 Expression of Antigens

Using both MRp and MIp vectors, a variety of foreign genes have been introduced into mycobacteria (19,40). Both the MRp and the MIp vectors have advantages and disadvantages. It is fairly simple to introduce foreign genes into *M. smegmatis* and *M. bovis* BCG with MRp vectors, and the MRp copy number is sufficiently high to permit a quick check for the presence of the plasmid with a rapid plasmid isolation procedure (29). However, plasmids that replicate autonomously with respect to the genome are notoriously unstable when foreign gene expression is deleterious to the growth rate of recombinant bacteria. The MIp vectors permit the stable replacement, addition, or deletion of genes in the mycobacterial genome (31,33,34).

A variety of mycobacterial gene promoters have been isolated and sequenced and some of these promoters have been incorporated into both MRp and MIp plasmids. The mycobacterial hsp60 and 70 promoters and translational start site have been employed to direct the expression of a variety of foreign genes. These regulatory elements were selected because they are among the most powerful in bacteria (41) and because hsp60 and hsp70 synthesis is induced to very high levels during phagocytosis of some bacteria by macrophage (10,42–47).

A variety of human immunodeficiency virus-1 (HIV-1) and simian immunodeficiency virus (SIV) polypeptides have been expressed in BCG recombinants, and these foreign polypeptides produced in BCG can induce antibody and T-cell responses in animal models (40,48–50,52). DNA fragments encoding HIV-1 Gag, Pol, and Env precursors were fused to the mycobacterial hsp70 promoter and translational start site so that they precisely replaced the hsp70 coding sequences (48), and the hybrid genes were inserted into the BCG autonomous replicating plasmid vector pYUB12 (29). When injected in mice, the BCG-HIV gag recombinants consistently induced T-cell responses to a variety of epitopes in the foreign protein (48). The Nef protein has also been expressed successfully in BCG under the control of the P_{AN} promoter from *Mycobacterium paratubercolosis* (50).

The *Leishmania major* surface protein gp63 has been expressed in BCG in an attempt to develop a recombinant vaccine against zoonotic cutaneous leishmaniasis (53,54). This protein was expressed intracellularly from a heat shock protein (hsp60) promoter or as a fusion with the N-terminal region of the *Mycobacterium fortuitum* β-lactamase.

The 28-kD glutathione S-transferase of *Shistosoma mansoni* has been expressed with or without the *M. tuberculosis* 85A antigen signal peptide from the hsp60 promoter. This protein that can stimulate production of protective antibody responses against the occurrence of shistosomiasis, and the BCG-produced antigen induced neutralizing antibodies among a variety of different isotypes in mice (55). The hsp60 promoter and other regulatory sequences were also used to express the full-length measles virus nucleoprotein gene in BCG (56).

The outer surface protein A (Osp A) antigen of *Borrelia burgdorferi* and the pneumococcal surface protein A (PspA) antigen of *Strepto-*

coccus pneumoniae have also been expressed in BCG in a variety of forms (57–60). These proteins were expressed as chimeras with the signal peptide of the *M. tuberculosis* 19-kDa lipoprotein antigen. They were also produced as secreted proteins fused to the BCG α antigen, a 32-kDa protein secreted in the media by BCG. In addition, these proteins have been expressed as intracellular proteins in BCG.

5.3.2 Expression of Cytokines

The profound immunostimulatory properties of BCG have been exploited in tubercolosis prevention and in therapy for certain human cancers, in particular, superficial bladder cancer (61,62). In both cases, BCG has limitations. The efficacy of BCG against tuberculosis is poor in many settings. Intravesical administration of BCG has a high efficacy against superficial bladder carcinomas, but large and frequent doses are required, occasionally leading to disseminated mycobacteriosis. The ability to genetically manipulate mycobacteria allowed investigators to explore the possibility that the inherent immunostimulatory properties of BCG could be modified or potentiated through the secretion of mammalian cytokines (63,64).

BCG strains have been constructed that produce a variety of cytokines fused to the BCG α antigen signal sequence, permitting the secretion of these cytokines in a functional form. BCG recombinants secreting functional interleukins (IL-2, IL-4, IL-6), granulocyte-macrophage colony-stimulating factor (GM-CSF) and interferon-γ (IFN-γ) have been generated and characterized (63,64). Cytokine-secreting BCG are substantially more potent stimulators of the cell-mediated immune response than are their normal BCG counterparts. The most profound effects were induced by BCG-secreting IL-2, IFN-γ, or GM-CSF (63). Mice injected with BCG strains secreting GM-CSF, IL-2, and IFN-γ exhibited an enhanced antigen-specific T-cell response, as measured by in vitro stimulation of splenocytes with PPD. The enhanced cell-mediated response to cytokine-secreting BCG strains was observed when mice were injected either by intravenous or by intraperitoneal routes, indicating that observed enhancement occurs independent of the route of inoculation. No signs of illness were observed with any BCG strains under any of the conditions used (63). Thus, cytokine-secreting BCG can enhance immune responses to mycobacterial antigens, and may be improved reagents for tuberculosis (TB) prophylaxis and cancer immunotherapy.

5.4 IN VIVO EXPERIMENTATION WITH rBCG

5.4.1 Persistence and Stability

The success of rBCG as a vaccine vehicle depends on engendering immune responses to the foreign antigen expressed in BCG. Persistence of the rBCG organisms in vivo and stable expression of the foreign gene are likely to be critical in eliciting the best response. Experiments carried out in mice indicate that, once injected in the animal, rBCG disseminates to multiple organs independent of the route of inoculation (65). Recombinant and nonrecombinant organisms can be isolated from lungs, spleen and liver two months after injection, although the bacterial recovery is substantially lower than the initial inoculum. The detection of rBCG months after injection indicates that at least a subset of the inoculated bacteria can stably retain the foreign DNA material, even in absence of antibiotic selection. Expression of proteins that are deleterious to BCG persistence may lead to suboptimal immunization.

The type of vector used for expressing foreign antigens can influence the level of antigen expression and thus, the ability to engender strong immune responses to the foreign antigen. In the case of episomal expression, in which the absence of selective pressure in vivo might lead to loss of the plasmid, BCG organisms might persist but might not continue to express the protein antigen of interest. In the case of integrated genes, in which the presence of a single-copy gene may produce lower level of the foreign antigen, it is critical to select gene expression signals that permit production of substantial amounts of the antigen of interest.

5.4.2 Immunogenicity

Recombinant BCG vaccine vehicles can induce immune responses to viral, bacterial, and parasite proteins produced by the bacillus, indicating that BCG can act simultaneously as an adjuvant and as a vehicle to produce and deliver selected antigens to the immune system. The tools now available for genetic manipulation of BCG make it possible that features of the BCG vaccine vehicle can be tailored to maximize the desired immune responses.

When tested in animal models, rBCG-expressing antigens from HIV, *Borrelia*, *Leishmania*, *Streptococcus pneumoniae*, *Shistosoma mansoni*, and rodent malaria all stimulated humoral and cell-mediated responses (40,48–51,53–60,66–69). The magnitude and type of response obtained in these cases are thought to depend on the intrinsic immunostimulatory properties of the antigen, on the site of its expression (whether intracellular, on the membrane surface or secreted), and on the immunization protocol.

In human vaccination, BCG is normally administered intradermally by scarification. The possibility of using rBCG in different immunization routes was tested in Guinea pigs by oral, respiratory, and intradermal exposure to rBCG (57,68). Humoral and cellular responses could be obtained through all routes of immunization. Mucosal exposure resulted in higher local and systemic responses than intradermal exposure. The oral route of immunization resulted in the presence of IgA both in the serum and in intestinal secretions.

5.4.3 Protective Immunity Elicited by rBCG Vaccines in Animal Models

The ability of rBCG expressing foreign antigens to engender protective immune responses has been established for a variety of pathogens (53,54,56–60,66,67). Protective responses have been documented in mice for two different bacterial pathogens, *Borrelia burgdorferi* (58,60) and *Streptococcus pneumoniae* (57,59), and for one parasite, *Leishmania* (53,54). The ability to elicit a protective antibody response against HIV was documented in mice with severe combined immunodeficiency (SCID) that had received passive immunotherapy with immunoglobulins induced by rBCG (67). An intranasal measles virus challenge of rhesus macaques that had been immunized with rBCG-expressing measles virus nucleoprotein failed to protect against the establishment of a systemic infection. However, virus clearance in the lung and peripheral blood mononuclear cells (PBMC) was accelerated, probably as a result of T-cell-mediated immunity. Although antigen-specific antibodies were produced by rBCG–nucleoprotein vaccination they were thought not to be protective because they were not directed to a coat protein (56).

In experiments designed to test the ability of rBCG to elicit protective immunity against *Borrelia burgdorferi*, the OspA antigen was expressed in BCG as a chimeric membrane-associated lipoprotein (58–60). High-titer humoral responses were elicited against OspA and were found to be protective against live challenge with *Borrelia*. Recombinant BCG expressing membrane-associated *Streptococcus pneumoniae* PspA antigen elicited protective immunity (50–80%)

against challenge with 100 LD_{50} of virulent pneumococci (57,59). On the basis of these preclinical studies, rBCG vaccines for Lyme and pneumococcal diseases are being developed for clinical trial in human subjects.

In the case of *Leishmania*, immunization with rBCG expressing the gene for gp63 antigen engendered protective immunity against challenge with either the promastigote or the amastigote form of *Leishmania mexicana* in BALB/c mice (54). The immunity induced by this vaccine was not sufficient to protect BALB/c mice from challenge with *Leishmania major*, a parasite whose disease course in mice is somewhat different from that with *L. Mexicana* (54). Vaccination with a rBCG expressing gp63 as a fusion with the N-terminal region of the *Mycobacterium fortuitum* β-lactamase induced immune responses that protected Balb/c mice from challenge with *Leishmania major* (53). It is possible that the difference in the outcome of these two different vaccination regimen depends on the stability and accumulation of the recombinant antigen in BCG.

Guinea pigs inoculated with rBCG secreting the V3 principal neutralizing epitope of HIV developed high-titer antibodies against the epitope (67). Their sera neutralized primary field isolates of HIV with matching V3 sequences in an in vitro assay. Furthermore, passive transfer of serum IgG from guinea pigs to SCID mice was effective in blocking HIV infection.

5.4.4 Safety

The safety of rBCG vaccination is dependent on the characteristics of BCG as a microbiological agent, on the genetic content of the recombinant DNA introduced in the bacterium and on the immunological status of the recipient host. BCG is actually a very safe vaccine. A review of its side effects in 5.5 million recipients (infants, children, and adolescents) indicated the risk of local lesions and regional suppurative lymphadenitis at 387 per million. The study showed that disseminated BCGosis occurred in 4.29 per million infants and was lower in subjects over one year of age (3–5). Although it was assumed that the risk of BCG dissemination should have been higher in immunocompromised hosts such as HIV-infected individuals, two controlled studies failed to show any increased risk of disseminated BCG infection in immunodeficient BCG recipients (6). In general, the side effects of BCG vaccination appeared to correlate with amount of dead BCG cells in the vaccine preparation (6).

The presence of antibiotic resistance markers in rBCG creates some additional safety issues for live recombinant vaccines, especially in light of the fact that rBCG can persist for months in mice in absence of drug selection (65). Vector-encoded kanamycin resistance may be transferable to other bacteria. BCG carrying the kanamycin resistance gene would be insensitive not only to kanamycin, but to neomycin as well. However, such recombinant BCG should retain sensitivity to clinically relevant antibiotics such as streptomycin, gentamycin, isoniazid, rifampin, and ethambutol.

5.5 PERSPECTIVES

5.5.1 rBCG for Immune Modulation

BCG-secreting cytokines, in particular GM-CSF, IL-2, and IFN-γ, can modify and potentiate the immune response to BCG antigens. These recombinants may be valuable for improved prophylactic and therapeutic vaccines and for further study of mycobacterial immune responses. BCG recombinants that express antigens of pathogens such as HIV (40,48–51,67), *Borrelia burgdorferi* (58,59) and *Leishmania* (53,54) engender long-lasting immune responses to the foreign antigens, and the coexpression of cytokines in these recombinants may further enhance desired immune responses. Cytokine-secreting BCG recombinants may also serve as improved reagents for bladder cancer immunotherapy, as there is a need for BCG strains that are effective at lower doses, and GM-CSF has already been shown to be a powerful cofactor in antitumor immunity experiments (70). Finally, BCG strains secreting cytokines may prove to be useful tools in dissecting the relationship between animals and mycobacteria, particularly in genetically altered mice which themselves are modified to create systems which are more amenable to analysis of complex immune responses.

5.5.2 Recombinant *Mycobacteria* as Improved Vaccines Against Tuberculosis

Among infectious diseases, tuberculosis remains the pre-eminent cause of death in most human societies. The World Health Organization (WHO) estimates that one in three human beings is infected with *Mycobacterium tuberculosis* (71,72). A small percentage of infected individuals develop clinical symptoms and succumb to the disease, accounting for the approximately 1 million deaths per annum (71). Furthermore, over the past decade, there has been a recent resurgence in the incidence of tuberculosis in developed countries that has coincided with the acquired immunodeficiency syndrome (AIDS) epidemic (73). In many cases, the host response to mycobacteria limits the proliferation of the pathogen, but does not produce sterilizing immunity. Because of their impact as human pathogens, and as a result of their profound immunostimulatory properties, mycobacteria have been widely used for basic immunological investigations and have become important tools for tuberculosis prophylaxis and cancer immunotherapy. The variable efficacy of BCG against TB observed in different vaccine trials, and the increase in drug-resistant TB cases worldwide, suggest the need for an improved vaccine against TB.

Among the approaches that are being used to generate an improved vaccine against tuberculosis are two that involve genetic manipulation of mycobacteria. BCG engineered to produce cytokines may prove to be more efficacious than BCG alone for TB prophylaxis (63). In addition, homologous recombination and gene replacement techniques are being used to attenuate *M. tuberculosis* itself (27,31).

5.6 CONCLUSIONS

BCG has many features that make it a particularly attractive live recombinant vaccine vehicle. BCG has a long record of safe use in humans, can be given at birth, and engenders long-lived immune responses with only a single dose; there is also a worldwide distribution network with experience in BCG vaccination. A variety of molecular genetic tools have been developed for mycobacteria that provide the means to introduce and express foreign genes in BCG. Recombinant BCG expressing a variety of viral, bacterial, and parasitic antigens have been demonstrated to elicit humoral and cellular immune responses, and some recombinant BCG vaccine candidates have been shown to elicit protective immunity in animal models. BCG that express and secrete cytokines have been shown to enhance the natural immune stimulatory properties of this mycobacterium. These results suggest that recombinant BCG vaccine vehicles will be useful for vaccination against a variety of important pathogens in humans.

5.7 REFERENCES

1. Bloom, B. R. 1989. Vaccines for the Third World. *Nature 342*:115.
2. Calmette, A., C. Guerin, and B. Weill-Halle. 1924. Essais de prémunition par le BCG contre l'infection tuberculeuse de l'homme et des animaux. *B. Bull. Acad. Natl. Med. (Paris) 91*:787.
3. Luelmo, F. 1982. BCG vaccination. *Am. Rev. Respir. Dis. 125*:70.
4. Lotte, A., O. Wasz-Hockert, N. Poisson, N. Dumitrescu, M. Verron, and E. Couvet. 1984. BCG complications. Estimates of the risks among vaccinated subjects and statistical analysis of their main characteristics. *Adv. Tuberc. Res. 21*:107.
5. Lotte, A., O. Wasz-Hockert, N. Poisson, H. Engbaek, H. Landmann, U. Quast, B. Andrasofszky, L. Lugosi, I. Vadasz, and P. Mihailescu. 1988. Second IUATLD study on complication induced by intradermal BCG vaccination. *Bull. Int. Union Tuberc. Lung Dis. 63*:1.
6. Milstien, J. B., and J. J. Gibson. 1990. Quality control of BCG vaccines by the World Health Organization: a review of factors that may influence vaccine effectiveness and safety. *Bull. World Health Organ. 68*(1):93–108.
7. Collins, F. N. 1982. The immunology of tuberculosis. *Am. Rev. Respir. Dis. 125*:42.
8. Husson, R., and R. A. Young. 1987. Genes for the major protein antigens of *M. tuberculosis*: the etiologic agents of tuberculosis and leprosy share a major protein antigen. *Proc. Natl. Acad. Sci. USA 84*:1679.
9. Kaplan, G., D. E. Weinstein, R. M. Steinman, W. R. Levis, U. Elvers, M. E. Patarroyo, and Z. A. Cohn. 1985. An analysis of in vitro T cell responsiveness in lepromatous leprosy. *J. Exp. Med. 162*:917.
10. Kaufmann, S. H. E. 1990. Heat shock protein and the immune response. *Immunol. Today 11*:129.
11. Wolfe, S. A., D. E. Tracey, and C. S. Henney. 1976. Induction of "natural killer" cells by BCG. *Nature 262*:584.
12. Young, D. B., and S. T. Cole. 1993. Leprosy, tuberculosis, and the new genetics. *J. Bacteriol. 175*:1.
13. Young, D. B., S. H. Kaufmann, P. W. Hermans, and J. E. Thole. 1992. Mycobacterial protein antigens: a compilation. *Mol. Microbiol. 6*:133.
14. Young, D., T. Garbe, R. Lathigra, and C. Abou-Zeid. 1990. Protein antigens: structure, function and regulation, p 1–35. *In* J. McFadden (ed.), Molecular biology of the Mycobacteria. Surrey University Press, London, UK.
15. Young, R. A., B. R. Bloom, C. M. Grosskinsky, J. Ivanyi, D. Thomas,

and R. W. Davis. 1985. Dissection of *Mycobacterium tuberculosis* antigens using recombinant DNA. *Proc. Natl. Acad. Sci. USA 82*:2583.

16. Telenti, A., P. Imboden, F. Marchesi, D. Lowrie, S. Cole, M. J. Colston, L. Matter, K. Schopfer, and T. Bodmer. 1993. Detection of rifampicin-resistance mutations in *Mycobacterium tuberculosis. Lancet 341*:647.
17. Zhang, Y., B. Heym, B. Allen, D. Young, and S. T. Cole. 1992. The catalase-peroxidase gene and isoniazid resistance of *Mycobacterium tuberculosis. Nature 358*:591.
18. Eiglmeier, K., N. Honore, S. A. Woods, B. Caudron, and S. T. Cole. 1993. Use of an ordered cosmid library to deduce genomic organisation of *Mycobacterium leprae. Mol. Microbiol. 7*:197.
19. Cirillo, J. D., C. K. Stover, B. R. Bloom, W. R. Jacobs, Jr., and R. G. Barletta. 1995. Bacterial vaccine vectors and bacillus Calmette-Guerin. *Clin. Infect. Dis. 20*:1001.
20. Donnelly-Wu, M. K., W. R. Jacobs, Jr., and G. F. Hatfull. 1993. Superinfection immunity of mycobacteriophage L5: applications for genetic transformation of mycobacteria. *Mol. Microbiol. 7*:407.
21. Hanson, M. S., C. V. Lapcevich, and S. Haun. 1995. Progress on development of the live BCG recombinant vaccine vehicle for combined vaccine delivery. *Ann. N.Y. Acad. Sci. 754*:214.
22. Husson, R. N., B. E. James, and R. A. Young. 1990. Gene replacement and expression of foreign DNA in mycobacteria. *J. Bacteriol. 172*:519.
23. Jacobs, W. R., Jr., R. Tuckman, and B. R. Bloom. 1987. Introduction of foreign DNA into mycobacteria using a shuttle plasmid. *Nature 327*:532.
24. Kalpana, G. V., B. R. Bloom, and W. R. Jacobs, Jr. 1991. Insertional mutagenesis and illegitimate recombination in mycobacteria. *Proc. Natl. Acad. Sci. USA 88*:5433.
25. Lee, M. H., L. Pascopella, W. R. Jacobs, Jr., and G. F. Hatfull. 1991. Site-specific integration of mycobacteriophage L5: integration-proficient vectors for *Mycobacterium smegmatis, Mycobacterium tuberculosis*, and bacille Calmette-Guérin. *Proc. Natl. Acad. Sci. USA 88*:3111.
26. Martin, C., J. Timm, J. Rauzier, R. Gomez-Lus, J. Davis, and B. Giquel. 1990. Transposition of an antibiotic resistance element in mycobacteria. *Nature 345*:739.
27. McFadden, J. 1996. Recombination in mycobacteria. *Mol. Microbiol. 21*:205.
28. Oka, A., H. Sugisaki, and M. Takanami. 1981. Nucleotide sequence of the kanamycin resistance transposon Tn903. *J. Mol. Biol. 147*:217.
29. Snapper, S. B., L. Lugosi, A. Jekkel, R. E. Melton, Z. T. Kieser, B. R. Bloom, and W. R. Jacobs, Jr. 1988. Lysogeny and transformation

in mycobacteria: stable expression of foreign genes. *Proc. Natl. Acad. Sci. USA 85*:6987.

30. Snapper, S. B., R. E. Melton, S. Mustafa, T. Kieser, and W. R. Jacobs, Jr. 1990. Isolation and characterization of efficient plasmid transformation mutants of *Mycobacterium smegmatis. Mol. Microbiol. 4*:1911.
31. Azad, A. K., Sirakova, T. D., Rogers, L. M., and P. E. Kolattukudy. 1996. Targeted replacement of the mycocerosic acid synthase gene in *Mycobacterium bovis* BCG produces a mutant that lacks mycosides. *Proc. Natl. Acad. Sci. USA 93*:4787.
32. Aldovini, A., Husson, R. N., and R. A. Young. 1993. The uraA locus and homologous recombination in *Mycobacterium bovis* BCG. *J. Bacteriol. 175*:7282.
33. Balasubramanian, V., M. S. Pavelka, Jr., S. S. Bardarov, J. Martin, T. R. Weisbrod, R. A. McAdam, B. R. Bloom, and W. R. Jacobs, Jr. 1996. Allelic exchange in *Mycobacterium tuberculosis* with long linear recombination substrates. *J. Bacteriol. 178*:273.
34. Reyrat, J. M., F. X. Berthet, and B. Gicquel. 1995. The urease locus of Mycobacterium tuberculosis and its utilization for the demonstration of allelic exchange in *Mycobacterium bovis* bacillus Calmette-Guérin. *Proc. Natl. Acad. Sci. USA 92*:8768.
35. Boeke, J., J. Truehart, B. Natsoulis, and G. R. Fink. 1987. 5-Flouro-orotic acid as a selective agent in yeast molecular genetics. *Methods Enzymol. 154*:164.
36. Botstein, D., and R. W. Davis. 1982. Principles and practice of recombinant DNA research with yeast, In: J. Strathern, E. Jones, and J. Broach, *The Molecular Biology of the Yeast Saccharomyces: Metabolism and Gene Expression*, edited by Strathern, J., Jones, E., and Broach, J. Cold Spring Harbor, N.Y.: Cold Spring Harbor Laboratory Press, p. 607.
37. Kimsey, H. H., and D. Kaiser. 1992. The orotidine-5′-monophosphate decarboxylase gene of *Myxococcus xanthus. J. Biol. Chem. 267*:819.
38. Sander, P., A. Meier, and E. C. Bottger. 1995. rpsL$^+$: a dominant selectable marker for gene replacement in mycobacteria. *Mol. Microbiol. 5*:991.
39. Baulard, A., L. Kremer, and C. Locht. 1996. Efficient homologous recombination in fast-growing and slow-growing mycobacteria. *J. Bacteriol. 178*:3091.
40. Stover, C. K., V. F. de la Cruz, T. R. Fuerst, J. W. Burlein, L. A. Benson, L. T. Bennett, G. P. Bansal, J. F. Young, M. H. Lee, G. F. Hatfull, S. B. Snapper, R. G. Barletta, W. R. Jacobs, Jr., and B. R. Bloom. 1991. New use of BCG for recombinant vaccines. *Nature 351*:456.
41. Neidhardt, F. C., and R. A. VanBogelen. 1987. In: *Escherichia coli and Salmonella typhimurium. Cellular and Molecular Biology*, edited

by Neidhardt, F. C., Ingraham, J. L., Low, K. B., Magasanik, B., and Schaechter, M. Washington, DC: American Society for Microbiology, 1654 pp.

42. Born, W., M. P. Happ, A. Dallas, C. Reardon, R. Kubo, T. Shinnick, P. Brennan, and R. O'Brien. 1990. Recognition of heat shock proteins and gd cell function. *Immunol. Today 11*:40.
43. Buchmeier, N. A., and F. Heffron. 1990. Induction of *Salmonella* stress proteins upon infection of macrophages. *Science 248*:730.
44. Lamb, J. R., and D. B. Young. 1990. T cell recognition of stress proteins. A link between infectious and autoimmune disease. *Mol. Biol. Med. 7*:311.
45. Murray, P. J., and R. A. Young. 1992. Stress and immunological recognition in host pathogen interactions. *J. Bacteriol. 174*:4193.
46. Shinnick, T. M. 1987. The 65-kilodalton antigen of *Mycobacterium tuberculosis. J. Bacteriol. 169*:1080.
47. Young, R. A. 1990. Stress protein and immunology. *Annu. Rev. Immunol. 8*:401.
48. Aldovini, A., and R. A. Young. 1991. Humoral and cell-mediated cell responses to live recombinant BCG-HIV vaccines. *Nature 351*:479.
49. Kameoka, M., Y. Nishino, K. Matsuo, N. Ohara, T. Kimura, A. Yamazaki, T. Yamada, and K. Ikuta. 1994. Cytotoxic T lymphocyte response in mice induced by a recombinant BCG vaccination which produces an extracellular alpha antigen that fused with the human immunodeficiency virus type 1 envelope immunodominant domain in the V3 loop. *Vaccine 12*:153.
50. Winter, N., M. Lagranderie, J. Rauzier, J. Timm, C. Leclerc, B. Guy, M. P. Kieny, M. Gheorghiu, and B. Gicquel. 1991. Expression of heterologous genes in *Mycobacterium bovis* BCG: induction of a cellular response against HIV-1 Nef protein. *Gene 109*:47.
51. Yasutomi, Y., S. Koenig, S. S. Haun, C. K. Stover, R. K. Jackson, P. Conard, A. J. Conley, E. A. Emini, T. R. Fuerst, and N. L. Letvin. 1993. Immunization with recombinant BCG-SIV elicits SIV-specific cytotoxic T lymphocytes in rhesus monkeys. *J. Immunol. 150*:3101.
52. Lim, E. M., M. Lagranderie, R. Le Grand, J. Rauzier, M. Gheorghiu, B. Gicquel, and N. Winter. 1997. Recombinant *Mycobacterium bovis* BCG producing the N-terminal half of SIVmac251 Env antigen induces neutralizing antibodies and cytotoxic T lymphocyte responses in mice and guinea pigs. *AIDS Res. Hum. Retroviruses 13*:1573.
53. Abdelhak, S., H. Louzir, J. Timm, L. Blel, Z. Benlasfar, M. Lagranderie, M. Gheorghiu, K. Dellagi, and B. Gicquel. 1995. Recombinant BCG expressing the leishmania surface antigen Gp63 induces protective im-

munity against Leishmania major infection in BALB/c mice. *Microbiology 141*:1585.

54. Connell, N. D., E. Medina-Acosta, W. R. McMaster, B. R. Bloom, and D. G. Russell. 1993. Effective immunization against cutaneous leishmaniasis with recombinant bacille Calmette-Guérin expressing the *Leishmania* surface proteinase gp63. *Proc. Natl. Acad. Sci. USA 90*:11473.
55. Kremer, L., G. Riveau, A. Baulard, A. Capron, and C. Locht. 1996. Neutralizing antibody responses elicited in mice immunized with recombinant bacillus Calmette-Guérin producing the *Schistosoma mansoni* glutathione S-transferase. *J. Immunol. 156*:4309.
56. Zhu, Y. D., G. Fennelly, C. Miller, R. Tarara, I. Saxe, B. Bloom, and M. J. McChesney. 1997. Recombinant bacille Calmette-Guérin expressing the measles virus nucleoprotein protects infant rhesus macaques from measles virus pneumonia. *Infect. Dis. 176*:1445.
57. Langermann, S., S. R. Palaszynski, J. E. Burlein, S. Koenig, M. S. Hanson, D. E. Briles, and C. K. Stover. 1994. Protective humoral response against pneumococcal infection in mice elicited by recombinant bacille Calmette-Guérin vaccines expressing pneumococcal surface protein A. *J. Exp. Med. 180*:2277.
58. Langermann, S., S. Palaszynski, A. Sadziene, C. K. Stover, and S. Koenig. 1994. Systemic and mucosal immunity induced by BCG vector expressing outer-surface protein A of *Borrelia burgdorferi. Nature 372*:552.
59. Stover, C. K., G. P. Bansal, S. Langerman, and M. S. Hanson. 1994. Protective immunity elicited by rBCG vaccines. *Dev. Biol. Stand. 82*:163.
60. Stover, C. K., G. P. Bansal, M. S. Hanson, J. E. Burlein, S. R. Palaszynski, J. F. Young, S. Koenig, D. B. Young, A. Sadziene, and A. G. Barbour. 1993. Protective immunity elicited by recombinant bacille Calmette-Guérin (BCG) expressing outer surface protein A (OspA) lipoprotein: a candidate Lyme disease vaccine. *J. Exp. Med. 178*:197.
61. Lamm, D. L. 1992. Long-term results of intravesical therapy for superficial bladder cancer. *Urol. Clin. North Am. 19*:573.
62. Morales, A., and J. C. Nickel. 1992. Immunotherapy for superficial bladder cancer. A developmental and clinical overview. *Urol. Clin. North Am. 19*:549.
63. Murray, P. J., Aldovini, A., and Young, R. A. 1996. Manipulation and potentiation of anti-mycobacterial immunity using recombinant BCG secreting murine cytokines. *Proc. Natl. Acad. Sci. USA 93*:934.
64. O'Donnell, M. A., A. Aldovini, R. B. Duda, H. Yang, A. Szilvasi, R. A. Young, and W. C. DeWolf. 1994. Recombinant BCG secreting functional IL-2 can modulate cytokine production by lymphocytes. *Infect. Immun. 62*:2508.

65. Hanson, M. S., G. P. Bansal, S. Langermann, C. K. Stover, and I. Orme. 1995. Efficacy and safety of live recombinant BCG vaccines. *Dev. Biol. Stand. 84*:229.

66. Baumgart, K. W., H. R. McKenzie, A. J. Radford, I. Ramshaw, W. J. Britton. 1996. Immunogenicity and protection studies with recombinant mycobacteria and vaccinia vectors coexpressing the 18-kilodalton protein of *Mycobacterium leprae. Infect. Immun. 64*:2274.

67. Honda, M., K. Matsuo, T. Nakasone, Y. Okamoto, H. Yoshizaki, K. Kitamura, W. Sugiura, K. Watanabe, Y. Fukushima, and S. Haga. 1995. Protective immune responses induced by secretion of a chimeric soluble protein from a recombinant Mycobacterium bovis bacillus Calmette-Guérin vector candidate vaccine for human immunodeficiency virus type 1 in small animals. *Proc. Natl. Acad. Sci. USA 92*:10693.

68. Lagranderie, M., A. M. Balazuc, B. Gicquel, and M. Gheorghiu. 1997. Oral immunization with recombinant *Mycobacterium bovis* BCG simian immunodeficiency virus nef induces local and systemic cytotoxic T-lymphocyte responses in mice. *J. Virol. 71*:2303.

69. Matsumoto, S., T. Yanagi, N. Ohara, N. Wada, H. Kanbara, and T. Yamada. 1996. Stable expression and secretion of the B-cell epitope of rodent malaria from *Mycobacterium bovis* BCG and induction of long-lasting humoral response in mouse. *Vaccine 14*:54.

70. Dranoff, G., E. Jaffee, A. Lazenby, P. Golumbek, H. Levitsky, K. Brose, V. Jackson, H. Hamada, D. Pardoll, and R. C. Mulligan. 1993. Vaccination with irradiated tumor cells engineered to secrete murine granulocyte-macrophage colony-stimulating factor stimulates potent, specific, and long-lasting antitumor immunity. *Proc. Natl. Acad. Sci. USA 90*:3539.

71. Bloom, B. R., and C. Murray. 1992. Tuberculosis: commentary on an emergent killer. *Science 257*:1055.

72. Styblo, K. 1989. Overview and epidemiological assessment of the current global tuberculosis situation with an emphasis on control in developing countries. *Rev. Infect. Dis. 11*(Suppl 2):S339–46.

73. Snider, D. E., and W. L. Roper. 1992. The new tuberculosis. *N. Engl. J. Med. 326*:703.

CHAPTER 6

MUCOSAL VACCINATION WITH *Salmonella* VACCINE VECTORS

DAVID M. HONE, MOHAMED T. SHATA, DAVID W. PASCUAL, and GEORGE K. LEWIS

6.1 INTRODUCTION

The importance of mucosal immunity in vaccine development was established by the discovery of secretory component and evidence showing that mucosal surfaces and the lymphoid tissue associated with these surfaces constitute an immune compartment that is distinct from the systemic immune compartment (1–9). Although there are several routes by which vaccines that target the mucosal immune compartment are administered, there are imposing reasons for selecting an oral vaccination strategy to induce mucosal immunity. First, the oral route has been the most widely used mucosal vaccination route; it has proved both practical and reliable in large-scale public health vaccination programs (10–19). Moreover, the currently licensed oral

Abbreviations: AIDS, acquired immunodeficiency syndrome; CDC, Centers for Disease Control; CFA/I, colonization factor antigen I; CFU, colony-forming unit; CHO, Chinese hamster ovary; CMV, cytomegalovirus; CSP, circumsporozoite protein; CTL, cytotoxic T lymphocyte; DHB, 2,3-dihydroxybenzoate; ELISA, enzyme-linked immunosorbent assay; ELISPOT, enzyme-linked immunosorbent SPOT; ETEC, enterotoxigenic *Escherichia coli*; GALT, gut-associated lymphoid tissue; Hfr, high frequency of recombination; HIV, human immunodeficiency virus; HSV-1, herpes simplex virus type 1; IFN-γ, interferon-γ; IL, interleukin; LTB, heat-labile toxin; LLO, listeriolysin O; LPS, lipopolysaccharide; MHC, major histocompatibility complex; PABA, *p*-aminobenzoic acid; S-IgA, secretory immunoglobulin A; SIV, simian immunodeficiency virus; TCR, T-cell receptor; Th, T helper; TNF, tumor necrosis factor; UDF, uridine diphosphate; Vi, virulence antigen = capsular polysaccharide = (α-1,4 2-deoxy-2-*N*-acetylgalacturonic acid)$_n$.

Intracellular Bacterial Vaccine Vectors, Edited by Yvonne Paterson.
ISBN 0-471-17278-2

polio (10,11), adenovirus (18,19), and typhoid (14–17) vaccines were efficacious in phase III field trials and in large-scale vaccination programs. Another significant factor in favor of using the oral route is the high level of compliance displayed by clinical cohorts enrolled in oral vaccine field trials (10–19). Despite this successful background, the poor immunogenicity of most antigens when given orally has hindered the development of oral vaccines against other pathogens. By contrast, live oral *Salmonella* vaccine vectors traverse the natural defenses of the gastrointestinal tract and target antigens to inductive sites in the mucosal immune compartment (Fig. 6.1). Further, live oral *Salmonella* vaccines possess attributes that make them well suited for large-scale use in developed and developing countries (20).

Any general discussion of *Salmonella* vectors is complicated by the nomenclature of this family of organisms. Members of the *Salmon-*

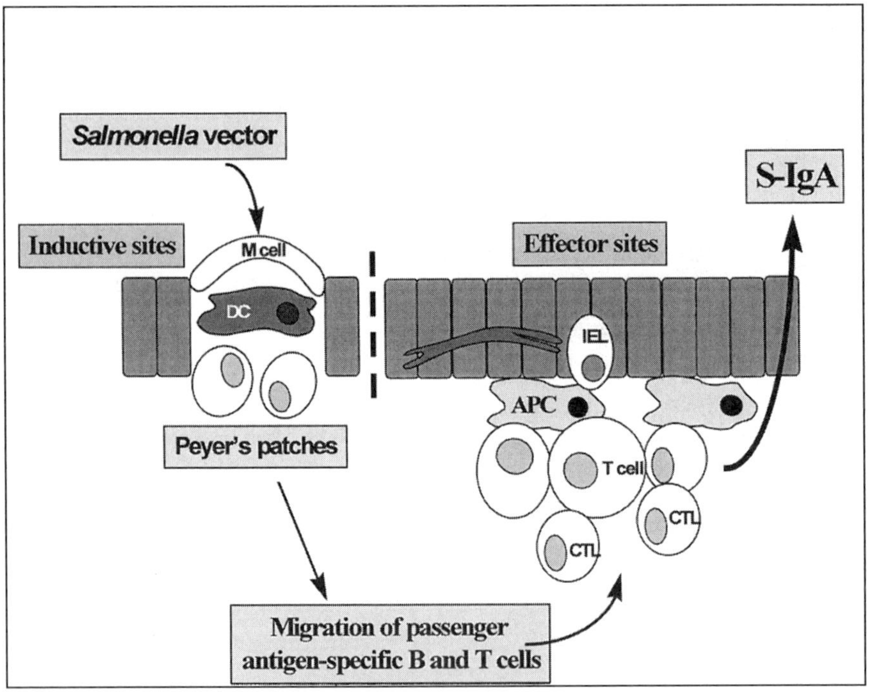

Figure 6.1 Induction of passenger antigen-specific mucosal responses with *Salmonella* vectors.

ella family, now considered a single species called *Salmonella enterica* (21), display an immense array of biochemical and antigenic variation. In the currently accepted *Salmonella* classification scheme, each organism that expresses a unique combination of biotype and serotype, although once afforded species status, is called an *S. enterica* variant (21). For example, *Salmonella typhi*, the causative agent of typhoid fever, is now referred to as *S. enterica* var. Typhi (Typhi) and *Salmonella typhimurium*, which causes acute gastroenteritis, is now designated *S. enterica* var. Typhimurium (Typhimurium) (21).

Another issue complicating interpretation of the *Salmonella* vector literature is the fact that a number of *Salmonella enterica* variants have been used to characterize this vector system. This complexity is driven by the animal models employed to evaluate each specific vector construct and the host specificity of individual *S. enterica* variants. Most of the documented experience with *Salmonella* vectors, however, has been generated using the mouse typhoid model. This model was developed to avoid costly volunteer studies with Typhi (22–24) and, since its inception, has been instrumental in answering questions related to *Salmonella* pathogenesis and immunity (25–34). For the most part, mouse typhoid studies use members of the *Salmonella* family that are virulent in mice, including Typhimurium, *S. enterica* var. Enteritidis (Enteritidis), *S. enterica* var. Dublin (Dublin), and *S. enterica* var. Cholerae-suis (Cholerae-suis). In light of the parallels between the behavior of mouse-virulent *Salmonella* in this model and the behavior of human-specific *Salmonella* variants, we and others have used the mouse typhoid model to characterize the immunogenicity of a variety of prototype *Salmonella* vector strains (Table 6.1). In this role, the mouse typhoid model creates an invaluable tool with which to investigate basic questions related to passenger antigen immunogenicity. Furthermore, since the mouse typhoid model is the only established small laboratory animal model for *Salmonella* that allows rigorous assessment of passenger antigen immunogenicity after oral vaccination, most documented *Salmonella* vector data were developed using this model (Table 6.1). Therefore, this chapter mainly details the findings of experiments using the mouse typhoid model to evaluate Typhimurium, Enteritidis, Dublin and Cholerae-suis vector constructs. Where appropriate, experiments with Typhi vectors in laboratory animals and volunteers are also discussed.

TABLE 6.1 Murine Studies With Prototype *Salmonella* Vectors

Salmonella Mutant	Passenger Antigen	Type of Immune Response	Functional Assay	References
A. Viral antigens				
Typhimurium *aroA*	Influenza virus HA and NP proteins	Humoral; Cellular (Th1)	CTLs	(37–41)
Typhimurium or Typhi; Δ*cya*/Δ*crp*, *phoP*^{c}, or *aroA*	HBV pre-S, core, and peptide antigens	Humoral (mucosal and systemic IgG and IgA)	ND	(42–48)
Typhimurium or Dublin; Δ*aroA*	HIV-1 and -2 gp120, gp41, and Gag proteins and peptides	Humoral (mucosal and systemic IgG and IgA); Cellular (Th1)	ND	(49–58)
Typhimurium or Dublin; Δ*aroA*	SIV Nef and Gag proteins	Humoral; Cellular	CTLs	(59,60)
Typhimurium Δ*cya*/Δ*crp*	Gastroenteritis virus S protein	Humoral (musocal and systemic IgG and IgA)	ND	(61)
Typhimurium Δ*aroA*	Poliovirus VP1 peptide	Humoral	ND	(46,47)
Typhimurium Δ*aroA*	Human papillomavirus type 16	Humoral; Cellular	Virus neutralization	(62)
Typhimurium Δ*htrA*	HSV gpD peptide	Humoral	Virus neutralization and protection	(63)
B. Bacterial antigens				
Typhi, Typhimurium, Enteritidis, and Dublin; *galE*, *aroA*, or *aroA*/*purA*	ETEC β subunit of LT (LTB)	Humoral (musocal and systemic IgG and IgA); Cellular	Toxin neutralization	(64–71)

Typhimurium, Enteritidis, or Typhi; *aroA* or *galE*	ETEC CFA/I, CS3, K88, and K99 fimbriae	Humoral (mucosal and systemic IgG and IgA); Cellular	Protection	(72–78)
Typhi *galE*	*Shigella* spp. O antigen	Humoral	Partial protection	(36,79–83)
Typhi *galE*	*Vibrio cholerae* O antigen	Humoral	ND	(84–88)
Typhimurium *aroA* or $\Delta cya/\Delta crp$	*E. coli* β-galactosidase	Humoral (mucosal and systemic IgG and IgA); Cellular (DTH)	ND	(89,90)
Typhimurium or Typhi; $\Delta aroA$; $\Delta aroC/\Delta aroD$	Tetanus toxin fragment C	Humoral (mucosal and systemic IgG and IgA); Cellular (Th1; DTH)	Protection	(91–97)
Typhimurium $\Delta aroA$	*Bordetella pertussis* pertactin and pertussis toxin S1 subunit	Humoral; Cellular	Protection	(95,98)
Typhimurium $\Delta aroA$	*Yersinia invasin*, F1 and V antigens	Humoral; Cellular	Partial protection	(99–101)
Typhimurium or Dublin; $\Delta aroA$ and $\Delta cya/\Delta crp$	*Streptococcus* spp. SpaA and M proteins	Humoral (mucosal and systemic IgG and IgA); Cellular	Protection	(102–107)
Typhimurium $\Delta aroA$	*E. coli* alkaline phosphatase	Humoral	ND	(108)
Typhimurium $\Delta cya/\Delta crp$	*Porphyromonas gingivalis* HA	Humoral	ND	(109–111)
Typhimurium or Dublin *aroA*	*Pseudomonas aerouginosa* exoprotein A and outer membrane protein I	Humoral (mucosal IgA)	Protection	(112,113)

TABLE 6.1 (*Continued*)

Salmonella Mutant	Passenger Antigen	Type of Immune Response	Functional Assay	References
B. Bacterial antigens (*Continued*)				
Typhimurium Δ*aroA*	*Listeria monocytogenes* p60, Hly, and SOD	Cellular	$CD8^+$ CTL; Protection	(114–118)
Typhimurium *phoP*^{c}	*Helicobacter pylori* urease	Humoral; Cellular	Protection	(119)
Typhimurium Δ*aroA*	*Chlamydia trachomatis* MOMP	Humoral	ND	(120)
C. Eukaryote antigens				
Typhimurium, Dublin, or Typhi Δ*aroA*	*Plasmodium* CSP, MSP, and RESA proteins and peptides	Humoral (IgG and IgA); Cellular	$CD8^+$ CTL; Protection	(121–127)
Typhi Δ*cya*/Δ*crp*	Serine-rich *Entamoeba histolytica* protein (SREHP)	Humoral	ND	(128)
Typhimurium Δ*aroA*	*Echinococcus granulosus* fatty acid-binding protein	Humoral; Cellular (Th1 and Th2)	ND	(129)
Typhimurium Δ*aroA*	*Schistosoma mansoni* glutathione S-transferase	Humoral	ND	(130–132)
Typhimurium Δ*cya*/Δ*crp*	Human sperm antigen	Humoral (mucosal and systemic IgG and IgA)	ND	(133)

D. Cytokines				
Typhimurium *ΔaroA/ΔaroD*	IL-2, IFN-γ, and TNF-α	Nonspecific immune activation	Increased nonspecific protection against *Leishmania major*	(134)
Typhimurium *ΔaroA*	TGF-β		Reduced inflammation, IL-2, and IFN-γ, but enhanced IL-10, in carrageenin-induced edema	(135)
Typhimurium *ΔaroA*	IL-1β and IL-4	Altered survival in host tissue	ND	(136–138)
Typhimurium *aroA*	IL-5	Adjuvant affect	ND	
Typhimurium *aroA*	Nonapeptide of murine IL-1β	Cellular (adjuvant affect)	ND	(139)
Typhimurium *Δcya/Δcrp*	Human IL-2	ND	Antitumor immunity	(140)

6.2 LESSONS FROM THE PAST TO THE PRESENT

6.2.1 Laboratory Animal Studies with *Salmonella* Vectors: Establishing the Paradigm

Although the advent of recombinant DNA technology was necessary for the development of most *Salmonella* vectors, the first such report described the immunogenicity of a Typhimurium vector into which the *Escherichia coli* 08 *rfb* genes were introduced by Hfr transfer. The resultant Typhimurium hybrid expressed the 08 antigen of *Escherichia coli*, in place of the Typhimurium O-antigen (35). Analysis of the humoral responses generated by oral vaccination of mice with the Typhimurium-08 recombinant, demonstrated that it induced mucosal and systemic antibodies against the passenger 08 antigen (35). Independently, Formal et al. (36) constructed a hybrid Typhi vector strain by mobilizing the virulence plasmid of *Shigella sonnei*, that expressed the form 1 0-antigen, into attenuated Typhi strain Ty21a. Mice immunized parenterally with this latter hybrid developed impressive humoral responses against *S. sonnei* O-antigen and were protected against subsequent challenge with *S. sonnei* (36). The ensuing studies employed recombinant DNA techniques to introduce a broad array of bacterial, viral and protozoan antigens into attenuated Typhimurium vectors, the overwhelming majority of which proved to be immunogenic in mice (Table 6.1).

Besides inducing mucosal and systemic antibodies against passenger antigens, *Salmonella* vectors are capable of inducing protective antibody responses against targeted pathogens or toxins. Direct evidence along this vein was reported by Attridge et al. (141), who showed that an attenuated Typhimurium expressing K88 or K99 fimbriae elicited colostral and milk antibodies against the fimbrial antigens in pregnant sows following oral immunization and afforded protection to suckling piglets via the passive transfer of protective antibodies (141). Similarly, mice immunized orally with an attenuated Typhimurium vector expressing a 50-kDa fragment of tetanus toxin (designated fragment c induced tetanus toxin-specific serum IgG responses that correlated with protection against a lethal tetanus toxin challenge (91,142). Other bacterial pathogens against which protective antibody responses were generated using *Salmonella* vectors include *Yersinia pseudotuberculosis* (101) and *Borrelia burgdorferi* (143). Viral neutralizing antibodies have also been induced using a *Salmonella* vector expressing a contiguous B-cell epitope of herpes simplex virus type 1 (HSV-1) (63). Furthermore, *Salmonella* vector-induced virus-specific antibody responses correlated with protection against influenza virus (144) and HSV-1 (63) in laboratory animals. Overall, therefore, these data present compelling evidence that *Salmonella* vectors are capable of eliciting protective humoral responses against bacterial, protozoan, and viral pathogens.

In addition, *Salmonella* vectors also induce passenger antigen-specific $CD4^+$ and $CD8^+$ T-cell responses (Table 6.1). A lion's share of attention has been devoted toward the characterization of the passenger antigen specific $CD4^+$ T-cell responses. In most reports, passenger antigen-specific splenocytes produced IFN-γ but did not produce detectable levels of T-helper type 2 (Th2) cytokines (37,49,145,146), lending support to the notion that the responses were predominated by passenger antigen-specific T-helper type 1 (Th1) cells. These findings have been confirmed using cytokine-specific enzyme-linked immunosorbent SPOT (ELISPOT) assays, which show a predominance of passenger antigen-specific, IFN-γ-secreting, $CD4^+$ T cells in mice orally vaccinated with *Salmonella* vectors (51,94).

Occasionally, Th2 responses have also been noted (94,129). However, the specific role played by individual T-cell subsets in passenger antigen-specific humoral and cell-mediated responses has not been fully delineated. Nonetheless, evidence documented to date suggests that *Salmonella* vectors elicit distinct mucosal $CD4^+$ T cells subsets compared to those induced by soluble antigens mixed with cholera toxin (94,147). Hence, oral immunization of IL-$4^{-/-}$ knockout mice with a *Salmonella* vector that expressed tetanus toxin fragment C as a passenger antigen developed comparable secretory IgA (S-IgA) responses to those that developed in IL-$4^{+/+}$ mice (94,147). Conversely, IL-$4^{-/-}$ knockout mice failed to develop a tetanus-specific S-IgA response after vaccination with tetanus toxoid mixed with cholera toxin, whereas IL-$4^{+/+}$ mice developed strong S-IgA responses to this vaccine formulation (94,147). This finding implied that the development of S-IgA responses after vaccination with *Salmonella* vectors may be regulated by distinct Th2-cell subsets and is IL-4 independent (94,147). Before conclusions can be drawn, however, definitive characterization of these Th1- and Th2-cell subsets and their role in regulating responses against passenger antigens must be completed.

The capacity of live *Salmonella* vectors to stimulate major histocompatibility complex (MHC) class I restricted $CD8^+$ T-cell responses has also received some attention. Since *Salmonella* is believed to remain endosome-bound throughout infection (148–151), this organism was not thought to directly access MHC class I presentation pathways in the cytoplasm of host cells (152). Nonetheless, passenger antigen-specific MHC class I-restricted cytotoxic T lymphocytes (CTLs) after vaccination with live *Salmonella* vaccine vectors have now been documented by several independent groups (39,60,122,123,126,153,154). Further, these CTL responses were shown to be MHC class I restricted and were eliminated after depletion of $CD8^+$ T cells (39,60,122,123,126,153,154). In one instance a *Salmonella* construct expressing full-length SIV Gag was shown to elicit Gag-specific $CD8^+$ CTLs that were detected 70 days after immunization (60), suggesting that these responses may persist after vaccination. In several examples, CTLs were not detected after vaccination with *Salmonella* vectors (37,49,54,155). Thus, the rules that govern the development of CTL responses following vaccination with *Salmonella* vectors need further characterization.

A variety of laboratory animal models have shown that *Salmonella* vectors induce protection against the target pathogen from which the passenger antigen originated through $CD4^+$ and $CD8^+$ T-cell-mediated mechanisms. $CD4^+$ T-cell-mediated protection was inferred by data showing protection against *L. major* in highly susceptible BALB/c mice after oral vaccination with a *Salmonella* vector expressing *Leishmania major* gp63. This *Salmonella*-gp63 vector was shown to induce *Leishmania*-specific $CD4^+$ Th1 cell responses, which presumably mediated the observed protection against *Leishmania* (145,146). In addition, Aggarwal and colleagues in collaboration with our group (122) provided evidence that *Salmonella* vectors may engender protection through passenger antigen-specific $CD8^+$ T-cell responses. We showed that oral vaccination of mice with a Typhimurium-malaria vector that expressed the circumsporozoite protein (CSP) of *Plasmodium berghei* induced protection against a *P. berghei* challenge that was abrogated by the elimination of $CD8^+$ T cells before challenge (122). When compiled with the above-cited examples, these results firmly established that *Salmonella* vectors are capable of eliciting cellular immunity in the mucosal and systemic compartments against polysaccharide and protein passenger antigens.

6.2.2 Properties of Immunogenic *Salmonella* Vectors

The results cited above suggest that *Salmonella* vectors possess specialized delivery properties for the induction of immune responses to passenger antigens. To address this question, we compared the immunogenicity of *Salmonella* and *E. coli* vectors that expressed enterotoxigenic *Escherichia coli* (ETEC) fimbrial antigen, colonization factor antigen I (CFA/I) (73). Accordingly, a balanced lethal-stabilized plasmid carrying ETEC *cfaABCE* genes, called pJGX15C-*asd*$^+$ was constructed and introduced into attenuated Typhimurium Δ*aro* Δ*asd* strain H683 and nonpathogenic laboratory *E. coli* Δ*asd* strain χ6212. The resultant Typhimurium and *E. coli* transformants stably expressed comparable levels of CFA/I. To appraise the immunogenicity of these constructs, BALB/c mice were immunized orally with a single 10^9 CFU dose of either Typhimurium strain H683(pJGX15C-*asd*$^+$) or *E. coli* strain χ 6212(pJGX15C-*asd*$^+$); the responses to CFA/I were measured enzyme-linked immunosorbent assay (ELISA) and IgA-specific ELISPOT (73). The results indicated that mice immunized with a single dose of the Typhimurium construct developed a 10^5-fold increase in CFA/I-specific serum IgG and significantly elevated numbers of CFA/I-specific, IgA-secreting B cells in the intestinal lamina propria and mesenteric lymph nodes (73). By contrast, mice immunized in parallel with the *E. coli*–CFA/I construct did not develop significant serum or mucosal responses against CFA/I (73). Since the virulence properties of the *Salmonella* and *E. coli* vectors significantly differed, the above results implied that *Salmonella* may possess specialized properties that facilitate the induction of passenger antigen-specific mucosal and systemic humoral responses.

To date, studies that characterized the specific virulence properties of *Salmonella* that enable effective delivery of passenger antigens to the gut-associated lymphoid tissue (GALT) have been infrequent. Typhimurium *htrA* mutants, which are defective in their capacity to survive in murine macrophages and to persist in murine lymphoid tissue (156), retain the capacity to elicit humoral responses against passenger antigens (63). Similarly, Typhimurium strains that lack the virulence plasmid and are greatly diminished in their ability to colonize the systemic compartment after oral immunization, have also been shown to function as vaccine vectors (157). By contrast, PurA-negative mutants of Typhimurium, which are defective in their capacity to colonize the small intestine and Peyer's patches of mice, were shown to be poorly immunogenic (65). By and large, these results suggest that the capacity of *Salmonella* to colonize the small intestine and Peyer's patches may be critical elements of the immunogenicity of these vectors, whereas persistence in host tissues and spread to the systemic compartment may be less important attributes.

6.2.3 Improved Passenger Antigen Expression Systems

Reports of the ineffectiveness of *Salmonella* vectors may be found in the literature. In one such instance, an attenuated *typhi* strain that expressed the circumsporozoite (CSP) of *Plasmodium falciparum* induced only modest immunity against CSP in a small number of vaccine recipients (126). Analogous to this finding, Nardelli-Haeflinger et al. (44) found that a *Salmonella* recombinant that expressed hepatitis B surface antigen in the cytoplasm of the vector infrequently elicited humoral responses against the passenger antigen. A similar occurrence was reported by Franchini et al. (54), who found that a *Salmonella* recombinant expressing HIV antigens cytoplasmically was poorly immunogenic in Rhesus monkeys. Since the development of these early constructs several advances in this technology have been made. Two decades of research with *Salmonella* vectors have provided a basis for this variability and suggest that, in addition to the virulence properties of the vector, the immunogenicity of *Salmonella* vector-delivered passenger antigens appears to be controlled by at least three expression parameters: in vivo stability, the characteristics of the expression cassette, and the location of the passenger antigen within the vector.

There are two facets to in vivo passenger antigen stability in *Salmonella* vectors: genetic stability and product stability. The genetic stability of passenger antigen expression cassettes in the absence of antibiotic selection markers is in part restored using chromosomal integration systems (75,158) and the balanced-lethal plasmid stabilization system (159). Methods designed to increase product stability have only begun to emerge since this form of in vivo instability may not be pertinent to all passenger antigens (49,50,93,95). Thus, some passenger antigens are resistant to the proteases present in the cytoplasm of *Salmonella* and are immunogenic when expressed in this compartment (93,95). Other antigens, such as diphtheria toxin and the S1 subunit of *Bordetella pertussis* toxin, were found to be susceptible to proteolytic degradation when expressed in the cytoplasm of *Salmonella* vectors (93,95). These antigens were "rescued" by creating chimeric fusions with fragment C of tetanus toxin (93,95). The configuration of the fusion proteins was crucial and fragment C fusions that displayed the highest level of resistance to proteolytic degradation also induced the strongest immune responses (95). Additionally, other cytoplasmically expressed passenger antigens form inclusion bodies as a result of misfolding (49,50). Abnormal proteins, such as those that partition into this insoluble fraction, have short half-lives within the bacterial cytoplasm (160,161). Fouts and associates (49, 50), therefore, proposed that passenger antigens that form inclusion bodies may also exhibit poor immunogenicity, as a result of epitope degradation. Although it is unclear whether fragment C fusions would eliminate this problem, passenger antigen secretion was shown to alleviate the formation of inclusion bodies by gp120 of HIV-1 (51).

Techniques to elevate the expression of recombinant proteins in bacterial host strains include the use of high-copy plasmids, strong promoters, RNA stabilization techniques, strong ribosome binding sites, and modification of the host strain to eliminate endogenous proteases (162). To date, however, passenger antigen expression in *Salmonella* has been manipulated using high-copy plasmids (42,49,133), strong promoters (163–165) and by expressing tandem repeats of the antigen (63,104,131). The sum of these experiences suggested a direct association between passenger antigen expression level and immunogenicity. Under some circumstances, however, high level passenger antigen was found to be toxic to the vector. The development of expression cassettes incorporating a strong promoter located on an inverting sequence, may resolve this form of passenger antigen toxicity (163–165). These systems employ an invertase that inverts sequences encoding a strong promoter to an orientation in-frame with sequences encoding the passenger antigen. This results in strains that produce mixed cultures, composed of expression-negative and expression-positive populations. Since these biphasic expression systems employ strong promoters, the quantity of passenger antigen expressed as a function of the total cell protein rivals levels achieved using constitutive promoters (163–165). Furthermore, strains bearing these expression systems induced humoral responses against the passenger antigens in mice (163–165).

Another potential solution to passenger antigen toxicity is the use of in vivo-induced promoters, which express the passenger antigen in response to environmental signals encountered in the host (91,108,166,167). The potential of this approach was elegantly demonstrated using a Typhimurium vector bearing a single chromosomal gene copy of the *E. coli phoA* gene under the control of the *pagC* promoter, which is activated after *Salmonella* enters macrophages (108). The development of strong PhoA-specific humoral responses in mice vaccinated with this construct suggested that, in addition to reducing passenger antigen toxicity, in vivo-induced promoters may provide a general tool to improve the immunogenicity of passenger antigens in *Salmonella*. The effectiveness of these promoters has not been extensively analyzed in side-by-side comparisons with other high-level expression systems and, therefore, it is difficult to judge the universality of this approach.

Other experimentation suggests that the timing of passenger antigen expression may be critical to passenger antigen immunogenicity for mucosal responses. This facet was well illustrated by Ervin et al. (90), who used a controlled expression system based on two incompatible plasmids; one plasmid that expressed β-galactosidase and the second that repressed the expression of β-galactosidase expression by the first plasmid (90). Expression of β-galactosidase occurred only after the repressor plasmid was lost by segregation in vivo (90). Oral inoculation of mice with a Typhimurium vector containing both plasmids induced serum IgG but not nasal, salivary, or biliary IgA antibody to β-galactosidase (90). A strain carrying the β-galactosidase-encoding plasmid alone, however, induced serum and mucosal antibodies against β-galactosidase. Since the strain bearing both plasmids expressed β-galactosidase only after a period of replication in the host, these results suggest that early passenger antigen expression may be necessary for the induction of mucosal responses.

Passenger antigen placement within the vector is another expression parameter that is believed to influence passenger antigen immunogenicity. Although humoral immunity is not restricted to secreted antigens, a large proportion of secreted antigens induce responses during bacterial infection. By inference, therefore, secreted passenger antigens might be more immunogenic than cytoplasmic passenger antigens. Accordingly, a number of passenger antigen secretion systems have been developed for *Salmonella* vectors. These include the periplasmic secretion systems: *malE* (periplasmic maltose-binding protein; (46,47,56)), and *eltB* (encodes the β-subunit of heat-labile toxin (LTB) (61,105,127). Membrane-associated passenger antigens genetically fused to outer membrane proteins, such as LamB (46,56) and OmpA (51), have also been reported. To secrete passenger antigens externally, several groups have successfully employed fusion to the flagellin subunit (106,153,168,169) or hemolysin A secretion system of *E. coli* (115,117,118). The size of the passenger antigen in these fusions was largely dependent on the host carrier protein, so that the *fla* and *lamB* secretion systems have been used to express short peptide sequences (46,56,106,153,168,169) and may be unstable with larger inserts, whereas *eltB*, *malE*, *hlyA*, and *ompA* have been used successfully to secrete large passenger antigens (115,117,118,127).

Numerous lines of evidence indicate that secreted passenger antigens may be more immunogenic than their cytoplasmic counterparts (51,117,118,153,169) (G. K. Lewis, unpublished observations). For example, a *Salmonella* vector that expressed a chimeric gp120–LTB fusion in the periplasm induced significant levels of serum IgG against gp120, whereas an analogous construct that expressed recombinant gp120 in the cytoplasm did not induce a significant gp120-specific IgG response (G. K. Lewis, unpublished observations). Similarly, a single dose of a *Salmonella* vector that expressed recombinant gp120 in the periplasm elicited a fivefold greater level of gp120-specific proliferation, compared to three doses of an analogous cytoplasmic construct (51). The enhanced immunogenicity of secreted passenger antigens may not be restricted to humoral and $CD4^+$ T-cell responses, since periplasmic, but not cytoplasmic, expression influenza virus nucleoprotein by a *Salmonella* vector induced a nucleoprotein-specific CTL response in mice. In agreement, Hess and coworkers, (117,118) provided evidence that *Salmonella* constructs that externally secreted *L. monocytogenes* antigens elicited stronger CTL responses and protection against *L. monocytogenes* in mice, than *Salmonella* constructs bearing these analogous *L. monocytogenes* antigens in the cytosol.

6.2.4 Evaluation of Attenuated Typhi Strains in Volunteers

A substantive safety issue associated with the use of live vectors is their potential for spread to nontarget hosts. While several *S. enterica* variants display promiscuous host specificities, some are highly host restricted (27,170,171). One such host restricted *S. enterica* var., Typhi, is human-specific and, with the exception of chimpanzees, does not colonize domestic or wild animals (170,171). The use of an attenuated Typhi strain as the "corner stone" of a live oral vaccine vector, therefore, reduces the risk of spread beyond the initial vaccinee via an intermediate host thereby providing a safety advantage over other live oral bacterial vectors (172–178). However, while the aforementioned murine studies clearly showed that *Salmonella* vectors were capable of eliciting immune responses against passenger antigens, the characterization of this vector system in humans was hindered by the availability of Typhi strains that were well tolerated and immunogenic in volunteers. Nonetheless, a number of mutations that attenuate *Salmonella* were identified using the mouse typhoid model (Table 6.2). As discussed below, some of these mutations also attenuate Typhi in humans.

During the early phases of *Salmonella* vector development, the

TABLE 6.2 Attenuated Strains of *Salmonella*

Gene	Phenotype	Virulence	Immunogenicity	References
LPS mutants				
galE	Rough LPS	Attenuated in mice but retain some virulence in humans	Humoral and cellular responses Protection against *Salmonella* in mice	(179,180)
pmi	Rough LPS	Partially attenuated in mice	Protection against *Salmonella* in mice	(181)
rfc	Rought LPS	Attenuated in mice	Protection against *Salmonella* in mice	(181)
htrB	Defective lipid A	Attenuated in mice	Protection against *Salmonella* in mice	
Auxotrophic mutants				
aro	Auxotrophic for aromatic amino acids, PABA, and DHB	Attenuated in mice, sheep, cattle, and humans	Humoral and cellular responses Protection against *Salmonella* in mice	(4–8)
pur	Auxotrophic for purines	Attenuated in mice	Poor immunogenicity	(65, 185–187)
thyA	Auxotrophic for thymidine (unstable phenotype)	Mutants with high thymidine requirement are partially attenuated in mice	ND	(188)
pab	Auxotrophic for PABA	Attenuated in mice	ND	(189)
gua	Auxotrophic for	Partially attenuated in mice	ND	(185)

Defective regulatory genes				
cya + *crp*	Defective regulation in response to catabolites	Completely attenuated in mice but retain some virulence in humans	Strong humoral and cellular responses. Protection against *Salmonella* in mice	(190–192)
phoPQ or *PhoP*[c]	Diminished survival in macrophages	Attenuated in mice and humans	Humoral and cellular responses Protection against *Salmonella* in mice	(28,193)
ompR	Defective osmoregulation Defective Vi expression in *typhi*	Completely attenuated in mice	Humoral and cellular responses Protection against *Salmonella* in mice	(194,195)
htrA	Defective macrophage survival	Attenuated in mice	Humoral and cellular responses Protection against *Salmonella* in mice	(156, 196,197)
recA	Recombination deficient	Partially attenuated in mice	ND	
rpoS	Defective sigma factor S (σ^s or σ^{38})	Partially attenuated in mice	Protection against *Salmonella* in mice when combined with an *aroA* mutation	(198,199)
Defective virulence determinant				
pag	Defective survival in macrophages	Partial attenuation	ND	(193)
cdt	Defective colonization of deep tissue	Partial attenuation	Protection against *Salmonella* in mice when combined with *crp cya* mutations	(45,190, 200)
inv, sip	Defective invasion	Partial attenuation	ND	(29,201,202)

only available live oral Typhi vaccine strain that was well tolerated in humans was strain Ty21a. A series of controlled small-scale and large-scale trials conducted with Ty21a during the 1970s and early 1980s showed that it was well tolerated when given as freshly harvested or lyophilized preparations (14–17, 203–205). This strain also afforded significant levels of protection against typhoid in double-blind field trials conducted in Alexandria, Egypt (203), and Santiago, Chile (14,17,205). However, although Ty21a has proved effective as a typhoid vaccine, this strain displayed deficiencies that make it less attractive as a vector. First, Ty21a has only modest immunogenicity and three to four doses of 10^9 Ty21a colon-forming units (CFU) are required to elicit significant serum IgG against Typhi O-antigen in little more than one-half of recipients (14,16,17,204,205). Furthermore, the basis for the attenuation and safety of Ty21a remain undefined, since Ty21a was made by nonspecific chemical and ultraviolet (UV) mutagenesis (206). The most notable of these, the loss of galactose-4-epimerase activity, was originally thought to be central to the safety and attenuation of Ty21a in humans (179,206,207). However, we showed that a genetically defined *galE* mutant of Typhi retained virulence in volunteers (208). Similarly, restoration of Vi expression in Ty21a not increase virulence or increase the immunogenicity of this organism in volunteers (209).

These shortfalls and discrepancies, therefore, renewed interest in developing genetically defined attenuated Typhi strains that mimicked the safety of Ty21a but that were significantly more immunogenic. By screening auxotrophic Typhi strains for attenuation in mice, Bacon and coworkers (210) found that a *p*-aminobenzoic acid (PABA)-dependent strain of Typhi was attenuated when given in large doses by the intraperitoneal route to mice. This work did not receive much attention, however, until Hoiseth and Stocker (182) showed that an *aroA* mutant of Typhimurium, which was dependent on aromatic amino acids, PABA, and 2,3-dihydroxybenzoate (DHB) for growth was 10^6-fold less virulent in mice (DHB restores the ability to synthesize the iron chelator enterochelin). In further studies, *Salmonella aro* mutants were demonstrably attenuated in bovine and ovine models of salmonellosis (183,184,211–215). Moreover, these strains were highly immunogenic, so that oral and parenteral vaccination of mice, cattle, and sheep with *Salmonella aro* mutants engendered protection against virulent *Salmonella* (183,212,213,215).

Building on their initial observations, Edwards and Stocker (216) carefully constructed a nonreverting aromatic-dependent mutant (*aroA*) of Typhi strain CDC 10–80. At that time, attenuated Typhi oral vaccine candidates for use in humans were not considered safe unless they possessed at least two well-separated and well-defined mutations that independently cause attenuation, thereby virtually eliminating the chance of in vivo reversion (216). In this light, a nonreverting *purA* deletion mutation (causing adenine and/or adenosine dependence) was introduced into their aromatic-dependent derivative for added safety (216). In clinical trials, two such Typhi *aroA purA* strains, 541Ty and 543Ty (a Vi-negative derivative of 541Ty), were remarkably well tolerated by volunteers and elicited cell-mediated immunity in nearly all volunteers (217,218). Unfortunately, Typhi *aroA purA* strains induced only meager humoral responses in a small percentage of volunteers even when two 10^9-organism doses were given (218).

The desirability of well-defined double mutants taken together with the poor immunogenicity of *aro*, *pur* mutants of Typhi in volunteers, suggested that Typhi mutants with only a single auxotrophic requirement should be evaluated as live oral typhoid vaccines. The fact that the *aro* genes are well separated on the *Salmonella* chromosome and several individual *aro* genes have been shown to be equally attenuating (182,187,219–221), taken together with data showing that the *purA* mutation either alone or in combination with *aroA* results in poorly immunogenic Typhimurium vaccine strains (65,186,187,217,218), suggested that evaluation of Typhi *aro* mutants was the direction of choice.

To investigate this avenue, we constructed two double *aro* mutants of Typhi: the first, CVD 906, was derived from wild-type Typhi strain ISP 1820, and the second, CVD 908, was derived from wild-type Typhi strain Ty2 (219). Strains CVD906 and CVD908 differed from all preceding *aro* mutants of Typhi as no antibiotic-resistance genes, plasmid sequences or Typhimurium DNA sequences were introduced during the construction of these strains (219). This precision was the result of the recombinant DNA techniques used to introduce the *aro* mutations into ISP 1820 and Ty2. In each case, the deletion mutations were introduced into the *aroC* and *aroD* genes by allelic exchange, resulting in genetically defined nonreverting *aro* mutations (219). Analysis of the growth requirements of CVD 908 and CVD 906 showed that these mutants were incapable of replicating in defined medium in the absence of PABA and DHB and replicated only for a few generations in pooled human serum (219,222).

The clinical acceptability of CVD 906 was evaluated in a phase 1 clinical trial in which volunteers ingested doses ranging from 5 ×

10^3 to 5×10^7 CVD 906 CFU, preceded by bicarbonate (222). Of 11 volunteers who ingested a single dose of 5×10^3 CVD 906 bacilli, 27% developed significant serum responses to Typhi lipopolysaccharide (LPS) (222). Volunteers who received the 5×10^7 dose CVD 906 developed remarkable systemic and mucosal immune responses (222); 89% of volunteers developed marked serum antibody levels to Typhi antigens and high numbers of antigen-specific gut-derived antibody secreting cells (222). Four (44%) volunteers developed asymptomatic vaccinemia at 4–10 days at this dose and all volunteers excreted CVD 906 on at least one occasion. However, two volunteers developed febrile adverse reactions, one on the day of vaccination and the other on day 4 (222). We concluded that although strain CVD 906 was attenuated and highly immunogenic, the occasional febrile reactions at high doses indicated that further attenuation of this strain was necessary.

By contrast, CVD 908 did not produce febrile responses or other significant adverse reactions in Phase 1 adult volunteer studies when given oral doses of 5×10^4 to 5×10^7 organisms with sodium bicarbonate (192,223). This study showed that a single 5×10^7 CFU oral dose of CVD 908 induced IgG seroconversion to Typhi LPS in 83% of vaccinees and high levels of Typhi-specific IgA-secreting gut-derived lymphocytes in 100% of vaccinees, without causing untoward clinical symptoms (192,223). Oral immunization of volunteers with CVD 908 also elicited the development of increased T-cell proliferative responses in peripheral blood mononuclear cells (PBMCs) taken up to four weeks after vaccination (224). These phase 1 studies with strain CVD 908, therefore, provided an important breakthrough, demonstrating that it was possible to attenuate Typhi without significantly impairing immunogenicity.

Further derivatives of Typhi strains CVD 906 and CVD 908 were developed that harbor a deletion in *htrA* (156,225). The *htrA* mutation was shown to impair the capacity of Typhimurium to survive in host tissues (156,196). In a phase 1 volunteer study, doses ranging from 5×10^7 to 5×10^9 CFU of both CVD 906-*htrA* and CVD 908-*htrA* were well tolerated and only caused diarrhea in 3 of 36 volunteers and fever in one volunteer at the upper end of the dose response curve (225). An important finding from this study, was that the vaccine strains were not detected in blood cultures, suggesting that these strains may possess a greater margin of safety than that of the parent strains CVD 906 and CVD 906 (225).

Additional candidate live oral Typhi vaccine strains have been described that have been evaluated in volunteers (Table 6.3). One such

TABLE 6.3 Characteristics of Candidate Live Oral Typhi Vaccines in Volunteers

Strain	Parent	Mutation(s)	Phase 1 Safety	Responses	Ref.
CVD 906	ISP 1820	Δ*aroC*, Δ*aroD*	Febrile reactions	Good	(222)
CVD 908	Ty2	Δ*aroC*, Δ*aroD*	Well tolerated	Good	(192,223)
CVD 906-*htrA*	Ty2	Δ*aroC*, Δ*aroD*, Δ*htrA*	Well tolerated	Good	(225)
CVD 908-*htrA*					
χ3927	Ty2	Δ*cya*, Δ*crp*	Febrile reactions	Good	(192)
χ4073	Ty2	Δ*cya*, Δ*crp*, Δ*cdt*	Well tolerated	Modest	(45)
Ty800	Ty2	Δ*phoP*/*Q*	Well tolerated	Modest	(226)

strain, strain Ty800, displayed safety characteristics similar to those of CVD 908-*htrA* (226). Ty800 was constructed by introducing a deletion into the *phoPQ* virulence regulatory genes of Typhi strain Ty2 (226). In a phase 1 volunteer trial, small groups of volunteers were vaccinated orally with 10^7, 10^8, 10^9, or 10^{10} CFU of strain Ty800. The vaccine was well tolerated and only volunteers who received the 10^{10}-CFU dose displayed mild self-limiting adverse effects (226). Of note, Ty800 was not detected in blood cultures collected sequentially after vaccination (226).

Although freshly harvested formulations of strains CVD 908, CVD 906-*htrA*, CVD 908-*htrA*, and Ty800 were well tolerated and immunogenic in phase 1 volunteer studies, each of these strains displays potential shortfalls. With respect to CVD908, some formulations of this strain caused febrile reactions (C. O. Tacket, M. Stein, G. Losonsky, S. Cryz, D. M. Hore and M. M. Levine, unpublished observations). Also, the basis for the safety of this strain is not fully understood, as introduction of identical *aroC* and *aroD* mutations into Typhi strain ISP 1820 did not result in complete attenuation (222). This finding suggests that as yet undefined mutations outside *aro* may contribute to the attenuation of CVD 908. The main difference between CVD 906 and CVD 908 is the nature of the parent Typhi isolates from which these strains were developed (219). CVD 906 was derived from Typhi strains ISP 1820, which underwent minimal laboratory passage before the construction of CVD 906. CVD 908, on the other hand, was derived from Typhi strain Ty2, which in turn is derived from a 1913 typhoid outbreak in Russia and represents a laboratory adapted Typhi strain (219). Therefore, Ty2 may have acquired one or more attenuating mutations during the many years of laboratory culture and storage that this strain underwent before being used to construct CVD 908.

By contrast, strains CVD 906-*htrA*, CVD 908-*htrA*, and Ty800 display improved safety characteristics in volunteers over CVD 908 (225,226). A major difference in the behavior of these strains in volunteers compared to CVD 908 is that they were not detected in blood cultures after vaccination (225,226). However, a single dose of 10^9 Ty800 bacilli only induced elevated serum antibody responses against Typhi LPS in 25% of volunteers (226). Similarly, CVD 906-*htrA*, CVD 908-*htrA*, induced significantly lower levels of serum IgG against LPS than were displayed by parent strain CVD 908 and was only modestly immunogenic for T-cell responses (225). Thus, the increased margin of safety exhibited by CVD 908-*htrA* and Ty800 may have decreased the immunogenicity of these strains. Further volunteer studies will resolve this question. In the interim, there is a need to continue the search for attenuated Typhi strains that have the safety attributes of CVD 906-*htrA*, CVD 908-*htrA*, and Ty800 but that are significantly more immunogenic.

6.2.5 Evaluation of Prototype *Salmonella* Vectors in Volunteers

The first prototype *Salmonella* vector to be evaluated in volunteers were derivatives of Ty21a expressing *S. sonnei* O antigen (36,82,227). Volunteers who received three to four oral doses containing 10^9 CFU of this construct developed modest levels of protection against *S. sonnei* (82). This vaccine, unfortunately, was not investigated further when manufactured preparations were found to display substantial lot-to-lot variation (82). Further disappointment was experienced with a Ty21a-*Vibria cholerae* O antigen hybrid, which induced modest rises in vibriocidal antibody in only 36% of the vaccinees and no substantive protection against *V. cholerae* (85). A reason for the poor immunogenicity of these early constructs may have been the modest immunogenicity of Ty21a. This strain only induces modest increases in serum IgG against homologous *S. typhi* O antigen in 60–70% of vaccinees after four oral 10^9 CFU doses (14,204,205,228). However, the immunogenicity of a new generation Typhi vector (Table 6.3) expressing either the *Shigella* or *V. cholerae* O antigens has not as yet been explored.

A phase 1 volunteer study, however, was conducted to evaluate the immunogenicity of a derivative of CVD 908 that expressed the circumsporozoite (CSP) of *P. falciparum*. Although this construct only induced modest immune responses against CSP in volunteers (126), it is important to note that this prototype recombinant strain, CVD 908-CSP, expressed extremely low levels of CSP (<0.01% of the total protein) in the cytoplasm of the vector. Despite this low-level cytoplasmic expression and the notoriously poor immunogenicity of CSP in humans, oral immunization with CVD 908-CSP induced detectable responses in 3 of 10 individuals and one of these responders displayed a CSP-specific $CD8^+$ CTL activity (126). In a similar manner, Nardelli-Haeflinger et al. (44) found that a *Salmonella* recombinant that expressed hepatitis B surface antigen in the cytoplasm of the vector elicited modest humoral responses against the passenger antigen in a small percentage of volunteers. Since these early constructs were developed, many advances have been made in *Salmonella* vector technology (discussed above). It remains a high priority to investigate whether these improved passenger antigen expression systems will increase the immunogenicity of Typhi-delivered passenger antigens in volunteers.

6.3 FUTURE DIRECTIONS

6.3.1 *Salmonella* Vaccine Vectors Targeted Against Specific Pathogens

While the bulk of evidence indicates that *Salmonella* vectors are proficient at eliciting Th1-driven cell-mediated immunity, recent evidence from our group suggests that it may be possible to develop *Salmonella* vectors that induce T-helper type 2 (Th2) responses ((52); D. W. Pascual and D. M. Hone, unpublished data). Thus, a *Salmonella* vaccine vector expressing CFA/I induced predominantly IL-4- and IL-5-secreting Th2 cells in the Pever's patches and spleen shortly after immunization. Furthermore, mice vaccinated with this *Salmonella*–CFA/I vector construct developed a serum IgG response against CFA/I composed predominantly of IgG1 and low levels of IgG2a and potent CFA/I-specific S-IgA responses ((52); D. W. Pascual and D. M. Hone, unpublished data). It is our hope that by delineating the mechanism to this phenomenon future *Salmonella* vectors might be developed that preferentially tilt the host response toward the development of S-IgA (Th2). Circumstances under which it may be advantageous to develop a *Salmonella* vaccine vector that induce a Th2-driven S-IgA response against a passenger antigen include *Salmonella* recombinants expressing *V. cholerae* or *Shigella* O antigens, or the colonization factor antigens of enterotoxigenic *E. coli*.

Alternatively, *Salmonella* vaccine vectors that preferentially elicit MHC class I-restricted $CD8^+$ CTLs may be preferred. This is likely to be the case for the development of *Salmonella*–malaria (122) and *Salmonella*–HIV-1 vectors (51,52,60). Moreover, although *Salmonella* vectors expressing *Plasmodium* (122) and SIV (60) antigens elicited MHC class I-restricted $CD8^+$ CTLs in mice, this vector has not reproducibly induced MHC class I restricted T-cell responses (38,53,54). Since *Salmonella* remains in the endosomal compartment of infected cells, this vector may not efficiently deliver antigen to the MHC class I antigen presentation pathway. This is in contrast to *L. monocytogenes* vectors, which naturally escape the endosome and replicate in the cytoplasm of infected host cells and are effective at generating $CD8^+$ T-cell responses against passenger antigens in mice (172–177). However, the promiscuous host specificity of *L. monocytogenes* and the complexity of establishing the safety of this vector in high-risk groups, comprising pregnant females, neonates, and immunosuppressed individuals (229–235), may significantly hinder the egress of this vector beyond the laboratory.

Beyond the use of improved expression systems described above, another solution to this dilemma may be to construct a Typhi vector that accesses the cytoplasm of infected cells and thereby mimics the intracellular tropism of *Listeria* vectors. The advantage of this approach is that such live oral Typhi vectors with altered intracellular tropism may possess the immunogenic properties of *Listeria*, while retaining the safety properties and host restriction of Typhi. Supporting evidence for this contention was obtained by showing that a genetically modified *Salmonella* vector, which expressed listeriolysin O (LLO) of *L. monocytogenes* and escaped the endosomal compartment elicited superior $CD8^+$ T-cell-mediated protection against *L. monocytogenes* than an analogous construct that remained phagosome-bound (30,114,117). More importantly, this strain did not display enhanced virulence in H-2 I-Aβ-deficient mice, which lack MHC class II molecules and are devoid of mature $CD4^+$ TCR-$\alpha\beta$ cells (30). This finding provides strong support for this direction; however, volunteer studies are needed to extend these findings to humans.

6.3.2 Typhi Vectors for Use in Typhoid-Endemic Regions

A practical consideration for large-scale vaccination programs is the possibility that pre existing immunity to the vector may prevent or hinder subsequent vaccine vector "take" and diminish the immune response to the passenger antigen. While Bao and Clements (236) showed that pre-exposure of mice with a Typhimurium strain did not diminish the subsequent immunogenicity of a Typhimurium-delivered passenger antigen (236), others have reported results to the contrary (78). Interestingly, the poor responsiveness in vector-primed mice was virtually overcome by changing the serotype of the strain subsequently used to deliver the passenger antigen (78). This latter observation has repercussions, given the fact that exposure to Typhi is common in many regions of the world.

To bypass this potential obstacle, we developed an allelic exchange procedure that alters the O-antigen of Typhi, by introducing *rfb* genes from other *S. enterica* serovariants (237). To realize this O-antigen conversion a 7.5-kb *Kpn*I-generated fragment from within the *rfb* cluster of Typhimurium that expressed the O4 antigen was inserted into suicide vector pKTN701 (237). Using an allelic exchange technique, the *rfb* genes of Typhimurium were substituted into the *rfb* clusters of Typhi (237). Immunoblot analysis of LPS purified from the resultant strains demonstrated that the recombinant strain expressed smooth 04,12 LPS instead of smooth O9,12 LPS (Fig. 6.2). Furthermore, DNA hybridization analysis of chromosomal DNA from such recombinants confirmed that a precise recombination event within sequences flanking *rfbSE* of Typhi (that encodes the enzymes necessary for O9 synthesis) replaced *rfbSE* with *rfbJ* of Typhimurium (that encodes the enzyme necessary for O4 synthesis). Since the inhibition of *Salmonella* vector pre-exposed mice was shown to be serotype specific (78), these and other variants may have value as vectors in regions in which typhoid remains endemic or in individuals who have been vaccinated with a typhoid vaccine.

6.3.3 *Salmonella* and *Shigella* DNA Vaccine Vectors: A New Paradigm

A common feature of the conventional live oral *Salmonella* vaccine vectors discussed above is that they all carry the passenger antigens

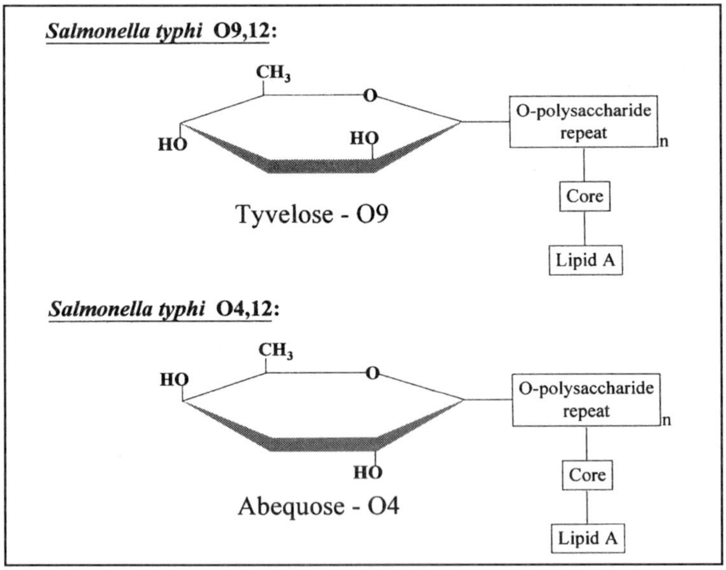

Figure 6.2 Expression of an altered O antigen by Typhi.

on prokaryotic expression cassettes (Table 6.1). However, some passenger antigens are likely to form non-native antigenic conformations when expressed in heterologous bacterial system. This was clearly demonstrated by the analysis of cytoplasmically expressed rgp120 in *Salmonella* (50). Normally the V3 loop is surface-exposed in native Chinese hamster ovary (CHO)-cell-produced HIV-1 envelope but upon heat denaturation of this glycoprotein the V3 loop becomes embedded within gp120. By contrast, the V3 loop is concealed within native *Salmonella*-expressed rgp120 indicating that this protein is incorrectly folded compared with native HIV-1 envelope gp120 (50). Since passenger antigen folding greatly influences the specificity of humoral immunity to discontiguous epitopes, vectors that express misfolded passenger antigens, such as viral glycoprotein envelope proteins, would induce humoral immunity against contiguous epitopes and irrelevant discontiguous epitopes. Therefore, although these vectors may prove to be effective at eliciting humoral responses against bacterial antigens and cell-mediated responses against a broad array of pathogens, their inability to express conformational epitopes of surface glycoproteins limits their value (49,50).

As a remedy to this limitation, we proposed that invasive bacterial vectors may be capable of delivering nucleic acid vaccines and eliciting humoral and cellular responses against the antigens that are encoded by the nucleic acid vaccine (238). In support of this hypothesis, we presented data showing that an invasive attenuated *Shigella* strain CVD 1203, was capable of delivering a eukaryotic expression cassette encoding β-galactosidase to HeLa cells (238). Conversion of HeLa cells to a β-galactosidase-positive phenotype in this system was dependent on the presence of an SV40 promoter in the reporter gene expression cassette (238). We also obtained similar results in mice inoculated intratracheally with CVD 1203 bearing the β-galactosidase reporter gene with or without the SV40 promoter (D. M. Hone, G. K. Lewis and R. J. Powell, unpublished data). Subsequent reports from other groups supported our findings (Table 6.4).

To investigate the feasibility of using bacterial vectors to deliver nucleic acid vaccines we (238) and others (239,240) initially chose to use *Shigella* as the vector. The rationale for this decision was prompted by the capacity of *Shigella* to efficiently escape the endosome and access the cytoplasm of host cells (Fig. 6.3). *Salmonella*, as discussed above, is thought to remain endosome bound in host cells (148–151) and may not efficiently deliver nucleic acid vac-

TABLE 6.4 Experimental Results With Bacterial Nucleic Acid Vaccine Vectors

Organism	Foreign Gene	Promoter	Results	Environment	References
Shigella flexneri	*IacZ*	SV40	P_{SV40}-dependent LacZ expression	*in vitro* (HeLa cells)	(52, 238)
Shigella flexneri	*IacZ*	CMV	Direct staining and LacZ activity assays of cultured cells	*in vitro* (BHK cells)	(239, 240)
			Detection of LacZ expression in guinea pig tissue	*in vivo* (guinea pigs)	
Shigella flexneri	*lacZ*	SV40 or CMV	Staining for LacZ expression	*in vitro* (HeLa, CHO, COS cells)	(241)
Escherichia coli	*lacZ*	SV40 or CMV	Staining for LacZ expression	*in vitro* (HeLa, CHO, COS cells)	
Typhimurium	*lacZ*	CMV	Induced CTLs against LacZ	*in vivo* (mice)	(242)
	actA (from *Listeria monocytogenes*)	CMV	Induced CTLs against Act A	*in vivo* (mice)	
Typhimurium	*llo* (from *Listeria monocytogenes*)	CMV	Induced CTL's against L10 and affords protection against *Listeria*	*in vivo* (mice)	

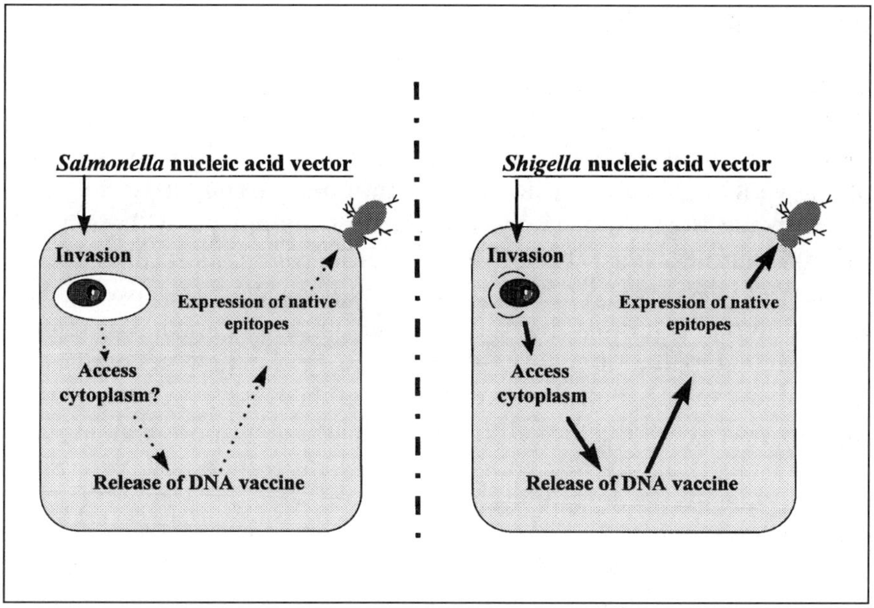

Figure 6.3 Bacterial vector-mediated delivery of nucleic acid vaccines.

cines to host cells (Fig. 6.3). Nonetheless, a recent report by Darji et al. (242) showed that *Salmonella* vectors were capable of delivering eukaryotic expression cassettes to mammalian cells both in vitro and in vivo (242). These investigators demonstrated that oral immunization of mice with a Typhimurium *aro* mutant bearing the *E. coli lacZ* gene under the control of the cytomegalovirus (CMV) promoter elicited β-galactosidase-specific antibodies, T-cell proliferation and CTL activity (242). They also reported that oral vaccination of mice with a *Salmonella* vector carrying the *L. monocytogenes llo* gene under the control of the CMV promoter induced similar humoral and cellular responses against LLO and afforded protection against *L. monocytogenes* (242). While the pathway by which the *Salmonella* vector delivered the nucleic acid vaccines to the host was not resolved and the efficiency of *Salmonella* compared with *Shigella* was not examined, these pilot studies demonstrated that *Salmonella* vectors possess the capacity to deliver nucleic acid vaccines. As such, these findings have opened a new horizon for *Salmonella* vectors by broadening the scope of the delivery properties of this vector system.

6.4 CONCLUSIONS

With this strong foundation laid, the future for *Salmonella* vectors looks very promising. The potential of *Salmonella* vectors to elicit protection against bacterial, viral, protozoan, and metazoan pathogens, along with their capacity to induce antitumor immunity, may have a significant impact on mucosal vaccine development. Although significant hurdles must be traversed before the widespread use of *Salmonella* vectors is realized, the remaining problems are dwarfed by the numerous solutions that have already been obtained. We remain hopeful that before the turn of the century the first generation of *Salmonella* vectors will be ready for phase three trials. Another exciting prospect is the likelihood that the construction of *Salmonella* vectors, which is rapidly becoming an accessible technology, will occur more frequently in developing countries.

ACKNOWLEDGMENTS

This work was supported by National Institutes of Health grants AI41914 (to D.M.H.), AI42603 (to D.M.H.), and AI40288 (to D.W.P.), U.S. Department of Agriculture grant 9602195 (to D.W.P.), and Montana Agriculture Station research award J-5196 (to D.W.P.).

6.5 REFERENCES

1. Brandtzaeg, P. 1968. Hidden antigenic determinant in secretory immunoglobulin A. *Nature 220*:292.
2. Mach, J. P., J. J. Pahud, and H. Isliker. 1969. IgA with "secretory piece" in bovine colostrum and saliva. *Nature 223*:952.
3. Halpern, M. S., and M. E. Koshland. 1970. Noval subunit in secretory IgA. *Nature 228*:1276.
4. Brandtzaeg, P. 1971. Human secretory immunoglobulins. VI. Association of free secretory piece with serum IgA in vitro. *Immunology 21*:323.
5. Brandtzaeg, P. 1971. Human secretory immunoglobulins. 3. Immunochemical and physicochemical studies of secretory IgA and free secretory piece. *Acta Pathol. Microbiol. Scand. Sect. B Microbiol. Immunol. 79*:165.

6. Shuster, J. 1971. Pepsin hydrolysis of IgA—delineation of two populations of molecules. *Immunochemistry 8*:405.
7. Brandtzaeg, P. 1973. Two types of IgA immunocytes in man. *Nature New Biol. 243*:142.
8. Lindh, E. 1975. Increased resistance of immunoglobulin A dimers to proteolytic degradation after binding of secretory component. *J. Immunol. 114*:284.
9. Brandtzaeg, P., and H. Prydz. 1984. Direct evidence for an integrated function of J chain and secretory component in epithelial transport of immunoglobulins. *Nature 311*:71.
10. Sabin, A. B. 1984. Strategies for elimination of poliomyelitis in different parts of the world with use of oral poliovirus vaccine. *Rev. Infect. Dis. 6*:S391.
11. Sabin, A. B. 1985. Oral poliovirus vaccine: history of its development and use and current challenge to eliminate poliomyelitis from the world. *J. Infect. Dis. 151*:420.
12. Nagaraj, K., and B. V. Babu. 1997. Field trial of oral cholera vaccine in Vietnam [letter; comment]. *Lancet 349*:1253.
13. van Loon, F. P., J. D. Clemens, J. Chakraborty, M. R. Rao, B. A. Kay, D. A. Sack, M. Yunus, M. Ali, A. M. Svennerholm, and J. Holmgren. 1996. Field trial of inactivated oral cholera vaccines in Bangladesh: results from 5 years of follow-up. *Vaccine 14*:162.
14. Black, R. E., M. M. Levine, C. Ferreccio, M. L. Clements, C. Lanata, J. Rooney, and R. Germanier. 1990. Efficacy of one or two doses of Ty21a *Salmonella typhi* vaccine in enteric-coated capsules in a controlled field trial. *Chilean Typhoid Comm. Vaccine 8*:81.
15. Cryz, S. J., Jr., N. Vanprapar, U. Thisyakorn, T. Olanratmanee, G. Losonsky, M. M. Levine, and S. Chearskul. 1993. Safety and immunogenicity of *Salmonella typhi* Ty21a vaccine in young Thai children. *Infect. Immun. 61*:1149.
16. Murphy, J. R., L. Grez, L. Schlesinger, C. Ferreccio, S. Baqar, C. Munoz, S. S. Wasserman, G. Losonsky, J. G. Olson, and M. M. Levine. 1991. Immunogenicity of *Salmonella typhi* Ty21a vaccine for young children. *Infect. Immun. 59*:4291.
17. Levine, M. M., C. Ferreccio, S. Cryz, and E. Ortiz. 1990. Comparison of enteric-coated capsules and liquid formulation of Ty21a typhoid vaccine in randomised controlled field trial. *Lancet 336*:891.
18. Gurwith, M. J., G. S. Horwith, C. A. Impellizzeri, A. R. Davis, M. D. Lubeck, and P. P. Hung. 1989. Current use and future directions of adenovirus vaccine. *Semin. Respir. Infect. 4*:299.
19. Ogra, P. L., M. Fishaut, and M. R. Gallagher. 1980. Viral vaccination via the mucosal routes. *Rev. Infect. Dis. 2*:352.

20. Levine, M. M., D. Hone, C. Tacket, C. Ferreccio, and S. Cryz. 1990. Clinical and field trials with attenuated *Salmonella typhi* as live oral vaccines and as "carrier" vaccines. *Res. Microbiol. 141*:807.
21. Le Minor, L., and M. Y. Popoff. 1987. Designation of *Salmonella enterica* sp. nov., nom. rev., as the type and only species of the genus *Salmonella. Int. J. Syst. Bacteriol. 37*:465.
22. Blanden, R. V., G. B. Mackaness, and F. M. Collins. 1966. Mechanisms of acquired resistance in mouse typhoid. *J. Exp. Med. 124*:585.
23. Collins, F. M., G. B. Mackaness, and R. V. Blanden. 1966. Infection-immunity in experimental salmonellosis. *J. Exp. Med. 124*:601.
24. Mackaness, G. B., R. V. Blanden, and F. M. Collins. 1966. Host-parasite relations in mouse typhoid. *J. Exp. Med. 124*:573.
25. Francis, C. L., T. A. Ryan, B. D. Jones, S. J. Smith, and S. Falkow. 1993. Ruffles induced by *Salmonella* and other stimuli direct macropinocytosis of bacteria. *Nature 364*:639.
26. Jones, B., L. Pascopella, and S. Falkow. 1995. Entry of microbes into the host: using M cells to break the mucosal barrier. *Curr. Opin. Immunol. 7*:474.
27. Pascopella, L., B. Raupach, N. Ghori, D. Monack, S. Falkow, and P. L. Small. 1995. Host restriction phenotypes of *Salmonella typhi* and *Salmonella gallinarum. Infect. Immun. 63*:4329.
28. Galan, J. E., and R. d. Curtiss. 1989. Virulence and vaccine potential of phoP mutants of *Salmonella typhimurium. Microbial Pathog. 6*:433.
29. Galan, J. E., and R. d. Curtiss. 1989. Cloning and molecular characterization of genes whose products allow *Salmonella typhimurium* to penetrate tissue culture cells. *Proc. Natl. Acad. Sci. USA 86*:6383.
30. Hess, J., C. Ladel, D. Miko, and S. H. Kaufmann. 1996. *Salmonella typhimurium aroA*$^-$ infection in gene-targeted immunodeficient mice: major role of CD4$^+$ TCR-alpha beta cells and IFN-γ in bacterial clearance independent of intracellular location. *J. Immunol. 156*:3321.
31. Eisenstein, T. K., L. M. Killar, B. A. Stocker, and B. M. Sultzer. 1984. Cellular immunity induced by avirulent *Salmonella* in LPS-defective C3H/H3] mice. *J. Immunol. 133*:958.
32. Killar, L. M., and T. K. Eisenstein. 1985. Immunity to *Salmonella typhimurium* infection in C3H/H3J and C3H/HeNcrlBr mice: studies with an aromatic-dependent live *S. typhimurium* strain as a vaccine. *Infect. Immun. 47*:605.
33. Lee, J. C., C. W. Gibson, and T. K. Eisenstein. 1985. Macrophage-mediated mitogenic suppression induced in mice of the C3H lineage by a vaccine strain of *Salmonella typhimurium. Cell. Immunol. 91*:75.
34. Killar, L. M., and T. K. Eisenstein. 1986. Delayed-type hypersensitivity and immunity to *Salmonella typhimurium. Infect. Immun. 52*:504.

35. Hohmann, A., G. Schmidt, and D. Rowley. 1979. Intestinal and serum antibody responses in mice after oral immunization with *Salmonella, Escherichia coli*, and *Salmonella, Escherichia coli*, and *Salmonella–Escherichia coli* hybrid strains. *Infect. Immun. 25*:27.

36. Formal, S. B., L. S. Baron, D. J. Kopecko, O. Washington, C. Powell, and C. A. Life. 1981. Construction of a potential bivalent vaccine strain: introduction of *Shigella sonnei* form I antigen genes into the *galE Salmonella typhi* Ty21a typhoid vaccine strain. *Infect. Immun. 34*:746.

37. Tite, J. P., X. M. Gao, C. M. Hughes-Jenkins, M. Lipscombe, O. C. D, G. Dougan, and F. Y. Liew. 1990. Anti-viral immunity induced by recombinant nucleoprotein of influenza A virus. III. Delivery of recombinant nucleoprotein to the immune system using attenuated *Salmonella typhimurium* as a live carrier. *Immunology 70*:540.

38. Brett, S. J., J. Rhodes, F. Y. Liew, and J. P. Tite. 1993. Comparison of antigen presentation of influenza A nucleoprotein expressed in attenuated AroA-negative *Salmonella typhimurium* with that of live virus. *J. Immunol. 150*:2869.

39. Gao, X. M., J. P. Tite, M. Lipscombe, S. Rowland-Jones, D. J. Ferguson, and A. J. McMichael. 1992. Recombinant *Salmonella typhimurium* strains that invade nonphagocytic cells are resistant to recognition by antigen-specific cytotoxic T lymphocytes. *Infect. Immun. 60*:3780.

40. Brett, S. J., X. M. Gao, F. Y. Liew, and J. P. Tite. 1991. Selection of the same major T cell determinants of influenza nucleoprotein after vaccination or exposure to infectious virus. *J. Immunol. 147*:1647.

41. Brett, S. J., L. Dunlop, F. Y. Liew, and J. P. Tite. 1993. Influence of the antigen delivery system on immunoglobulin isotype selection and cytokine production in response to influenza A nucleoprotein. *Immunology 80*:306.

42. Schodel, F., S. M. Kelly, D. L. Peterson, D. R. Milich, and R. Curtiss, III. 1994. Hybrid hepatitis B virus core-pre-S proteins synthesized in avirulent *Salmonella typhimurium* and *Salmonella typhi* for oral vaccination. *Infect. Immun. 62*:1669.

43. Hopkins, S., J. P. Kraehenbuhl, F. Schodel, A. Potts, D. Peterson, P. de Grandi, and D. Nardelli-Haefliger. 1995. A recombinant *Salmonella typhimurium* vaccine induces local immunity by four different routes of immunization. *Infect. Immun. 63*:3279.

44. Nardelli-Haefliger, D., J. P. Kraehenbuhl, R. Curtiss, 3rd, F. Schodel, A. Potts, S. Kelly, and P. De Grandi. 1996. Oral and rectal immunization of adult female volunteers with a recombinant attenuated *Salmonella typhi* vaccine strain. *Infect. Immun. 64*:5219.

45. Tacket, C. O., S. M. Kelly, F. Schodel, G. Losonsky, J. P. Nataro, R.

Edelman, M. M. Levine, and R. Curtiss, III. 1997. Safety and immunogenicity in humans of an attenuated *Salmonella typhi* vaccine vector strain expressing plasmid-encoded hepatitis B antigens stabilized by the Asd-balanced lethal vector system. *Infect. Immun. 65*:3381.

46. O'Callaghan, D., A. Charbit, P. Martineau, C. Leclerc, S. van der Werf, C. Nauciel, and M. Hofnung. 1990. Immunogenicity of foreign peptide epitopes expressed in bacterial envelope proteins. *Res. Microbiol. 141*:963.
47. O'Callaghan, D., P. Martineau, C. Fayolle, C. Leclerc, J. G. Guillet, A. Charbit, and M. Hofnung. 1993. Immune responses to hybrid maltose-binding proteins. *Vaccine 11*:140.
48. Charbit, A., S. M. Newton, P. E. Klebba, J. M. Clement, C. Fayolle, R. Lo-Man, C. Leclerc, and M. Hofnung. 1997. Expression and immune response to foreign epitopes in bacteria. Perspectives for live vaccine development. *Behring Inst. Mitteil. 98*:135.
49. Fouts, T. R., R. G. Tuskan, S. Chada, D. M. Hone, and G. K. Lewis. 1995. Construction and immunogenicity of *Salmonella typhimurium* vaccine vectors that express HIV-1 gp120. *Vaccine 13*:1697.
50. Fouts, T. R., G. K. Lewis, and D. M. Hone. 1995. Construction and characterization of a *Salmonella typhi*-based human immunodeficiency virus type 1 vector vaccine. *Vaccine 13*:561.
51. Wu, S., D. W. Pascual, G. K. Lewis, and D. M. Hone. 1997. Induction of mucosal and systemic responses against human immunodeficiency virus type 1 glycoprotein 120 in mice after oral immunization with a single dose of a *Salmonella*–HIV vector. *AIDS Res. Hum. Retroviruses 13*:1187.
52. Pascual, D. W., R. J. Powell, G. K. Lewis, and D. M. Hone. 1997. Oral bacterial vaccine vectors for the delivery of subunit and nucleic acid vaccines to the organized lymphoid tissue of the intestine. *Behring Inst. Mitteil. 98*:143.
53. Berggren, R. E., A. Wunderlich, E. Ziegler, M. Schleicher, R. C. Duke, D. Looney, and F. C. Fang. 1995. HIV gp120-specific cell-mediated immune responses in mice after oral immunization with recombinant *Salmonella. J. Acquir. Immune Defic. Syndr. Hum. Retrovirol. 10*:489.
54. Franchini, G., M. Robert-Guroff, J. Tartaglia, A. Aggarwal, A. Abimiku, J. Benson, P. Markham, K. Limbach, G. Hurteau, J. Fullen, K. Aldrich, N. Miller, J. Sadoff, E. Paoletti, and R. C. Gallo. 1995. Highly attenuated HIV type 2 recombinant poxviruses, but not HIV-2 recombinant *Salmonella* vaccines, induce long-lasting protection in rhesus macaques. *AIDS Res. Hum. Retroviruses 11*:909.
55. Cattozzo, E. M., B. A. Stocker, A. Radaelli, C. De Giuli Morghen, and M. Tognon. 1997. Expression and immunogenicity of V3 loop epitopes

of HIV-1, isolates SC and WMJ2, inserted in *Salmonella* flagellin. *J. Biotechnol. 56*:191.

56. Charbit, A., P. Martineau, J. Ronco, C. Leclerc, R. Lo-Man, V. Michel, O. C. D., and M. Hofnung. 1993. Expression and immunogenicity of the V3 loop from the envelope of human immunodeficiency virus type 1 in an attenuated *aroA* strain of *Salmonella typhimurium* upon genetic coupling to two *Escherichia coli* carrier proteins. *Vaccine 11*:1221.
57. Newton, S. M., P. E. Klebba, M. Hofnung, and A. Charbit. 1995. Studies of the anaerobically induced promoter P*nirB* and the improved expression of bacterial antigens. *Res. Microbiol. 146*:193.
58. Newton, S. M., T. M. Joys, S. A. Anderson, R. C. Kennedy, M. E. Hovi, and B. A. Stocker. 1995. Expression and immunogenicity of an 18-residue epitope of HIV1 gp41 inserted in the flagellar protein of a *Salmonella* live vaccine. *Res. Microbiol. 146*:203.
59. Cattozzo, E. M., and B. A. Stocker. 1994. Immunogenicity of Nef protein of SIVSMM-PBj14 expressed in a live vaccine strain of *Salmonella* species. *AIDS Res. Hum. Retroviruses 10*:1011.
60. Valentine, P. J., K. Meyer, M. M. Rivera, C. Lipps, D. Pauza, R. T. Maziarz, M. So, and F. Heffron. 1996. Induction of SIV capsid-specific CTL and mucosal sIgA in mice immunized with a recombinant *S. typhimurium aroA* mutant. *Vaccine 14*:138.
61. Smerdou, C., I. M. Anton, J. Plana, R. Curtiss, III, and L. Enjuanes. 1996. A continuous epitope from transmissible gastroenteritis virus S protein fused to *E. coli* heat-labile toxin B subunit expressed by attenuated *Salmonella* induces serum and secretory immunity. *Virus Res. 41*:1.
62. Nardelli-Haefliger, D., R. B. Roden, J. Benyacoub, R. Sahli, J. P. Kraehenbuhl, J. T. Schiller, P. Lachat, A. Potts, and P. De Grandi. 1997. Human papillomavirus type 16 virus-like particles expressed in attenuated *Salmonella typhimurium* elicit mucosal and systemic neutralizing antibodies in mice. *Infect. Immun. 65*:3328.
63. Chabalgoity, J. A., C. M. Khan, A. A. Nash, and C. E. Hormaeche. 1996. A *Salmonella typhimurium htrA* live vaccine expressing multiple copies of a peptide comprising amino acids 8–23 of herpes simplex virus glycoprotein D as a genetic fusion to tetanus toxin fragment C protects mice from herpes simplex virus infection. *Mol. Microbiol. 19*:791.
64. Clements, J. D., and S. El-Morshidy. 1984. Construction of a potential live oral bivalent vaccine for typhoid fever and cholera–*Escherichia coli*-related diarrheas. *Infect. Immun. 46*:564.
65. Sigwart, D. F., B. A. Stocker, and J. D. Clements. 1989. Effect of a

purA mutation on efficacy of *Salmonella* live-vaccine vectors. *Infect. Immun. 57*:1858.

66. Clements, J. D., F. L. Lyon, K. L. Lowe, A. L. Farrand, and S. el-Morshidy. 1986. Oral immunization of mice with attenuated *Salmonella enteritidis* containing a recombinant plasmid which codes for production of the B subunit of heat-labile *Escherichia coli* enterotoxin. *Infect. Immun. 53*:685.
67. Dougan, G., C. E. Hormaeche, and D. J. Maskell. 1987. Live oral *Salmonella* vaccines: potential use of attenuated strains as carriers of heterologous antigens to the immune system. *Parasite Immunol. 9*:151.
68. Maskell, D. J., K. J. Sweeney, O. C. D, C. E. Hormaeche, F. Y. Liew, and G. Dougan. 1987. *Salmonella typhimurium aroA* mutants as carriers of the *Escherichia coli* heat-labile enterotoxin B subunit to the murine secretory and systemic immune systems. *Microb. Pathog. 2*:211.
69. Takahashi, I., H. Kiyono, R. J. Jackson, K. Fujihashi, H. F. Staats, S. Hamada, J. D. Clements, K. L. Bost, and J. R. McGhee. 1996. Epitope maps of the *Escherichia coli* heat-labile toxin B subunit for development of a synthetic oral vaccine. *Infect. Immun. 64*:1290.
70. Cardenas, L., U. Dasgupta, and J. D. Clements. 1994. Influence of strain viability and antigen dose on the use of attenuated mutants of *Salmonella* as vaccine carriers. *Vaccine 12*:833.
71. Cardenas, L., and J. D. Clements. 1992. Oral immunization using live attenuated *Salmonella* spp. as carriers of foreign antigens. *Clin. Microbiol. Rev. 5*:328.
72. Yamamoto, T., Y. Tamura, and T. Yokota. 1985. Enteroadhesion fimbriae and enterotoxin of *Escherichia coli*: genetic transfer to a streptomycin-resistant mutant of the *galE* oral-route live-vaccine *Salmonella typhi* Ty21a. *Infect. Immun. 50*:925.
73. Wu, S., D. W. Pascual, J. L. VanCott, J. R. McGhee, D. R. Maneval, Jr., M. M. Levine, and D. M. Hone. 1995. Immune responses to novel *Escherichia coli* and *Salmonella typhimurium* vectors that express colonization factor antigen I (CFA/I) of enterotoxigenic *E. coli* in the absence of the CFA/I positive regulator *cfaR*. *Infect. Immun. 63*:4933.
74. Giron, J. A., J. G. Xu, C. R. Gonzalez, D. Hone, J. B. Kaper, and M. M. Levine. 1995. Simultaneous expression of CFA/I and CS3 colonization factor antigens of enterotoxigenic *Escherichia coli* by delta aroC, delta aroD *Salmonella typhi* vaccine strain CVD 908. *Vaccine 13*:939.
75. Hone, D., S. Attridge, L. van den Bosch, and J. Hackett. 1988. A chromosomal integration system for stabilization of heterologous genes in *Salmonella*-based vaccine strains. *Microb. Pathog. 5*:407.
76. Morona, R., J. K. Morona, A. Considine, J. A. Hackett, L. van den

Bosch, L. Beyer, and S. R. Attridge. 1994. Construction of K88- and K99-expressing clones of *Salmonella typhimurium* G30: immunogenicity following oral administration to pigs. *Vaccine 12*:513.

77. Bertram, E. M., S. R. Attridge, and I. Kotlarski. 1994. Immunogenicity of the *Escherichia coli* fimbrial antigen K99 when expressed by *Salmonella enteritidis* 11RX. *Vaccine 12*:1372.
78. Attridge, S. R., R. Davies, and J. T. LaBrooy. 1997. Oral delivery of foreign antigens by attenuated *Salmonella*: consequences of prior exposure to the vector strain. *Vaccine 15*:155.
79. Seid, R. C., Jr., D. J. Kopecko, J. C. Sadoff, H. Schneider, L. S. Baron, and S. B. Formal. 1984. Unusual lipopolysaccharide antigens of a *Salmonella typhi* oral vaccine strain expressing the Shigella sonnei form I antigen. *J. Biol. Chem. 259*:9028.
80. Baron, L. S., D. J. Kopecko, S. B. Formal, R. Seid, P. Guerry, and C. Powell. 1987. Introduction of *Shigella flexneri* 2a type and group antigen genes into oral typhoid vaccine strain *Salmonella typhi* Ty21a. *Infect. Immun. 55*:2797.
81. Van de Verg, L., D. A. Herrington, J. R. Murphy, S. S. Wasserman, S. B. Formal, and M. M. Levine. 1990. Specific immunoglobulin A-secreting cells in peripheral blood of humans following oral immunization with a bivalent *Salmonella typhi–Shigella sonnei* vaccine or infection by pathogenic *S. sonnei. Infect. Immun. 58*:2002.
82. Black, R. E., M. M. Levine, M. L. Clements, G. Losonsky, D. Herrington, S. Berman, and S. B. Formal. 1987. Prevention of shigellosis by a *Salmonella typhi–Shigella sonnei* bivalent vaccine. *J. Infect. Dis. 155*:1260.
83. Tramont, E. C., R. Chung, S. Berman, D. Keren, C. Kapfer, and S. B. Formal. 1984. Safety and antigenicity of typhoid–*Shigella* sonnei vaccine (strain 5076-1C). *J. Infect. Dis. 149*:133.
84. Morona, R., J. Yeadon, A. Considine, J. K. Morona, and P. A. Manning. 1991. Construction of plasmid vectors with a non-antibiotic selection system based on the *Escherichia coli* thyA^+ gene: application to cholera vaccine development. *Gene 107*:139.
85. Tacket, C. O., B. Forrest, R. Morona, S. R. Attridge, J. LaBrooy, B. D. Tall, M. Reymann, D. Rowley, and M. M. Levine. 1990. Safety, immunogenicity, and efficacy against cholera challenge in humans of a typhoid–cholera hybrid vaccine derived from *Salmonella typhi* Ty21a. *Infect. Immun. 58*:1620.
86. Attridge, S. R., C. Dearlove, L. Beyer, L. van den Bosch, A. Howles, J. Hackett, R. Morona, J. LaBrooy, and D. Rowley. 1991. Characterization and immunogenicity of EX880, a *Salmonella typhi* Ty21a-

based clone which produces *Vibrio cholerae* O antigen. *Infect. Immun. 59*:2279.

87. Attridge, S. 1991. Oral immunization with *Salmonella typhi* Ty21a-based clones expressing *Vibrio cholerae* O-antigen: serum bactericidal antibody responses in man in relation to pre-immunization antibody levels. *Vaccine 9*:877.

88. Attridge, S. R., D. Daniels, J. K. Morona, and R. Morona. 1990. Surface co-expression of *Vibrio cholerae* and *Salmonella typhi* O-antigens on Ty21a clone EX210. *Microb. Pathog. 8*:177.

89. Brown, A., C. E. Hormaeche, R. Demarco de Hormaeche, M. Winther, G. Dougan, D. J. Maskell, and B. A. Stocker. 1987. An attenuated *AroA Salmonella typhimurium* vaccine elicits humoral and cellular immunity to cloned beta-galactosidase in mice. *J. Infect. Dis. 155*:86.

90. Ervin, S. E., P. A. Small, Jr., and P. A. Gulig. 1993. Use of incompatible plasmids to control expression of antigen by *Salmonella typhimurium* and analysis of immunogenicity in mice. *Microb. Pathog. 15*:93.

91. Chatfield, S. N., I. G. Charles, A. J. Makoff, M. D. Oxer, G. Dougan, D. Pickard, D. Slater, and N. F. Fairweather. 1992. Use of the *nirB* promoter to direct the stable expression of heterologous antigens in *Salmonella* oral vaccine strains: development of a single-dose oral tetanus vaccine. *Bio/Technology 10*:888.

92. Jackson, R. J., H. F. Staats, J. Xu-Amano, I. Takahashi, H. Kiyono, M. E. Hudson, R. M. Gilley, S. N. Chatfield, and J. R. McGhee. 1994. Oral vaccine models: multiple delivery systems employing tetanus toxoid. *Ann. NY Sci. 730*:217.

93. Gomez-Duarte, O. G., J. Galen, S. N. Chatfield, R. Rappuoli, L. Eidels, and M. M. Levine. 1995. Expression of fragment C of tetanus toxin fused to a carboxyl-terminal fragment of diphtheria toxin in *Salmonella typhi* CVD 908 vaccine strain. *Vaccine 13*:1596.

94. Okahashi, N., M. Yamamoto, J. L. Vancott, S. N. Chatfield, M. Roberts, H. Bluethmann, T. Hiroi, H. Kiyono, and J. R. McGhee. 1996. Oral immunization of interleukin-4 (IL-4) knockout mice with a recombinant *Salmonella* strain or cholera toxin reveals that CD4+ Th2 cells producing IL-6 and IL-10 are associated with mucosal immunoglobulin A responses. *Infect. Immun. 64*:1516.

95. Barry, E. M., O. Gomez-Duarte, S. Chatfield, R. Rappuoli, M. Pizza, G. Losonsky, J. Galen, and M. M. Levine. 1996. Expression and immunogenicity of pertussis toxin S1 subunit-tetanus toxin fragment C fusions in *Salmonella typhi* vaccine strain CVD 908. *Infect. Immun. 64*:4172.

96. Jackson, R. J., M. Marinaro, J. L. VanCott, M. Yamamoto, N. Okahashi, K. Fujihashi, H. Kiyono, S. N. Chatfield, and J. R. McGhee.

1996. Mucosal immunity: regulation by helper T cells and a novel method for detection. *J. Biotechnol. 44*:209.

97. VanCott, J. L., H. F. Staats, D. W. Pascual, M. Roberts, S. N. Chatfield, M. Yamamoto, M. Coste, P. B. Carter, H. Kiyono, and J. R. McGhee. 1996. Regulation of mucosal and systemic antibody responses by T helper cell subsets, macrophages, and derived cytokines following oral immunization with live recombinant *Salmonella. J. Immunol. 156*:1504.
98. Strugnell, R., G. Dougan, S. Chatfield, I. Charles, N. Fairweather, J. Tite, J. L. Li, J. Beesley, and M. Roberts. 1992. Characterization of a *Salmonella typhimurium aro* vaccine strain expressing the P.69 antigen of *Bordetella pertussis. Infect. Immun. 60*:3994.
99. Leary, S. E., S. M. Eley, E. D. Williamson, and R. W. Titball. 1995. Expression of *Yersinia pestis* V antigen in attenuated *Salmonella typhimurium*: development of a novel vaccine for plague. *Contrib. Microbiol. Immunol. 13*:216.
100. Leary, S. E. C., K. F. Griffin, H. S. Garmory, E. D. Williamson, and R. W. Titball. 1997. Expression of an F1/V fusion protein in attenuated *Salmonella typhimurium* and protection of mice against plague. *Microb. Pathog. 23*:167.
101. Simonet, M., N. Fortineau, J. L. Beretti, and P. Berche. 1994. Immunization with live *aroA* recombinant *Salmonella typhimurium* producing invasin inhibits intestinal translocation of *Yersinia pseudotuberculosis. Infect. Immun. 62*:863.
102. Harokopakis, E., G. Hajishengallis, T. E. Greenway, M. W. Russell, and S. M. Michalek. 1997. Mucosal immunogenicity of a recombinant *Salmonella typhimurium*-cloned heterologous antigen in the absence or presence of coexpressed cholera toxin A2 and B subunits. *Infect. Immun. 65*:1445.
103. Curtiss, R. d., R. M. Goldschmidt, N. B. Fletchall, and S. M. Kelly. 1988. Avirulent *Salmonella typhimurium* delta *cya* delta *crp* oral vaccine strains expressing a streptococcal colonization and virulence antigen. *Vaccine 6*:155.
104. Doggett, T. A., E. K. Jagusztyn-Krynicka, and R. d. Curtiss. 1993. Immune responses to *Streptococcus sobrinus* surface protein antigen A expressed by recombinant *Salmonella typhimurium. Infect. Immun. 61*:1859.
105. Jagusztyn-Krynicka, E. K., J. E. Clark-Curtiss, and R. d. Curtiss. 1993. Escherichia coli heat-labile toxin subunit B fusions with *Streptococcus sobrinus* antigens expressed by *Salmonella typhimurium* oral vaccine strains: importance of the linker for antigenicity and biological activities of the hybrid proteins. *Infect. Immunity 61*:1004.

106. Newton, S. M., M. Kotb, T. P. Poirier, B. A. Stocker, and E. H. Beachey. 1991. Expression and immunogenicity of a streptococcal M protein epitope inserted in *Salmonella* flagellin. *Infect. Immun. 59*:2158.

107. Hajishengallis, G., E. Harokopakis, S. K. Hollingshead, M. W. Russell, and S. M. Michalek. 1996. Construction and oral immunogenicity of a *Salmonella typhimurium* strain expressing a streptococcal adhesion linked to the A2/B subunits of cholera toxin. *Vaccine 14*:1545.

108. Hohmann, E. L., C. A. Oletta, W. P. Loomis, and S. I. Miller. 1995. Macrophage-inducible expression of a model antigen in *Salmonella typhimurium* enhances immunogenicity. *Proc. Natl. Acad. Sci. USA 92*:2904.

109. Dusek, D. M., A. Progulske-Fox, J. Whitlock, and T. A. Brown. 1993. Isolation and characterization of a cloned *Porphyromonas gingivalis* hemagglutinin from an avirulent strain of *Salmonella typhimurium. Infect. Immun. 61*:940.

110. Dusek, D. M., A. Progulske-Fox, and T. A. Brown. 1994. Systemic and mucosal immune responses in mice orally immunized with avirulent *Salmonella typhimurium* expressing a cloned *Porphyromonas gingivalis* hemagglutinin. *Infect. Immun. 62*:1652.

111. Dusek, D. M., A. Progulske-Fox, and T. A. Brown. 1995. Expression and immunogenicity of a cloned *Porphyromonas gingivalis* hemagglutinin in *Salmonella typhimurium. Adv. Exp. Med. Biol. 371B*:1119.

112. von Specht, B. U., H. Domdey, F. Schodel, B. Blum, C. Lucking, B. Knapp, G. Muth, K. D. Hungerer, and M. Broker. 1994. Outer membrane proteins of *Pseudomonas aeruginosa* as vaccine candidates. *Behring Inst. Mitteil. 95*:85.

113. von Specht, B., B. Knapp, K. Hungerer, C. Lucking, A. Schmitt, and H. Domdey. 1996. Outer membrane proteins of *Pseudomonas aeruginosa* as vaccine candidates. *J. Biotechnol. 44*:145.

114. Gentschev, I., Z. Sokolovic, H. J. Mollenkopf, J. Hess, S. H. Kaufmann, M. Kuhn, G. F. Krohne, and W. Goebel. 1995. *Salmonella* strain secreting active listeriolysin changes its intracellular localization. *Infect. Immun. 63*:4202.

115. Gentschev, I., H. Mollenkopf, Z. Sokolovic, J. Hess, S. H. Kaufmann, and W. Goebel. 1996. Development of antigen-delivery systems, based on the *Escherichia coli* hemolysin secretion pathway. *Gene 179*:133.

116. Hess, J., I. Gentschev, G. Szalay, C. Ladel, A. Bubert, W. Goebel, and S. H. Kaufmann. 1995. *Listeria monocytogenes* p60 supports host cell invasion by and in vivo survival of attenuated *Salmonella typhimurium. Infect. Immun. 63*:2047.

117. Hess, J., I. Gentschev, D. Miko, M. Welzel, C. Ladel, W. Goebel, and

S. H. Kaufmann. 1996. Superior efficacy of secreted over somatic antigen display in recombinant *Salmonella* vaccine induced protection against listeriosis. *Proc. Natl. Acad. Sci. USA 93*:1458.

118. Hess, J., G. Dietrich, I. Gentschev, D. Miko, W. Goebel, and S. H. Kaufmann. 1997. Protection against murine listeriosis by an attenuated recombinant *Salmonella typhimurium* vaccine strain that secretes the naturally somatic antigen superoxide dismutase. *Infect. Immun. 65*:1286.

119. Corthesy-Theulaz, I. E., S. Hopkins, D. Bachmann, P. F. Saldinger, N. Porta, R. Haas, Y. Zheng-Xin, T. Meyer, H. Bouzourene, A. L. Blum, and J. P. Kraehenbuhl. 1998. Mice are protected from Helicobacter pylori infection by nasal immunization with attenuated *Salmonella typhimurium* phoPc expressing urease A and B subunits. *Infect. Immun. 66*:581.

120. Hayes, L. J., J. W. Conlan, J. S. Everson, M. E. Ward, and I. N. Clarke. 1991. *Chlamydia trachomatis* major outer membrane protein epitopes expressed as fusions with LamB in an attenuated *aroA* strain of *Salmonella typhimurium*; their application as potential immunogens. *J. Gen. Microbiol. 137*:1557.

121. Sadoff, J. C., W. R. Ballou, L. S. Baron, W. R. Majarian, R. N. Brey, W. T. Hockmeyer, J. F. Young, S. J. Cryz, J. Ou, G. H. Lowell, and J. D. Chulay. 1988. Oral *Salmonella typhimurium* vaccine expressing circumsporozoite protein protects against malaria. *Science 240*:336.

122. Aggarwal, A., S. Kumar, R. Jaffe, D. Hone, M. Gross, and J. Sadoff. 1990. Oral *Salmonella*: malaria circumsporozoite recombinants induce specific $CD8^+$ cytotoxic T cells. *J. Exp. Med. 172*:1083.

123. Flynn, J. L., W. R. Weiss, K. A. Norris, H. S. Seifert, S. Kumar, and M. So. 1990. Generation of a cytotoxic T-lymphocyte response using a *Salmonella* antigen-delivery system. *Mol. Microbiol . 4*:2111.

124. Schorr, J., B. Knapp, E. Hundt, H. A. Kupper, and E. Amann. 1991. Surface expression of malarial antigens in *Salmonella typhimurium*: induction of serum antibody response upon oral vaccination of mice. *Vaccine 9*:675.

125. Haddad, D., S. Liljeqvist, S. Kumar, M. Hansson, S. Stahl, H. Perlmann, P. Perlmann, and K. Berzins. 1995. Surface display compared to periplasmic expression of a malarial antigen in *Salmonella typhimurium* and its implications for immunogenicity. *FEMS Immunol. Med. Microbiol. 12*:175.

126. Gonzalez, C., D. Hone, F. R. Noriega, C. O. Tacket, J. R. Davis, G. Losonsky, J. P. Nataro, S. Hoffman, A. Malik, E. Nardin, and et al. 1994. *Salmonella typhi* vaccine strain CVD 908 expressing the circum-

sporozoite protein of *Plasmodium falciparum*: strain construction and safety and immunogenicity in humans. *J. Infect. Dis. 169*:927.

127. Toebe, C. S., J. D. Clements, L. Cardenas, G. J. Jennings, and M. F. Wiser. 1997. Evaluation of immunogenicity of an oral *Salmonella* vaccine expressing recombinant *Plasmodium berghei* merozoite surface protein-1. *Am. J. Trop. Med. Hyg. 56*:192.

128. Zhang, T., and S. L. Stanley, Jr. 1997. Expression of the serine rich *Entamoeba* histolytica protein (SREHP) in the avirulent vaccine strain *Salmonella typhi* TY2 chi 4297 (delta *cya* delta *crp* delta *asd*): safety and immunogenicity in mice. *Vaccine 15*:1319.

129. Chabalgoity, J. A., J. A. Harrison, A. Esteves, R. Demarco de Hormaeche, R. Ehrlich, C. M. Khan, and C. E. Hormaeche. 1997. Expression and immunogenicity of an *Echinococcus granulosus* fatty acid-binding protein in live attenuated *Salmonella* vaccine strains. *Infect. Immun. 65*:2402.

130. Khan, C. M., B. Villarreal-Ramos, R. J. Pierce, G. Riveau, R. Demarco de Hormaeche, H. McNeill, T. Ali, N. Fairweather, S. Chatfield, A. Capron, G. Dougan, and C. E. Hormaeche. 1994. Construction, expression, and immunogenicity of the *Schistosoma mansoni* P28 glutathione S-transferase as a genetic fusion to tetanus toxin fragment C in a live *aro* attenuated vaccine strain of *Salmonella*. *Proc. Natl. Acad. Sci. USA 91*:11261.

131. Khan, C. M., B. Villarreal-Ramos, R. J. Pierce, R. Demarco de Hormaeche, H. McNeill, T. Ali, S. Chatfield, A. Capron, G. Dougan, and C. E. Hormaeche. 1994. Construction, expression, and immunogenicity of multiple tandem copies of the *Schistosoma mansoni* peptide 115-131 of the P28 glutathione S-transferase expressed as C-terminal fusions to tetanus toxin fragment C in a live *aro*-attenuated vaccine strain of *Salmonella*. *J. Immunol. 153*:5634.

132. Chabalgoity, J. A., B. Villareal-Ramos, C. M. Khan, S. N. Chatfield, R. D. de Hormaeche, and C. E. Hormaeche. 1995. Influence of preimmunization with tetanus toxoid on immune responses to tetanus toxin fragment C-guest antigen fusions in a *Salmonella* vaccine carrier. *Infect. Immun. 63*:2564.

133. Srinivasan, J., S. Tinge, R. Wright, J. C. Herr, and R. Curtiss, 3rd. 1995. Oral immunization with attenuated *Salmonella* expressing human sperm antigen induces antibodies in serum and the reproductive tract. *Biol. Reprod. 53*:462.

134. Cox, F. E. 1997. Designer vaccines for parasitic diseases. *Int. J. Parasitol. 27*:1147.

135. Ianaro, A., D. Xu, C. A. O'Donnell, M. Di Rosa, and F. Y. Liew. 1995. Expression of TGF-beta in attenuated *Salmonella typhimurium*: oral

administration leads to the reduction of inflammation, IL-2 and IFN-gamma, but enhancement of IL-10, in carrageenin-induced oedema in mice. *Immunology 84*:8.

136. Carrier, M. J., S. N. Chatfield, G. Dougan, U. T. Nowicka, D. O'Callaghan, J. E. Beesley, S. Milano, E. Cillari, and F. Y. Liew. 1992. Expression of human IL-1 beta in *Salmonella typhimurium*. A model system for the delivery of recombinant therapeutic proteins in vivo. *J. Immunol. 148*:1176.
137. Denich, K., P. Borlin, P. D. O'Hanley, M. Howard, and A. W. Heath. 1993. Expression of the murine interleukin-4 gene in an attenuated aroA strain of *Salmonella typhimurium*: persistence and immune response in BALB/c mice and susceptibility to macrophage killing. *Infect. Immun. 61*:4818.
138. Whittle, B. L., R. M. Smith, K. I. Matthaei, I. G. Young, and N. K. Verma. 1997. Enhancement of the specific mucosal IgA response in vivo by interleukin-5 expressed by an attenuated strain of *Salmonella* serotype Dublin. *J. Med. Microbiol. 46*:1029.
139. Beckers, W., L. Villa, S. Gonfloni, L. Castagnoli, S. M. Newton, G. Cesareni, and P. Ghiara. 1993. Increasing the immunogenicity of protein antigens through the genetic insertion of VQGEESNDK sequence of human IL-1 beta into their sequence. *J. Immunol. 151*:1757.
140. Saltzman, D. A., E. Katsanis, C. P. Heise, D. E. Hasz, V. Vigdorovich, S. M. Kelly, R. Curtiss, III, A. S. Leonard, and P. M. Anderson. 1997. Antitumor mechanisms of attenuated *Salmonella typhimurium* containing the gene for human interleukin-2: a novel antitumor agent? *J. Pediatr. Surg. 32*:301.
141. Attridge, S., J. Hackett, R. Morona, and P. Whyte. 1988. Towards a live oral vaccine against enterotoxigenic *Escherichia coli* of swine. *Vaccine 6*:387.
142. Fairweather, N. F., S. N. Chatfield, A. J. Makoff, R. A. Strugnell, J. Bester, D. J. Maskell, and G. Dougan. 1990. Oral vaccination of mice against tetanus by use of a live attenuated *Salmonella* carrier. *Infect. Immun. 58*:1323.
143. Dunne, M., B. K. al-Ramadi, S. W. Barthold, R. A. Flavell, and E. Fikrig. 1995. Oral vaccination with an attenuated *Salmonella typhimurium* strain expressing *Borrelia burgdorferi* OspA prevents murine Lyme borreliosis. *Infect. Immun. 63*:1611.
144. McEwen, J., R. Levi, R. J. Horwitz, and R. Arnon. 1992. Synthetic recombinant vaccine expressing influenza haemagglutinin epitope in *Salmonella* flagellin leads to partial protection in mice. *Vaccine 10*:405.
145. Yang, D. M., N. Fairweather, L. L. Button, W. R. McMaster, L. P. Kahl, and F. Y. Liew. 1990. Oral *Salmonella typhimurium* (AroA-) vaccine

expressing a major leishmanial surface protein (gp63) preferentially induces T helper 1 cells and protective immunity against leishmaniasis. *J. Immunol. 145*:2281.

146. Xu, D., S. J. McSorley, S. N. Chatfield, G. Dougan, and F. Y. Liew. 1995. Protection against *Leishmania major* infection in genetically susceptible BALB/c mice by gp63 delivered orally in attenuated *Salmonella typhimurium* ($AroA^{-}$ $AroD^{-}$). *Immunology 85*:1.

147. Yamamoto, M., J. L. Vancott, N. Okahashi, M. Marinaro, H. Kiyono, K. Fujihashi, R. J. Jackson, S. N. Chatfield, H. Bluethmann, and J. R. McGhee. 1996. The role of Th1 and Th2 cells for mucosal IgA responses. *Ann. NY Acad. Sci. 778*:64.

148. Buchmeier, N. A., and F. Heffron. 1991. Inhibition of macrophage phagosome-lysosome fusion by *Salmonella typhimurium. Infect. Immun. 59*:2232.

149. Alpuche Aranda, C. M., J. A. Swanson, W. P. Loomis, and S. I. Miller. 1992. *Salmonella typhimurium* activates virulence gene transcription within acidified macrophage phagosomes. *Proc. Natl. Acad. Sci. USA 89*:10079.

150. Alpuche-Aranda, C. M., E. L. Racoosin, J. A. Swanson, and S. I. Miller. 1994. *Salmonella* stimulate macrophage macropinocytosis and persist within spacious phagosomes. *J. Exp. Med. 179*:601.

151. Alpuche-Aranda, C. M., E. P. Berthiaume, B. Mock, J. A. Swanson, and S. I. Miller. 1995. Spacious phagosome formation within mouse macrophages correlates with *Salmonella* serotype pathogenicity and host susceptibility. *Infect. Immun. 63*:4456.

152. Harding, C. V., and J. D. Pfeifer. 1994. Antigen expressed by *Salmonella typhimurium* is processed for class I major histocompatibility complex presentation by macrophages but not infected epithelial cells. *Immunology 83*:670.

153. Verma, N. K., H. K. Ziegler, M. Wilson, M. Khan, S. Safley, B. A. Stocker, and G. K. Schoolnik. 1995. Delivery of class I and class II MHC-restricted T-cell epitopes of listeriolysin of *Listeria monocytogenes* by attenuated *Salmonella. Vaccine 13*:142.

154. Turner, S. J., F. R. Carbone, and R. A. Strugnell. 1993. *Salmonella typhimurium* delta *aroA* delta *aroD* mutants expressing a foreign recombinant protein induce specific major histocompatibility complex class I-restricted cytotoxic T lymphocytes in mice. *Infect. Immun. 61*:5374.

155. Abimiku, A. G., G. Franchini, K. Aldrich, M. Myagkikh, P. Markham, E. Gard, R. C. Gallo, and M. Robert-Guroff. 1995. Humoral and cellular immune responses in rhesus macaques infected with human immunodeficiency virus type 2. *AIDS Res. Hum. Retroviruses 11*:383.

156. Chatfield, S. N., K. Strahan, D. Pickard, I. G. Charles, C. E. Hormaeche, and G. Dougan. 1992. Evaluation of *Salmonella typhimurium* strains harbouring defined mutations in *htrA* and *aroA* in the murine salmonellosis model. *Microb. Pathog. 12*:145.

157. Redman, T. K., C. C. Harmon, and S. M. Michalek. 1996. Oral immunization with recombinant *Salmonella typhimurium* expressing surface protein antigen A (SpaA) of *Streptococcus sobrinus*: effects of the *Salmonella* virulence plasmid on the induction of protective and sustained humoral responses in rats. *Vaccine 14*:868.

158. Strugnell, R. A., D. Maskell, N. Fairweather, D. Pickard, A. Cockayne, C. Penn, and G. Dougan. 1990. Stable expression of foreign antigens from the chromosome of *Salmonella typhimurium* vaccine strains. *Gene 88*:57.

159. Galan, J. E., K. Nakayama, and R. d. Curtiss. 1990. Cloning and characterization of the *asd* gene of *Salmonella typhimurium*: use in stable maintenance of recombinant plasmids in *Salmonella* vaccine strains. *Gene 94*:29.

160. Kandror, O., L. Busconi, M. Sherman, and A. L. Goldberg. 1994. Rapid degradation of an abnormal protein in *Escherichia coli* involves the chaperones GroEL and GroES. *J. Biol. Chem. 269*:23575.

161. Kowit, J. D., and A. L. Goldberg. 1977. Intermediate steps in the degradation of a specific abnormal protein in *Escherichia coli. J. Biol. Chem. 252*:8350.

162. Reznikoff, A. E. 1986. *Maximizing Gene Expression*. Stoneham, MA: Butterworths.

163. Tijhaar, E. J., Y. Zheng-Xin, J. A. Karlas, T. F. Meyer, M. J. Stukart, A. D. Osterhaus, and F. R. Mooi. 1994. Construction and evaluation of an expression vector allowing the stable expression of foreign antigens in a *Salmonella typhimurium* vaccine strain. *Vaccine 12*:1004.

164. Yan, Z. X., F. Reuss, and T. F. Meyer. 1990. Construction of an invertible DNA segment for improved antigen expression by a hybrid *Salmonella* vaccine strain. *Res. Microbiol. 141*:1003.

165. Yan, Z. X., and T. F. Meyer. 1996. Mixed population approach for vaccination with live recombinant *Salmonella strains. J. Biotechnol. 44*:197.

166. Everest, P., G. Frankel, J. Li, P. Lund, S. Chatfield, and G. Dougan. 1995. Expression of LacZ from the *htrA*, *nirB* and *groE* promoters in a *Salmonella* vaccine strain: influence of growth in mammalian cells. *FEMS Microbiol. Lett. 126*:97.

167. McSorley, S. J., D. Xu, and F. Y. Liew. 1997. Vaccine efficacy of *Salmonella* strains expressing glycoprotein 63 with different promoters. *Infect. Immun. 65*:171.

168. Wu, J. Y., S. Newton, A. Judd, B. Stocker, and W. S. Robinson. 1989. Expression of immunogenic epitopes of hepatitis B surface antigen with hybrid flagellin proteins by a vaccine strain of *Salmonella. Proc. Natl. Acad. Sci. USA 86*:4726.

169. Verma, N. K., H. K. Ziegler, B. A. Stocker, and G. K. Schoolnik. 1995. Induction of a cellular immune response to a defined T-cell epitope as an insert in the flagellin of a live vaccine strain of *Salmonella. Vaccine 13*:235.

170. Gaines, S., J. G. Tully, and W. D. Tigertt. 1968. Studies on infection and immunity in experimental typhoid fever. 8. Intravenous and intra-lymph node challenge of chimpanzees with *Salmonella typhi. J. Infect. Dis. 118*:393.

171. Gaines, S., H. Sprinz, J. G. Tully, and W. D. Tigertt. 1968. Studies on infection and immunity in experimental typhoid fever. VII. The distribution of *Salmonella typhi* in chimpanzee tissue following oral challenge, and the relationship between the numbers of bacilli and morphologic lesions. *J. Infect. Dis. 118*:293.

172. Schafer, R., D. A. Portnoy, S. A. Brassell, and Y. Paterson. 1992. Induction of a cellular immune response to a foreign antigen by a recombinant *Listeria monocytogenes* vaccine. *J. Immunol. 149*:53.

173. Ikonomidis, G., D. A. Portnoy, W. Gerhard, and Y. Paterson. 1997. Influenza-specific immunity induced by recombinant *Listeria monocytogenes* vaccines. *Vaccine 15*:433.

174. Paterson, Y., and G. Ikonomidis. 1996. Recombinant *Listeria monocytogenes* cancer vaccines. *Curr. Opin. Immunol. 8*:664.

175. Frankel, F. R., S. Hegde, J. Lieberman, and Y. Paterson. 1995. Induction of cell-mediated immune responses to human immunodeficiency virus type 1 Gag protein by using *Listeria monocytogenes* as a live vaccine vector. *J. Immunol. 155*:4775.

176. Pan, Z. K., G. Ikonomidis, D. Pardoll, and Y. Paterson. 1995. Regression of established tumors in mice mediated by the oral administration of a recombinant *Listeria monocytogenes* vaccine. *Cancer Res. 55*:4776.

177. Pan, Z. K., G. Ikonomidis, A. Lazenby, D. Pardoll, and Y. Paterson. 1995. A recombinant *Listeria monocytogenes* vaccine expressing a model tumour antigen protects mice against lethal tumour cell challenge and causes regression of established tumours. *Nature Med. 1*:471.

178. Norton, P. M., R. W. F. Le Page, and J. M. Wells. 1995. Progress in the development of *Lactococcus lactis* as a recombinant mucosal vaccine delivery system. *Folia Microbiol. 40*:225.

179. Germanier, R., and E. Furer. 1971. Immunity in experimental salmonel-

losis. II. Basis for the avirulence and protective capacity of *gal E* mutants of *Salmonella typhimurium. Infect. Immun. 4*:663.

180. Hone, D., R. Morona, S. Attridge, and J. Hackett. 1987. Construction of defined *galE* mutants of *Salmonella* for use as vaccines. *J. Infect. Dis. 156*:167.
181. Collins, L. V., S. Attridge, and J. Hackett. 1991. Mutations at *rfc* or *pmi* attenuate *Salmonella typhimurium* virulence for mice. *Infect. Immun. 59*:1079.
182. Hoiseth, S. K., and B. A. Stocker. 1981. Aromatic-dependent *Salmonella typhimurium* are non-virulent and effective as live vaccines. *Nature 291*:238.
183. Robertsson, J. A., A. A. Lindberg, S. Hoiseth, and B. A. Stocker. 1983. *Salmonella typhimurium* infection in calves: protection and survival of virulent challenge bacteria after immunization with live or inactivated vaccines. *Infect. Immun. 41*:742.
184. Smith, B. P., M. Reina-Guerra, B. A. Stocker, S. K. Hoiseth, and E. Johnson. 1984. Aromatic-dependent *Salmonella dublin* as a parenteral modified live vaccine for calves. *Am. J. Vet. Res. 45*:2231.
185. McFarland, W. C., and B. A. Stocker. 1987. Effect of different purine auxotrophic mutations on mouse-virulence of a Vi-positive strain of *Salmonella dublin* and of two strains of *Salmonella typhimurium. Microb. Pathog. 3*:129.
186. O'Callaghan, D., D. Maskell, F. Y. Liew, C. S. Easmon, and G. Dougan. 1988. Characterization of aromatic- and purine-dependent *Salmonella typhimurium*: attention, persistence, and ability to induce protective immunity in BALB/c mice. *Infect. Immun. 56*:419.
187. O'Callaghan, D., D. Maskell, J. Tite, and G. Dougan. 1990. Immune responses in BALB/c mice following immunization with aromatic compound or purine-dependent *Salmonella typhimurium* strains. *Immunology 69*:184.
188. Nnalue, N. A., and B. A. Stocker. 1987. Test of the virulence and live-vaccine efficacy of auxotrophic and *galE* derivatives of *Salmonella choleraesuis. Infect. Immun. 55*:955.
189. Brown, R. F., and B. A. Stocker. 1987. *Salmonella typhi* 205aTy, a strain with two attenuating auxotrophic characters, for use in laboratory teaching. *Infect. Immun. 55*:892.
190. Kelly, S. M., B. A. Bosecker, and R. d. Curtiss. 1992. Characterization and protective properties of attenuated mutants of *Salmonella choleraesuis. Infect. Immun. 60*:4881.
191. Curtiss, R. d., and S. M. Kelly. 1987. *Salmonella typhimurium* deletion mutants lacking adenylate cyclase and cyclic AMP receptor protein are avirulent and immunogenic. *Infect. Immun. 55*:3035.

192. Tacket, C. O., D. M. Hone, R. d. Curtiss, S. M. Kelly, G. Losonsky, L. Guers, A. M. Harris, R. Edelman, and M. M. Levine. 1992. Comparison of the safety and immunogenicity of delta*aroC* delta*aroD* and delta*cya* delta*crp Salmonella typhi* strains in adult volunteers. *Infect. Immun. 60*:536.

193. Miller, S. I., A. M. Kukral, and J. J. Mekalanos. 1989. A two-component regulatory system (phoP phoQ) controls *Salmonella typhimurium* virulence. *Proc. Natl. Acad. Sci. USA 86*:5054.

194. Chatfield, S. N., C. J. Dorman, C. Hayward, and G. Dougan. 1991. Role of ompR-dependent genes in *Salmonella typhimurium* virulence: mutants deficient in both ompC and ompF are attenuated in vivo. *Infect. Immun. 59*:449.

195. Pickard, D., J. Li, M. Roberts, D. Maskell, D. Hone, M. Levine, G. Dougan, and S. Chatfield. 1994. Characterization of defined ompR mutants of *Salmonella typhi*: ompR is involved in the regulation of Vi polysaccharide expression. *Infect. Immun. 62*:3984.

196. Johnson, K., I. Charles, G. Dougan, D. Pickard, O. G. P, G. Costa, T. Ali, I. Miller, and C. Hormaeche. 1991. The role of a stress-response protein in *Salmonella typhimurium* virulence. *Mol. Microbiol. 5*:401.

197. Strahan, K., S. N. Chatfield, J. Tite, G. Dougan, and C. E. Hormaeche. 1992. Impaired resistance to infection does not increase the virulence of *Salmonella htrA* live vaccines for mice. *Microb. Pathog. 12*:311.

198. Coynault, C., V. Robbe-Saule, and F. Norel. 1996. Virulence and vaccine potential of *Salmonella typhimurium* mutants deficient in the expression of the RpoS (sigma S) regulon. *Mol. Microbiol. 22*:149.

199. Robbe-Saule, V., C. Coynault, and F. Norel. 1995. The live oral typhoid vaccine Ty21a is a *rpoS* mutant and is susceptible to various environmental stresses. *FEMS Microbiol. Lett. 126*:171.

200. Stabel, T. J., J. E. Mayfield, D. C. Morfitt, and M. J. Wannemuehler. 1993. Oral immunization of mice and swine with an attenuated *Salmonella choleraesuis* [delta cya-12 delta(crp-cdt)19] mutant containing a recombinant plasmid. *Infect. Immun. 61*:610.

201. Kaniga, K., D. Trollinger, and J. E. Galan. 1995. Identification of two targets of the type III protein secretion system encoded by the inv and spa loci of *Salmonella typhimurium* that have homology to the *Shigella* IpaD and IpaA proteins. *J. Bacteriol. 177*:7078.

202. Collazo, C. M., and J. E. Galan. 1996. Requirement for exported proteins in secretion through the invasion-associated type III system of *Salmonella typhimurium. Infect. Immun. 64*:3524.

203. Wahdan, M. H., C. Serie, Y. Cerisier, S. Sallam, and R. Germanier. 1982. A controlled field trial of live *Salmonella typhi* strain Ty 21a oral vaccine against typhoid: three-year results. *J. Infect. Dis. 145*:292.

204. Black, R., M. M. Levine, C. Young, J. Rooney, S. Levine, M. L. Clements, O. D. S, T. Hugues, and R. Germanier. 1983. Immunogenicity of Ty21a attenuated "*Salmonella typhi*" given with sodium bicarbonate or in enteric-coated capsules. *Dev. Biol. Stand. 53*:9.

205. Levine, M. M., C. Ferreccio, R. E. Black, and R. Germanier. 1987. Large-scale field trial of Ty21a live oral typhoid vaccine in enteric-coated capsule formulation. *Lancet 1*:1049.

206. Germanier, R., and E. Fuer. 1975. Isolation and characterization of *galE* mutant Ty 21a of *Salmonella typhi*: a candidate strain for a live, oral typhoid vaccine. *J. Infect. Dis. 131*:553.

207. Germanier, R. 1972. Immunity in experimental salmonellosis. 3. Comparative immunization with viable and heat-inactivated cells of *Salmonella typhimurium. Infect. Immun. 5*:792.

208. Hone, D. M., S. R. Attridge, B. Forrest, R. Morona, D. Daniels, J. T. LaBrooy, R. C. Bartholomeusz, D. J. Shearman, and J. Hackett. 1988. A *galE* via (Vi antigen-negative) mutant of *Salmonella typhi* Ty2 retains virulence in humans. *Infect. Immun. 56*:1326.

209. Tacket, C. O., G. Losonsky, D. N. Taylor, L. S. Baron, D. Kopecko, S. Cryz, and M. M. Levine. 1991. Lack of immune response to the Vi component of a Vi-positive variant of the *Salmonella typhi* live oral vaccine strain Ty21a in human studies. *J. Infect. Dis. 163*:901.

210. Bacon, B. A., T. W. Burrows, and M. Yates. 1950. The effects of biochemical mutation on the virulence of *Bacterium typhosum*: the virulence of mutants. *Br. J. Exp. Pathol. 31*:714.

211. Smith, B. P., M. Reina-Guerra, S. K. Hoiseth, B. A. Stocker, F. Habasha, E. Johnson, and F. Merritt. 1984. Aromatic-dependent *Salmonella typhimurium* as modified live vaccines for calves. *Am. J. Vet. Res. 45*:59.

212. Smith, B. P., M. Reina-Guerra, B. A. Stocker, S. K. Hoiseth, and E. H. Johnson. 1984. Vaccination of calves against *Salmonella dublin* with aromatic-dependent *Salmonella typhimurium. Am. J. Vet. Res. 45*:1858.

213. Mukkur, T. K., G. H. McDowell, B. A. Stocker, and A. K. Lascelles. 1987. Protection against experimental salmonellosis in mice and sheep by immunization with aromatic-dependent *Salmonella typhimurium. J. Med. Microbiol. 24*:11.

214. Mukkur, T. K., K. H. Walker, P. Baker, and D. Jones. 1995. Systemic and mucosal intestinal antibody response of sheep immunized with aromatic-dependent live or killed *Salmonella typhimurium. Comp. Immunol. Microbiol. Infect. Dis. 18*:27.

215. Jones, P. W., G. Dougan, C. Hayward, N. Mackensie, P. Collins, and S. N. Chatfield. 1991. Oral vaccination of calves against experimental

salmonellosis using a double *aro* mutant of *Salmonella typhimurium. Vaccine 9*:29.

216. Edwards, M. F., and B. A. Stocker. 1988. Construction of delta *aroA* his delta *pur* strains of *Salmonella typhi. J. Bacteriol. 170*:3991.

217. Stocker, B. A. 1988. Auxotrophic *Salmonella typhi* as live vaccine. *Vaccine 6*:141.

218. Levine, M. M., D. Herrington, J. R. Murphy, J. G. Morris, G. Losonsky, B. Tall, A. A. Lindberg, S. Svenson, S. Baqar, M. F. Edwards, and B. Stocker. 1987. Safety, infectivity, immunogenicity, and *in vivo* stability of two attenuated auxotrophic mutant strains of *Salmonella typhi*, 541Ty and 543Ty, as live oral vaccines in humans. *J. Clin. Invest. 79*:888.

219. Hone, D. M., A. M. Harris, S. Chatfield, G. Dougan, and M. M. Levine. 1991. Construction of genetically defined double *aro* mutants of *Salmonella typhi. Vaccine 9*:810.

220. Miller, I. A., S. Chatfield, G. Dougan, L. Desilva, H. S. Joysey, and C. Hormaeche. 1989. Bacteriophage P22 as a vehicle for transducing cosmid gene banks between smooth strains of *Salmonella typhimurium*: use in identifying a role for *aroD* in attenuating virulent *Salmonella* strains. *Mol. Gen. Genet. 215*:312.

221. Dougan, G., S. Chatfield, D. Pickard, J. Bester, D. O'Callaghan, and D. Maskell. 1988. Construction and characterization of vaccine strains of *Salmonella* harboring mutations in two different *aro* genes. *J. Infect. Dis. 158*:1329.

222. Hone, D. M., C. O. Tacket, A. M. Harris, B. Kay, G. Losonsky, and M. M. Levine. 1992. Evaluation in volunteers of a candidate live oral attenuated *Salmonella typhi* vector vaccine. *J. Clin. Invest. 90*:412.

223. Tacket, C. O., D. M. Hone, G. A. Losonsky, L. Guers, R. Edelman, and M. M. Levine. 1992. Clinical acceptability and immunogenicity of CVD 908 *Salmonella typhi* vaccine strain. *Vaccine 10*:443.

224. Sztein, M. B., S. S. Wasserman, C. O. Tacket, R. Edelman, D. Hone, A. A. Lindberg, and M. M. Levine. 1994. Cytokine production patterns and lymphoproliferative responses in volunteers orally immunized with attenuated vaccine strains of *Salmonella typhi. J. Infect. Dis. 170*:1508.

225. Tacket, C. O., M. B. Sztein, G. A. Losonsky, S. S. Wasserman, J. P. Nataro, R. Edelman, D. Pickard, G. Dougan, S. N. Chatfield, and M. M. Levine. 1997. Safety of live oral *Salmonella typhi* vaccine strains with deletions in *htrA* and *aroC aroD* and immune response in humans. *Infect. Immun. 65*:452.

226. Hohmann, E. L., C. A. Oletta, K. P. Killeen, and S. I. Miller. 1996. *phoP/phoQ*-deleted *Salmonella typhi* (Ty800) is a safe and immuno-

genic single-dose typhoid fever vaccine in volunteers. *J. Infect. Dis. 173*:1408.

227. Herrington, D. A., L. Van de Verg, S. B. Formal, T. L. Hale, B. D. Tall, S. J. Cryz, E. C. Tramont, and M. M. Levine. 1990. Studies in volunteers to evaluate candidate *Shigella* vaccines: further experience with a bivalent *Salmonella typhi–Shigella sonnei* vaccine and protection conferred by previous *Shigella sonnei disease. Vaccine 8*:353.
228. Gilman, R. H., R. B. Hornick, W. E. Woodard, H. L. DuPont, M. J. Snyder, M. M. Levine, and J. P. Libonati. 1977. Evaluation of a UDP-glucose-4-epimeraseless mutant of *Salmonella typhi* as a liver oral vaccine. *J. Infect. Dis. 136*:717.
229. Angulo, F. J., and D. L. Swerdlow. 1995. Bacterial enteric infections in persons infected with human immunodeficiency virus. *Clin. Infect. Dis. 21*:S84.
230. Rouquette, C., and P. Berche. 1996. The pathogenesis of infection by *Listeria monocytogenes. Microbiologia 12*:245.
231. Farber, J. M., W. H. Ross, and J. Harwig. 1996. Health risk assessment of *Listeria monocytogenes* in Canada. *Int. J. Food Microbiol. 30*:145.
232. Batt, C. A. 1997. Molecular diagnostics for dairy-borne pathogens. *J. Dairy Sci. 80*:220.
233. Low, J. C., and W. Donachie. 1997. A review of *Listeria monocytogenes* and listeriosis [see comments]. *Vet. J. 153*:9.
234. Anonymous. 1997. Food poisoning, listeriosis, and febrile gastroenteritis. *Nutr. Rev. 55*:57.
235. Rocourt, J., and J. Bille. 1997. Foodborne listeriosis. *World Health Stat. Q. Rapp. Trimest. Stat. Sanit. Mond. 50*:67.
236. Bao, J. X., and J. D. Clements. 1991. Prior immunologic experience potentiates the subsequent antibody response when *Salmonella* strains are used as vaccine carriers. *Infect. Immun. 59*:3841.
237. Hone, D. M., A. M. Harris, V. Lim, and M. M. Levine. 1994. Construction and characterization of isogenic O-antigen variants of *Salmonella typhi. Mol. Microbiol. 13*:525.
238. Powell, R. J., G. K. Lewis, and D. M. Hone. 1996. *Introduction of Eukaryotic Expression Cassettes into Animal Cells Using a Bacterial Vector Delivery System.* Cold Spring Harbor, N.Y.: Cold Spring Harbor Laboratory Press.
239. Sizemore, D. R., A. A. Branstrom, and J. C. Sadoff. 1995. Attenuated *Shigella* as a DNA delivery vehicle for DNA-mediated immunization. *Science 270*:299.
240. Sizemore, D. R., A. A. Branstrom, and J. C. Sadoff. 1997. Attenuated bacteria as a DNA delivery vehicle for DNA-mediated immunization. *Vaccine 15*:804.

241. Courvalin, P., S. Goussard, and C. Grillot-Courvalin. 1995. Gene transfer from bacteria to mammalian cells. *C. R. Acad. Sci. Ser. Iii Sci. Vie 318*:1207.

242. Darji, A., C. A. Guzman, B. Gerstel, P. Wachholz, K. N. Timmis, J. Wehland, T. Chakraborty, and S. Weiss. 1997. Oral somatic transgene vaccination using attenuated *S. typhimurium. Cell 91*:765.

CHAPTER 7

THE USE OF *Listeria monocytogenes* RECOMBINANTS AS VACCINE VECTORS IN INFECTIOUS AND NEOPLASTIC DISEASE

LARRY M. WEISKIRCH and YVONNE PATERSON

7.1 INTRODUCTION

Infection with the gram-positive facultative intracellular bacterium *Listeria monocytogenes* is kept under control by cells of the innate immune system, including neutrophils, natural killer (NK) cells, and $\gamma\delta$ T-cell receptor (TCR)-expressing lymphocytes (see Chapter 4, *this volume*). Antigen-specific $\alpha\beta$ TCR-expressing T cells, however, are required for the eradication of *L. monocytogenes* from the infected host. It is therefore appropriate that the immune response generated against *L. monocytogenes* consists principally of cell-mediated immunity.

L. monocytogenes is currently under investigation as a live vaccine vector because infection stimulates potent $CD8^+$ and $CD4^+$

Abbreviations: APC, antigen-presenting cell; CRPV, cottontail rabbit papillomavirus; CTL, cytotoxic T lymphocyte; DTH, delayed-type hypersensitivity; GM-CSF, granulocyte-macrophage colony-stimulating factor; HIV, human immunodeficiency virus; IFN, interferon; Ig, immunoglobulin; IL, interleukin; i.p., intraperitoneal; i.v., intravenous; kb, kilobase; kD, kilodalton; LCMV, lymphocytic choriomeningitis virus; LLO, *L. monocytogenes* hemolysin, listeriolysin O; Lm-Gag, *L. monocytogenes* mutant which secretes the Gag of HIV; Lm-NP, *L. monocytogenes* (Lm) mutant strain which secretes a fusion protein consisting of part of LLO and the nucleoprotein of influenza; Lm-WT, wild-type *L. monocytogenes*, strain 10403s; MHC, major histocompatibility complex; NK, natural killer; NP, nucleoprotein; PCR, polymerase chain reaction; RT, reverse transcription; s.c., subcutaneous; TCR, T-cell receptor; Th, T-helper lymphocyte; TNF-α, tumor necrosis factor-α.

Intracellular Bacterial Vaccine Vectors, Edited by Yvonne Paterson.
ISBN 0-471-17278-2

T-cell responses against secreted antigens. This chapter describes studies that have demonstrated that genetically engineered *L. monocytogenes* mutants are highly effective vectors for the induction of potent immune responses, and reviews methods designed to generate such mutants. In addition, we describe the underlying immunological principles believed to contribute to the success of *L. monocytogenes* as a vaccine vehicle. Finally, we discuss the strengths and weaknesses of *L. monocytogenes* as a vaccine vector.

7.2 *Listeria monocytogenes* INDUCES EFFICIENT ANTIGEN PROCESSING AND PRESENTATION

T cells recognize protein antigen as peptide fragments presented by class I or II MHC molecules (1,2). Whether the peptides are presented in the context of class I or II molecules is largely dependent on the source of the antigen: exogenous antigens entering antigen-presenting cells (APCs) via the endosomal system are primarily processed into peptides expressed on Class II molecules, whereas peptides from proteins found in the rough endoplasmic reticulum and cytoplasm of cells are expressed on MHC class I (3,4). The separate compartmentalization of antigen derived from exogenous versus endogenous sources results in the presentation of antigen to different T-cell subsets depending on which pathway the antigen utilizes: $CD4^+$ T cells, which provide paracrine "help" in the form of lymphokine secretion, recognize antigen in the context of MHC class II, whereas $CD8^+$ T cells, which mediate target cell-specific cytotoxic T-lymphocyte (CTL) lytic activity, recognize antigen presented on class I molecules. Thus, $CD8^+$ CTL lyse those cells that actively express foreign antigens, such as tumor cells, virus-infected cells, or cells that harbor intracellular pathogens. APCs, displaying peptides acquired from the extracellular environment in the context of class II MHC molecules, protect themselves from lysis by $CD8^+$ CTL while presenting antigen to $CD4^+$ "helper" T cells. However, the exogenous pathway of antigen presentation is apparently somewhat leaky: although the presentation of antigen acquired from the extracellular environment is primarily on class II molecules, presentation on class I molecules is also possible (5–7). Accordingly, presentation of antigen mediated by APCs in the context of MHC class I is apparently responsible for the generation of $CD8^+$ CTL in vivo against a class

I-deficient variant of the B16-F10 melanoma, and restoration of class I expression by transfection of the tumor cell did not improve the level of CTL generated (8).

L. monocytogenes is capable of infecting APCs, such as macrophages in vivo, and is actively phagocytosed by macrophages in vitro (9). Macrophage phagocytosis is facilitated by binding of *L. monocytogenes* to type I scavenger receptors, which recognize lipoteichoic acid (10). The complement system also aids uptake of *L. monocytogenes*: components C1q and C3b significantly increase phagocytosis, even when obtained from naive serum (11). Soon after uptake by nonactivated macrophages, *L. monocytogenes*-containing phagosomes are acidified as a consequence of fusion with lysosomes (12). Phagolysosome formation leads to killing of approximately 90% of the microorganisms (12), but also leads to activation of the hemolytic pore-forming protein listeriolysin O (LLO), which is active at acidic, but not at neutral, pH (13). As a consequence of LLO activation, some phagolysosomes are ruptured, allowing entry of the bacteria into the cytoplasm, where growth can occur (12,14). Thus, infection with *L. monocytogenes* leads to the infection of APCs and introduction of listerial proteins to both the endosomal and cytoplasmic antigen-processing pathways for presentation on class II and I MHC molecules, respectively.

Lysis of the phagolysosome is apparently required for the presentation of antigen by MHC class I molecules. A macrophage-derived cell line was rendered susceptible to lysis by antigen-specific $CD8^+$ CTL when infected with LLO-expressing, but not LLO-deficient, *L. monocytogenes* (15). In a more sensitive assay, interleukin-2 (IL-2) production by antigen-specific $CD8^+$ T-cell hybridomas was measured following culture with thioglycollate-elicited macrophages. The ability of the macrophages to present listerial antigens to the T-cell hybridomas was again associated with LLO expression. Although the LLO-deficient *L. monocytogenes* strain was capable of inducing levels of IL-2 production comparable to the level induced by macrophages infected with LLO-expressing *L. monocytogenes*, the dose of LLO-deficient *L. monocytogenes* required for comparable stimulation was 10,000-fold that of LLO^+ *L. monocytogenes* (16). Infection with LLO-deficient *L. monocytogenes* also failed to endue mice with the ability to form delayed-type hypersensitivity (DTH) reactions, as measured by footpad swelling in response to challenge with listerial antigen six days after i.v. infection, even though the dose tested was almost 1,000-

fold greater than the dose of LLO$^+$ *L. monocytogenes* required to induce a maximal DTH response (17).

In addition to escape from the phagolysosome, cell-to-cell spread by *L. monocytogenes* (18,19) (see Chapter 4, *this volume*) may actually be required for presentation of antigen on class II MHC molecules (16). Thioglycollate-elicited macrophages of one MHC haplotype were infected in vitro, washed, and then cultured with thioglycollate-elicited macrophages expressing a different MHC haplotype, in the presence of gentamicin to prevent extracellular growth of *L. monocytogenes*. By measuring the stimulation of *L. monocytogenes*-specific T-cell hybridomas restricted to one or the other MHC haplotype, Hiltbold and associates (16) were able to determine whether the cells infected by the extracellular route or through cell-to-cell spread were presenting antigen within the context of either MHC class I or II. These investigators found that while LLO-expressing *L. monocytogenes* delivered antigen to the class I pathway after both routes of infection, only macrophages infected by cell-to-cell spread presented antigen within the context of class II. If multiple cycles of infection are necessary in vivo for APCs to fully stimulate T cells, that may in part explain the ability of killed *L. monocytogenes* to immunize mice weakly or not at all (9,20–22). However, an ActA-deficient strain of *L. monocytogenes*, which lacks the ability to induce host cell actin polymerization and consequent cell-to-cell spreading from one infected cell directly to another, was shown to be capable of stimulating CD8$^+$ T-cell-mediated CTL, and perhaps also stimulation of CD4$^+$ T cells (23). This study did not compare the immunopotentiating activity of the actA mutant to wild-type *L. monocytogenes*.

7.3 VACCINES FOR THE INDUCTION OF CELL-MEDIATED IMMUNITY: THE IMPORTANCE OF APCs

For activation of cell-mediated immune responses, naive T cells must encounter the peptide–MHC complex in the presence of costimulatory signals such as CD80 or CD86, formerly known as B7-1 and B7-2 (24–26). Indeed, exposure to antigen in the absence of co-stimulation can actually lead to anergy or the generation of a Th2 pattern of cytokine production (27,28). Although it is possible for a T cell to recognize antigen on one cell while receiving costimulation from a different cell, optimal stimulation seems to occur when the peptide–MHC complex is on the same cell as the co-stimulatory ligand (29). APCs such as macrophages, which can present antigen within the context of MHC class I and II and express co-stimulatory ligands, are therefore important for the activation of antigen-specific T-cell clones.

A significant role for APC in generating cell-mediated immunity is demonstrated in cancer vaccination studies using irradiated B16-F10 melanoma cells transduced to express a panel of cytokine genes. These studies showed that granulocyte-macrophage colony-stimulating factor (GM-CSF)-secreting tumor cells can be considerably more effective at stimulating antitumor immunity than tumor cells secreting lymphokines such as IL-2, IL-4, or IL-6 (30). GM-CSF enhances the antigen-presenting function of APCs (31–36). Thus, one implication of these findings is that vaccine vectors intended to induce T-cell-mediated immune responses perhaps should be designed to enhance the function of APCs, in addition to T cells. Further evidence for the importance of APCs in the generation of CTL responses was obtained in a chimeric mouse model, using irradiated CT-26 colon carcinoma cells transduced to express influenza nucleoprotein (NP) (8). The MHC restriction of the NP-specific CTL generated was found to depend on the MHC haplotype of the bone marrow-derived APCs rather than on the MHC haplotype of the tumor cells, indicating that anti-NP T cells were induced in response to antigen presented by APC, not in response to antigen directly presented by tumor cells.

Dendritic cells have emerged as an important APC for the induction of antigen-reactive T cells, due in part to their ability to express high levels of CD80, CD86, and class II MHC (35–37). The ability of dendritic cells to provide co-stimulation and to secrete immunostimulatory cytokines is potentiated by GM-CSF (35). The expression of tumor antigens by dendritic cells leads to the generation of potent antitumor immunity and antigen-specific CTL responses (38,39). It is unclear whether dendritic cells participate in the generation of antilisterial T-cell responses, but it has been shown that the murine dendritic cell line CB-1 is efficiently infected by wild-type and even internalin-defective *L. monocytogenes* mutants (40). Moreover, transfer of immunogenic peptides from heat-killed *L. monocytogenes* has been reported to occur from interstitial lung macrophages to dendritic cells, which can then present antigen to T cells (41). In addition, GM-CSF, which is known to be an important stimulator and activator of dendritic cells (42,43), has been shown to be significantly upregulated as a consequence of experimentally induced *L. monocytogenes* infection, by both in situ hybridization (44) and semiquantitative polymerase chain reaction (PCR) (44,45). Interestingly, Klink and Rudnicka (46) reported that pregnant mice, which are much more susceptible to lethal infection with *L. monocytogenes*, have greatly reduced ability to form T-cell–dendritic cell clusters, relative to virgin females. These findings indicate that dendritic cells do have the potential to present listerial antigens to T cells. It remains to be established, however, whether dendritic cells actually participate in the presentation of listerial peptides to T cells after the delivery of *L. monocytogenes* either intraperitoneally or to the gut. Indeed, dendritic cell contact with *L. monocytogenes* might not necessarily result in enhanced antigen presentation: a splenic dendritic cell line undergoes apoptosis upon infection with LLO-expressing *L. monocytogenes* strains, or upon treatment with purified LLO (47).

Even if dendritic cells do not play an important role in the presentation of listerial antigens to the immune system, macrophages may be quite effective. Tissue macrophages are often class II negative and lack costimulatory molecules. However, infection with *L. monocytogenes* leads to rapid induction of co-stimulatory molecules (37,48). Moreover, the induction of IL-12 and tumor necrosis factor-α (TNF-α production by macrophages that occurs rapidly following infection with *L. monocytogenes* (see description in Chapter 4) activates NK cells to produce interferon-γ (IFN-γ), which can stimulate MHC Class II expression and further upregulates the expression of costimulatory molecules (37). In addition, IFN-γ can also upregulate expression of MHC class I and the antigen processing machinery (49).

7.4 *Listeria monocytogenes* IS A POTENT INDUCER OF Th1-TYPE RESPONSES

$CD4^+$ T-cell responses can be functionally divided into two categories characterized by somewhat distinct patterns of cytokine secretion (50). The Th1 subset is defined by production of IL-2, IFN-γ, and TNF-β, whereas Th2 cells produce IL-4, IL-5, IL-6, IL-10, and IL-13. Some cytokines, such as TNF-α, GM-CSF, and IL-3 are produced by both subsets (51–53). Th1 cytokine responses lead to the generation of cell-mediated immune responses and macrophage activation, while Th2 cytokine responses provide help for IgE production and eosinophil proliferative responses. Recently, $CD8^+$ cells have been shown to produce cytokines in patterns similar to those of $CD4^+$ cells, supporting the notion that the Th1 and Th2 cytokine secretion patterns are characteristic of all T cells (54).

Certain immunomodulatory cytokines associated with either the Th1 or Th2 responses are inhibitory for the reciprocal Th subset: IL-12, which upregulates Th1 responses, also downregulates Th2 responses, while IL-4 suppresses Th1 responses and stimulates Th2 responses (54–56). Likewise, IL-10 inhibits production of IL-12. As a consequence of this cross-regulation, immune responses can quickly become biased toward a Th1 or Th2 pattern of cytokine production.

Whether an immune response is protective against a particular pathogen can be determined by the type of T-helper cell response induced, as was demonstrated in experimental *Leishmania major* infections in mice (57–59). Infection of C57Bl/6 mice with *L. major* results in rapid clearance and a Th1-type response. By contrast, infection of BALB/c mice, which is fatal for this strain, leads to the generation of a Th2 response. The susceptibility of BALB/c mice to infection with *L. major* could be overcome by treatment with IL-12 (60), and treatment of infected BALB/c mice with anti-IL-4 neutralizing antibody significantly reduced the severity of infection (58). Conversely, in some instances, Th2 responses can be protective and Th1 responses associated with disease progression. For example, infection of resistant BALB/k mice with the helminth *Trichuris muris*, an enteric parasite, results in clearance of worms and protection against reinfection, whereas susceptible AKR mice develop persistent infections. Anti-IFN-γ antibody treatment or systemic IL-4 administration rendered susceptible mice resistant, whereas neutralization of IL-4 in resistant mice resulted in persistent infection (61). Likewise, the protective Th2-type immune response generated in BALB/c mice against the parasitic nematode *Nippostrongylus brasiliensis* can be reversed to a Th1 response by treatment with IL-12, exacerbating infection (62).

The Th1/Th2 dichotomy may actually be an oversimplification, since many T-cell clones produce patterns of cytokines inconsistent with the model (51). Nevertheless, it remains true that the general pattern of cytokine production can directly affect whether cell-mediated immune responses are generated. Moreover, the ability of Th2-associated cytokine responses to downregulate Th1 responses may account for some instances of immunosuppression (63–66).

IL-12 is a potent inducer of Th1-type responses and has been described as a Th1 inducing factor (67–69). Indeed, tumor bearing mice were cured simply by administration of IL-12, and this effect was mediated primarily by T cells (70,71). Infection with *L. monocytogenes* is associated with the rapid production of IL-12 and, as a consequence, strongly biases the development of immune responses toward a Th1-like pattern (67) (for a detailed description, see Chapter 4).

7.5 THE IMMUNE RESPONSE TO ORAL INFECTION WITH *Listeria monocytogenes:* ARE ANTIBODIES IMPORTANT?

L. monocytogenes can induce potent cell-mediated immune responses when delivered orally (72–74). However, even though the gut is the natural site of infection (75), most studies of experimental listeriosis have delivered the microorganism i.v. or i.p. Thus, comparatively little is known about the immune response to *L. monocytogenes* at the intestinal mucosa. Pathogenic strains of *L. monocytogenes* are believed to initially infect intestinal epithelium after endocytotic internalization, which results from binding of the *L. monocytogenes* surface proteins internalin A and internalin B to the E-cadherin receptor expressed on the lumenal surface of epithelial cells (18,76–78). After invasion of the epithelium, the infection apparently spreads to the Peyer's patches (79,80). Penetration beyond the epithelial layer, eventually leading to infection of mesenteric lymph nodes, the spleen, and the liver, requires the expression of hemolysin (81). Within the Peyer's patches, bacterial replication occurs in the cytoplasm of mononuclear cells, possibly macrophages or dendritic cells (80). It is conceivable that these infected cells leave the Peyer's patches and circulate to other lymphoid organs, perhaps spreading the infection at the same time.

Monoclonal antibody treatment studies indicate that neutralization of IFN-γ, TNF-α, or IL-6 increases the number of detectable bacteria in the mesenteric lymph nodes after intragastric delivery of *L. monocytogenes* (82). Conlan (83) reported that depletion of TNF-α or neutrophils greatly increased the number of bacteria recovered from all gastrointestinal tissues tested, including stomach, Peyer's patches, small and large intestine, and cecum, as well as the liver and spleen. Thus, the immunological mechanisms involved in control of listeriosis appear similar regardless of the route of initial infection (84) (for a review of the mechanisms of protection against listeriosis, see Chapter 4).

Although bacteremia can sometimes occur during listeriosis, growth of *L. monocytogenes* largely occurs within infected host cells, with direct cell-to-cell spread enabling the microorganism to avoid exposure to antibodies contained in the extracellular milieu. Oral infection with *L. monocytogenes* sometimes results in the generation of a serum antibody response (9,85,86), but the ability of antibodies to protect against oral infection has not been clearly demonstrated. Once an *L. monocytogenes* infection is established in the protected intracellular environment, antibodies are probably ineffective.

It is possible that a high anti-*L. monocytogenes* antibody titer in the lumen of the gut could block binding to intestinal epithelium, preventing initiation or infection. To block attachment, a humoral response would need to target surface proteins involved in binding to epithelial cells, such as internalin A and B (the role of these proteins for initiation of infection is reviewed in ref. 18). In a recent comparative study, LLO and IrpA protein were identified as the most commonly recognized proteins by serum antibodies from healthy individuals who had been exposed to *L. monocytogenes* (antibodies were not detected in serum from randomly selected donors) (87). IrpA is a recently described 30-kD secreted protein with sequence similarities to internalin A and B (88). It is unclear whether IrpA is involved in attachment and invasion, however, and four additional internalin-like proteins recently identified apparently are not required for invasion of various cell lines, based on studies with deletion mutants (89). The only healthy volunteer whose serum contained antibody to internalin B protein was a researcher studying the overexpression of this protein (87). Significantly, the serum antibodies specific for *L. monocytogenes*-derived proteins were IgG, and IgA antibodies were not detected in the serum samples, consistent with a polarized Th1 immune response. Taken together, these findings suggest that pre-existing antibody responses are not likely to be a significant obstacle to immunization with a live *L. monocytogenes* vaccine.

7.6 RATIONALE FOR THE USE OF *Listeria monocytogenes* AS AN EXPERIMENTAL LIVE VACCINE VECTOR

Cell-mediated immune responses are particularly important for clearance of viruses, tumors, and intracellular infections. Vaccines that selectively potentiate cell-mediated immunity are therefore of substantial interest (90–92). Taken together, the processes that occur during the course of infection with *L. monocytogenes* make it a "potentially ideal" live immunization vector for the generation of cell-mediated immune responses (92). Upon infection, *L. monocytogenes* enters the APCs, including macrophages. As a consequence of the escape of a fraction of the phagocytosed bacteria from the phagolysosome into the cytoplasm, listerial antigens are delivered to endosomes and also the cell cytoplasm. This allows the potential presentation of antigen secreted by *L. monocytogenes* within the context of both class I and II MHC molecules. The Th1-like pattern of cytokines induced upon infection of macrophages with *L. monocytogenes*, including IL-12, IFN-γ, and TNF-α, can enhance antigen presentation by these infected cells, and also bias the ensuing immune response in the direction of cell-mediated immunity. Moreover, a cell-mediated immune response can be induced by oral immunization, in addition to i.v. or i.p. routes of delivery, adding to the potential value of *L. monocytogenes* as a live vaccine vector.

7.7 EFFICACY OF *Listeria monocytogenes* AS A LIVE VACCINE VECTOR

The ability of a recombinant *L. monocytogenes* to function as a vaccine vector was first established in 1992, using a mutant strain transgenic for the β-galactosidase gene of *Escherichia coli* (72). Infection either orally or intraperitoneally was shown to induce a β-galactosidase-specific CTL response, as determined by MHC-restricted lysis of β-galactosidase-expressing tumor cells. A drawback of this system, however, was that the transgene was expressed at fairly low levels and was not secreted into the host cell cytoplasm. Although this report demonstrated that secretion of listerial antigens is not a strict requirement for the stimulation of cell-mediated immunity, the level of cytolytic activity generated was in fact quite weak, as the effector population required several weeks of in vitro stimulation before demonstrating a significant CTL response. (The probable importance of target antigen secretion to the construction of effective live *L. monocytogenes* vaccine vectors is discussed in detail in Chapter 4, *this volume*.) It should be noted, however, that secretion of antigen may not always be required. Shen and associates (93) demonstrated that an *L. monocytogenes* recombinant expressing a lymphocytic choriomeningitis virus (LCMV)-NP epitope can efficiently prime $CD8^+$ T-cell responses even in the absence of secretion of the antigen, although secretion does appear to be required for recognition of infected cells by CTL. Likewise, Paglia and colleagues (74) have shown that oral immunization with *L. monocytogenes* strains that express a model tumor antigen as either a secreted or as a cytoplasmic protein induce equivalent levels of protective antitumor immunity against tumor cells expressing the same antigen.

7.8 ANTIVIRAL RESPONSES INDUCED BY RECOMBINANT *Listeria monocytogenes* VACCINES

To maximize delivery of the target antigen to the cytoplasm of recombinant *L. monocytogenes*-infected cells, a fusion protein strategy was devised, using the first 420 amino acids of the secreted listerial protein, LLO, including the promoter and signal sequence fused to the NP gene of influenza (15). The fusion gene was cloned into a shuttle vector that was capable of replicating in gram-positive and gram-negative organisms. In order to force the retention of the plasmid in vivo, the gene coding for the transcriptional activator PrfA was included on the plasmid and the construct used to transform a replication defective *prfA*(−) *L. monocytogenes* strain. The transformant retained the plasmid stably in vivo and efficiently secreted the fusion protein. Infection of mice with the mutant *L. monocytogenes* secreting the LLO-NP fusion protein (Lm-NP) led to in vivo priming of CTL (15). More importantly, the anti-NP immune response induced by Lm-NP was found to be protective against viral infection at the mucosal surface of the lungs (94). Mice immunized with *L. monocytogenes* mutants expressing the influenza virus nucleoprotein were subsequently infected intranasally with influenza virus. Pulmonary viral titers were substantially reduced in immunized mice, relative to naive mice or mice infected with wild-type *L. monocytogenes*. Moreover, the magnitude of reduction of viral titer in the lungs was at least as large in Lm-NP immunized mice as in mice infected with a vaccinia virus carrying the influenza nucleoprotein gene.

Recombinant *L. monocytogenes* mutants have also been shown to effectively protect mice against challenge with lymphocytic choriomeningitis virus (LCMV) (23,95). Goosens and associates (23) constructed a plasmid encoding a fusion protein consisting of the NP gene of LCMV connected in-frame to the signal sequence of the *L. monocytogenes* hemolysin gene. Unlike the LLO-influenza fusion protein constructed by Ikonomidis and coworkers, no attempts were made to force the retention of the plasmid in vivo by including an essential virulence factor on the plasmid. Undoubtedly, this would result in loss of expression of the foreign protein in vivo. Nevertheless, attenuated *L. monocytogenes* mutants transfected with this construct were shown to induce a strong $CD8^+$ T-cell-mediated anti-LCMV cytolytic response, which was detectable in splenocytes and lymphoid cells isolated from the livers of i.v.-immunized mice. Moreover, mice immunized with LCMV-NP-secreting *L. monocytogenes* mutants were protected from a lethal intracerebral challenge with LCMV. This was the first demonstration that immunization with *L. monocytogenes* could induce protective immunity against a replicating pathogen.

Using the same viral antigen system, Shen and associates (95) also found that immunization with recombinant *L. monocytogenes* secreting the NP gene of LCMV induced protective antiviral immunity in vivo mediated by $CD8^+$ T cells. In addition, they described a system which allows site-specific integration of the transgene construct into the *L. monocytogenes* chromosome at a site between transcription regulons, thereby allowing the generation of stable mutants without disrupting expression of listerial genes. Subsequently, these investigators reported that the mice retained elevated numbers of CTL precursors for as long as 170 days after immunization with recombinant *L. monocytogenes* (96).

An exciting possibility is that protective CTL could be induced against the human immunodeficiency virus (HIV) by recombinant *L. monocytogenes* vectors. To date, most efforts to develop anti-HIV vaccines have focused on the induction of antibody responses, even though antibody responses are produced in vivo in response to infection and are not associated with clearance of the infection. Since HIV, like *L. monocytogenes*, is an intracellular pathogen which can spread through direct cell-to-cell contact (97), it is reasonable to expect that cell-mediated immunity is crucial for the control of HIV infection. In fact, cell-mediated immunity has been suggested as the pivotal determinant in controlling the progression of HIV infection (98). In this model, a switch from a predominantly Th1-type pattern of cytokine response to a Th2 pattern is responsible for increased susceptibility to HIV. Although quantitative differences in Th subsets were not detected as a function of disease progression (99), leading some investigators to challenge the Th1-to-Th2 model of HIV progression, it is nevertheless possible that a shift occurred but simply was not detectable (100). Longitudinal studies of anti-HIV CTL responses indicate a correlation between disease status and cell-mediated immunity: HIV-seropositive subjects undergoing progression to AIDS rapidly lost the ability to mount HIV-Gag-specific CTL responses, unlike long-term asymptomatic HIV-seropositive subjects (101). Likewise, Barker and associates (102) found that the $CD8^+$ T cells of long-term HIV seropositive subjects exhibited a threefold higher ability to suppress HIV replication in an in vitro viral infection assay. The ability of these $CD8^+$ cells to inhibit viral replication was enhanced by exposure to IL-2 and inhibited by exposure to IL-4 or IL-10 (102).

Because of the possibility that T cells may be important for controlling existing HIV infections, vaccine vectors capable of stimulating potent anti-HIV cell-mediated immune responses are of considerable interest (91). To test the ability of recombinant *L. monocytogenes* to induce anti-HIV CTL, mutants stably expressing the Gag protein of HIV type 1 were constructed by Frankel and colleagues (103). Consistent with the results from other antigen systems, these investigators found strong $CD8^+$ T-cell-mediated cytolytic responses against target cells expressing Gag or pulsed with synthesized Gag peptides. Because vaccination with *L. monocytogenes* can result in protective memory T cell responses (96), it is conceivable that prophylactic, as well as therapeutic, immunization could be achieved with this vector. Jonas Salk and colleagues (90) argued that effective prophylactic vaccines against HIV might preferentially target cell-mediated immunity, rather than an antibody response. Although immunization strategies do exist which induce both CTL and antibody responses (e.g., 104), it is generally true that vaccination conditions cannot be simultaneously optimized for both types of response (105). Thus, although systemic infection with *L. monocytogenes* can, in fact, lead to the generation of antibodies against not only listerial proteins (9,106), but also against an inserted target antigen (72,106), in general humoral responses to antigens delivered by *L. monocytogenes*, when immunized parenterally, are very weak. The inability of *L. monocytogenes* to induce strong antibody responses can be easily reconciled with its intracellular location and ability to spread from cell to cell, sequestering the organism from the humoral arm of the immune response.

7.9 ANTITUMOR IMMUNE RESPONSES INDUCED BY *Listeria monocytogenes*

The availability of tumor cells retrovirally transduced to express influenza NP (8) enabled evaluation of Lm-NP as an anticancer vaccine, in the CT26 colon tumor model and the Renca renal cell carcinoma model (106). Infection of mice with wild-type *L. monocytogenes* (Lm-WT) did not affect the growth rate of CT26-NP or Renca-NP. By contrast, mice previously immunized by infection with Lm-NP were completely protected against subsequent challenge with 100 times the minimal length tumor dose of Renca-NP cells. Most Lm-NP immunized mice challenged with CT26-NP also resisted challenge, and even the Lm-NP mice in which CT26-NP did grow exhibited substantially inhibited tumor growth. The parental tumor cell lines Renca and CT26, which lack NP expression, exhibited identical growth kinetics in mice previously infected with Lm-NP or Lm-WT, or in naive mice. Thus, infection with Lm-NP was shown to induce a potent anti-NP immune response capable of protecting mice against challenge with tumor cells expressing the model tumor antigen NP. This antitumor immunity was shown to be mediated principally by $CD8^+$ T cells, as depletion of these cells before tumor cell challenge abrogated the ability of Lm-NP-immunized mice to resist challenge with CT26-NP cells.

Infection with Lm-NP not only confers resistance to subsequent tumor challenge, but even leads to regression of established tumors (106). Mice bearing Renca-NP tumors were injected i.p. with Lm-NP, Lm-WT, or saline beginning 13 days after tumor inoculation. Infection with Lm-NP led to complete regression of tumors in 9 of 10 mice, whereas treatment with Lm-WT had no effect on the rate of tumor progression. Thus, *L. monocytogenes* represents an effective vector for cure of mice bearing established Renca tumors. The elimination of macroscopic tumors in the absence of an adjunctive treatment such as chemotherapy was an unprecedented result, illustrating the potency of *L. monocytogenes* as a therapeutic vaccine.

The Renca-NP-cured mice were subsequently challenged with Renca or Renca-NP and were found to resist challenge with Renca-NP completely, although Renca grew aggressively (106), indicating that the antitumor immunity that had been induced was specific for the model tumor antigen NP. The phenomenon of epitope spreading (107), in which an ongoing immune response leads to the recognition of additional epitopes other than those against which the immune response was initially induced, apparently did not occur after immunization with these live recombinant *L. monocytogenes* mutants. This is further evidenced by the outcome of experiments designed to test whether Lm-NP could induce regression of established CT26-NP tumors (106). Unlike Renca-NP, macroscopic CT26-NP tumors were not eradicated following treatment of the tumor bearers with Lm-NP. This was apparently due to loss of expression of NP by the tumor cells, which are removed from in vitro antibiotic selection for NP expression when they are injected into the mice. Nevertheless, in the CT26-NP model, unlike the Renca-NP model, Lm-NP immunization can result in some protection against the parental CT26 tumor line (Z.-K. Pan, L. M. Weiskirch, and Y. Paterson, unpublished observations). It is conceivable that the anti-NP immune response induced by immunization with Lm-NP provides "bystander" help for the generation of effector cells specific for endogenous tumor antigens expressed by the CT26 cells.

We have evaluated the role of cytokines in the antitumor immune response induced by immunization with Lm-NP (L. M. Weiskirch, Z.-K. Pan, G. Beatty, and Y. Paterson, unpublished observations). Initially, we measured cytokine production in the tumor nodules of Lm-NP treated mice by reverse transcription-polymerase chain reaction (RT-PCR). We found expression of a number of cytokines consistent with the generation of a cell-mediated immune response, including IL-12, IFN-γ, TNF-α, and IL-2. Interestingly, we also detected mRNA for IL-4. The production of these cytokines was at least partially non-specific, since they were also detectable in tumor nodules from mice treated with a recombinant strain of *L. monocytogenes*, Lm-Gag, which expresses an irrelevant viral antigen, the Gag protein of HIV. Nevertheless, Lm-NP treatment was far more effective at inhibiting tumor growth than Lm-Gag treatment. The cytokines induced by infection with *L. monocytogenes* appear to contribute to inhibition of tumor growth, which may explain why Lm-Gag-treated mice also exhibited a weak, but statistically significant, ability to slow tumor progression. The importance of these cytokines for the antitumor immune response was confirmed in mice that had previously been immunized with Lm-NP and were subsequently challenged with CT26-NP tumor cells. Cytokines were neutralized by treatment with specific monoclonal antibodies. In this way, the effect of the cytokine depletion on the anti-NP immune response could be dissociated from the clearance of the initial *L. monocytogenes* infection, which is known to require many of these cytokines. We found that depletion of IL-12, IFN-γ, TNF-α, IL-2 and even IL-4 abrogated or greatly reduced the ability of the previously immunized mice to resist the subsequent challenge. Although it is not yet known which cells in the tumor nodules are producing the cytokine message detected by RT-PCR, the tumor nodules are heavily infiltrated by T cells of both the CD8 and CD4 subsets (106).

Paglia and associates (74) have shown that in a second model tumor antigen system, vaccination with *L. monocytogenes* can protect mice against a subsequent tumor challenge. Mice were infected orally with strains of recombinant *L. monocytogenes* expressing an immunodominant epitope of *E. coli* β-galactosidase and then challenged with a fibrosarcoma retrovirally transduced to express β-galactosidase. Pre-immunization with recombinant *L. monocytogenes* was shown to be more protective against subsequent tumor challenge than either immunization with peptide in complete Freund's adjuvant or by loading dendritic cells with the peptide. Since Paglia and co-workers used a strain of *L. monocytogenes* deficient in the virulence-associated metalloprotease, this study also demonstrates the feasibility of using attenuated mutants to induce a protective antitumor immune response.

Immunization with *L. monocytogenes* recombinants can also protect animals from virus-induced tumor formation (108). Rabbits reproducibly undergo papilloma formation upon experimental infection with cottontail rabbit papillomavirus (CRPV). In this study, all rabbits initially developed papillomas after CRPV infection. However, the papillomas often regressed in rabbits previously immunized with *L. monocytogenes* recombinants secreting overlapping fragments of the CRPV E1 protein. By contrast, the papillomas continued to progress in size, and regression was not observed, in rabbits immunized with wild-type *L. monocytogenes*.

Although the number of examples of the use of *L. monocytogenes* as a vaccine vector is quite small compared with bacillus Calmette-Guérin (BCG) (see Chapter 5) or *Salmonella* (see Chapter 6), taken together the studies described above and summarized in Table 7.1 clearly demonstrate the efficacy of this vector.

7.10 GENETIC STRATEGIES USED TO GENERATE RECOMBINANT VACCINE STRAINS OF *Listeria monocytogenes*

The initial demonstration that *L. monocytogenes* could function as a vaccine vector employed a strain generated by transposon-mediated random chromsomal insertion of the β-galactosidase gene of *Escherichia coli* (72). As noted earlier, the β-galactosidase expression system did not induce optimal immunity, because fairly low levels of antigen were expressed, and the antigen was not secreted. Lm-NP was consequently designed to facilitate secretion of the transgene (15). A fusion gene was constructed consisting of the promoter, an upstream regulatory sequence, and the first 420 amino acids of LLO followed by NP. Thus, the LLO-NP fusion protein would be expected to be a secreted protein with regulation similar to that of LLO: strong expression in the phagolysosome and perhaps also in the host cell cytoplasm. The LLO-NP fusion protein was designed to be nonhemolytic; functional LLO would be made by the intact chromsomal copy of *hly* (Fig. 7.1). The gene encoding PrfA, a virulence regulator that controls the expression of *hly* and other genes required for intracellular replication (Table 7.2) was also cloned into this plasmid. The plasmid was then

TABLE 7.1 Know Vaccines Using *Listeria monocytogenes* As a Vector

Antigen Transgene	Location of Transgene	Regulation of Transgene	Reference
β-galactosidase, *Escherichia coli*	Chromosome (random insertion by transpon)	—	72
Gag, HIV	Chromosome (targeted recombinant)	*hly* promoter	103
Nucleoprotein, LCMV	Plasmid	*hly* promoter	23
Nucleoprotein, influenza	Plasmid	*hly* promoter	73,94,106
Nucleoprotein, LCMV	Chromosome (targeted recombinant)	*hly*, *actA* promoters	93,95,96
E1, Cottontail rabbit papillomavirus	Chromosome (targeted recombinant)	*hly* promoter	108
β-Galactosidase, *E. coli*	Plasmid	Streptococcal proteinase promoter	74
Green fluorescent protein, chloramphenicol acetyltransferase, ovalbumin peptide	Plasmid	Cytomegalovirus promoter	109

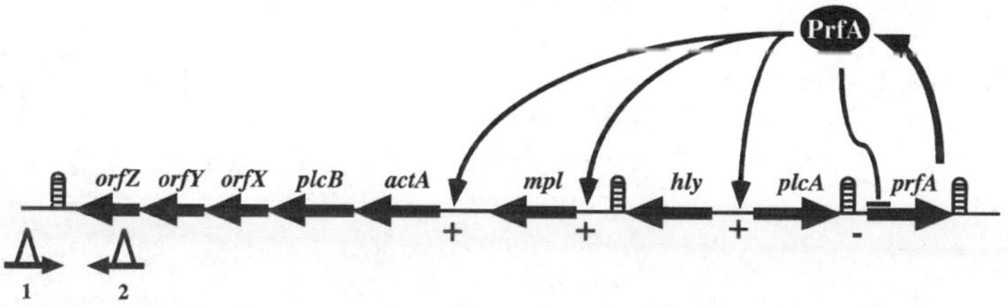

Figure 7.1 The PrfA regulon of *Listeria monocytogenes*. Adapted from Sheehan et al. (18). Expression of the virulence genes *actA*, *hly*, *mpl*, and *plcB*, along with *plcA* and open reading frames *X*, *Y*, and *Z* is upregulated by *prfA*, which also inhibits its own expression. Transcription termination signals follow *hly*, *orfZ*, *plcA*, and *prfA*. 1, site of insertion of expression cassette used by Shen and associates (95); 2, site of insertion of expression cassette, as depicted in Figure 7.2 (Z.-J. Yao and Y. Paterson, unpublished observations). The principal functions of the virulence factors of *L. monocytogenes* is described in Table 7.2

electroporated into a PrfA-deficient derivative of wild-type *L. monocytogenes*. Since PrfA is required for listerial escape from phagosomes and cell-to-cell spreading in infected host cells, it was thought that plasmid retention would be positively selected.

A disadvantage of the PrfA-expressing plasmid system developed by Ikonomidis and associates (15) is that loss of the transgene-containing plasmid remains a possibility. An alternative strategy to maintain retention of the transgene involves targeted recombination into the *L. monocytogenes* chromosome (Fig. 7.2). This approach allows the efficient generation of recombinants that have stable expression of the transgene, enabling construction of recombinant strains which lack antibiotic resistance markers. Targeted recombination was employed independently by Frankel and associates (103), who generated Lm-

TABLE 7.2 Principal Virulence Factors of *Listeria monocytogenes*

Virulence Factor Name	Gene	Principle Function(s)	Cellular Location	Reference
ActA	*actA*	Actin polymerization for cell-to-cell spreading	Cell surface	110,111
ClpC ATPase	*clpC*	Phagolysosome escape	—	112,113
InlA, B	*inlA, B*	Attachment	Cell surface	18,78
Listeriolysin O (LLO) (hemolysin)	*hly*	Phagolysosome escape	Secreted	114–116
Metalloprotease	*mpl*	Maturation of PC-PLC	Intracellular	117
PC-PLC; lecithinase	*plcB*	Escape from double-membrane vesicle during cell-to-cell spreading	Secreted	114
PI-PLC	*plcA*	Phagolysosome escape	Secreted	118
PrfA	*prfA*	Transcriptional regulator	Intracellular	114
p60	*iap*	Attachment, septation	Secreted	119,120

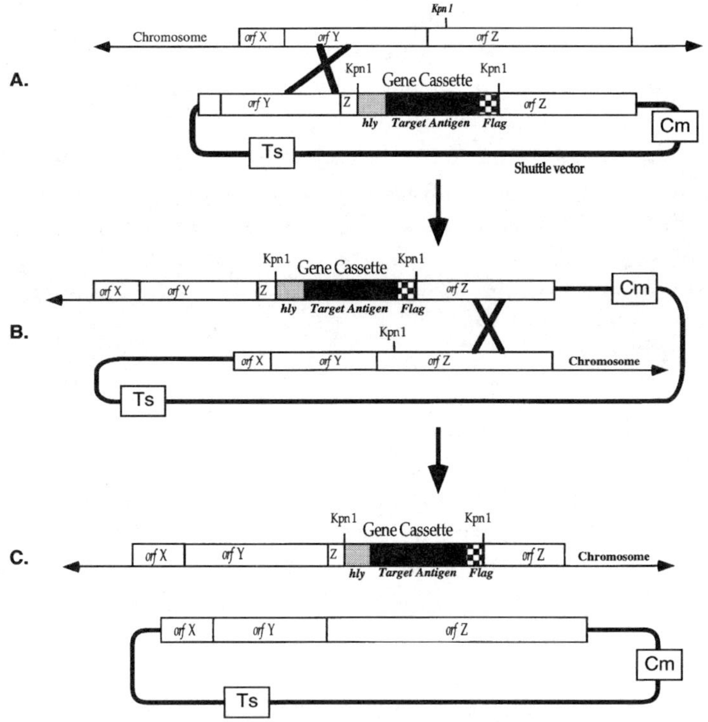

Figure 7.2 Targeted insertion of an expression cassette into the *Listeria monocytogenes* chromosome by homologous recombination. A shuttle vector, derived from pSKV7 contains an expression cassette consisting of a target antigen (*solid box)* connected in-frame to a portion of the *hly* gene, including the promoter and upstream elements as well as the 5′ portion of the coding region, including the signal sequence (*speckled box*). More recent constructs developed by Z.-J. Yao and Y. Paterson also feature an in-frame epitope tag, Flag (*checkered box*) at the C-terminal end, to facilitate detection of the transgenic protein produced by *L. monocytogenes* recombinants. The expression cassette is flanked on either side by sequences homologous to the *orfXYZ* region of the prfA regulon (Fig. 7.1). Integration of the expression cassette occurs when the plasmid undergoes two successive homologous recombination events, one on each side of the cassette (A, B). After the double recombination, the expression cassette remains on the *L. monocytogenes* chromosome, within *orfZ*, while the remainder of the shuttle vector is released from the chromosome (C). Successful insertion of the expression cassette is verified by (i) loss of chloramphenicol resistance; (ii) detection of the transgene in chromosomal DNA by PCR; (iii) demonstration of secretion of the target antigen by western blot. This process of targeted insertion is described in greater detail in the text (see Section 7.10).

Gag, an HIV-Gag-expressing *L. monocytogenes* recombinant, and Shen and associates (95), who generated a series of recombinant strains expressing the NP protein of lymphoid choriomeningitis virus (LCMV) or its immunodominant epitope. Frankel and associates targeted an uncharacterized region of the chromosome, which at the time was believed to be nonessential for replication of *L. monocytogenes*. Initially, this region, isolated as a 2.7-kilobase (kb) *hin*dIII restriction fragment, was inserted into a shuttle vector containing a temperature-sensitive origin of replication. Next, the expression cassette, consisting of the HIV-*gag* gene fused in-frame to the promoter and signal sequence of LLO, was inserted into the 2.7-kb region homologous to chromosomal DNA. Finally, this plasmid was electroporated into wild-type *L. monocytogenes*, and serial passages were performed under conditions of temperature or antibiotic selection, causing a two-step recombination process that inserts the 2.7-kb homology region plus the expression cassette into the *L. monocytogenes* chromosome. The plasmid, which carries the chloramphenicol resistance marker, was first positively selected by culture in the presence of chloramphenicol. Next, the chloramphenicol-resistant transfectants were grown at 40°C, preventing replication of the temperature-sensitive plasmid. Thus, *L. monocytogenes* cells in which the plasmid has recombined into the chromosome (most likely in the 2.7-kb homology region) are positively selected. Subsequently, the culture is passaged repeatedly in the absence of chloramphenicol, to allow a second recombination event to eliminate all the plasmid DNA, except for the region of homology containing the transgene expression cassette. Successful insertion was verified by determination of (i) loss of chloramphenicol resistance, indicating excision of the remainder of the plasmid; (ii) presence of the transgene expression cassette, as determined by PCR of chromosomal DNA; and (iii) secretion of the transgene, as determined by Western blot. A similar strategy of homologous recombination was employed by Shen and colleagues (95), targeting a more defined region of the *L. monocytogenes* chromosome adjacent to a predicted transcriptional terminator sequence between the convergent lecithinase and lactate dehydrogenase operons (Fig. 7.1).

In the development of newer generations of recombinant *L. monocytogenes* vaccines, an additional consideration may be which promoter and signal sequence facilitates optimal secretion of the transgene. To date, most investigators have used the LLO promoter and signal sequence. Shen and associates (95) generated LCMV-NP-expressing recombinants using the promoter and signal sequence either from *hly* or *act*A. The promoters of both of these virulence factors are upregulated by the transcriptional activator PrfA. Similar patterns of LCMV-NP transgene secretion were seen with either promoter/signal sequence. For both recombinants, transgene secretion was detected at 37°C but not 22°C, and at neutral but not acidic pH. Moreover, immunization with either construct protected mice against challenge with LCMV, and spleen cells from immunized mice generated potent virus-specific cytotoxic responses in vivo, after LCMV challenge. In addition to these inducible PrfA-controlled genes, constitutively expressed and secreted proteins such as p60 (121) might also be good candidates for targeting transgene secretion.

7.11 FEATURES OF VACCINATION WITH LIVE *Listeria monocytogenes*

Recombinant *L. monocytogenes* expressing specific target antigens can be a highly effective vector for induction of cell-mediated immune responses capable of protecting against challenge with virus or a lethal dose of tumor cells. Moreover, the potent immune response stimulated by infection with *L. monocytogenes* secreting a model tumor antigen was able to eradicate established tumors completely. Infection leads to the generation of transgene-specific CTL (23,72–74,94–96,103,106), as well as DTH responses (23,72). The generation of a potent $CD8^+$ CTL response has been shown against the transgene following immunization not only intraperitoneally (72,74,103,106), but also intravenously (23,94–96). More importantly, oral immunization is also effective (72–74), and levels of CTL generation are comparable after immunization by the oral versus the intraperitoneally route (72). Thus, immunization with *L. monocytogenes* is not only highly effective for the stimulation of CTL responses but may also be easily delivered. The effectiveness of immunization with *L. monocytogenes* recombinants may be due to its ability to induce a potent Th1-like cytokine response, thereby providing both adjuvant and targeted antigen delivery functions. Indeed, Paglia and associates (74) found that oral immunization with an attenuated *L. monocytogenes* recombinant was more effective at inducing antitumor immunity than either peptide immunization in complete Freund's adjuvant or by loading dendritic cells with the peptide.

The kinetics of clearance of recombinant *L. monocytogenes* were analyzed by Slifka and associates (96) after i.v. injection. *L. monocy-*

togenes recombinants persisted for approximately as long as wild-type *L. monocytogenes* in both the spleen and liver; bacteria levels were undetectable by the seventh day postinfection. Pan and associates (73) evaluated the persistence of Lm-NP and Lm-Gag in the gut after oral infection, and found that six days after infection, both recombinant strains of *L. monocytogenes* had been cleared from the liver, spleen, and mesenteric lymph nodes. In addition, elimination of Lm-NP, but not Lm-Gag, had been completed in Peyer's patches. Thus, recombinant *L. monocytogenes*, like wild-type *L. monocytogenes*, is effectively cleared after experimental infection.

7.12 PRACTICAL LIMITATIONS AND SAFETY CONCERNS OF *Listeria*-BASED VACCINES

Although *L. monocytogenes* is a potent inducer of a Th1-like pattern of cytokines and strong T-cell-mediated immune responses, this microorganism is also capable of causing severe, potentially fatal, bacteremia or meningitis, especially in immunocompromised humans (122,123) (see Chapter 4). Consequently, wild-type strains of *L. monocytogenes* engineered to express tumor antigens, although effective at stimulating protective antitumor immunity and even inducing the regression of palpable tumors, probably will not be satisfactory therapeutic vectors for human immunodeficiency virus (HIV) or immunosuppressed cancer patients, even though *L. monocytogenes* infections are readily eliminated by the use of appropriate antibiotics even in immunocompromised patients (124,125). The identification of mutants that retain the potent T-cell stimulatory capacity of wild-type *L. monocytogenes* without pathogenicity will be necessary before the efficacy of this strategy can be tested on humans. Naturally occurring mutants with reduced virulence that protect against subsequent infection with wild-type *L. monocytogenes* have been identified (74,126–128) and rationally attenuated mutants also exist (109,129–130). The safety of these attenuated mutants is unknown for immunocompromised hosts. Moreover, it remains unclear whether the ability of these strains to stimulate anti-listerial immunity will be diminished along with their virulence. *L. monocytogenes* recombinants of reduced virulence do appear to be competent to induce potent CTL responses (15,103). In the case of Lm-NP, which secretes a hemolysin/influenza nucleoprotein fusion protein, the virulence of this organism was about 3 logs lower than wild-type strains. Nevertheless, this mutant was shown to be a potent anticancer and antiviral immunotherapeutic (73,94,106). Paglia and associates (74) reported that pre-immunization with either metalloprotease-deficient or wild-type *L. monocytogenes* strains that express a model tumor antigen induced comparable antitumor immunity when administered orally, but slightly weaker antitumor immunity after i.p. delivery.

The potential clearly exists for the development of rationally attenuated *L. monocytogenes* mutants as well. Goossens and associates (23) have demonstrated that a transposon-insertion mutant defective for the *act*A gene is capable of inducing protective antiviral immunity. More recently, Thompson and associates (130) described the construction of a crippled *L. monocytogenes* mutant which is unable to synthesize D-alanine, an essential cell wall component. These investigators identified two genes, *dal* and *dat*, required for D-alanine synthesis. By inactivating both of these genes, an *L. monocytogenes* strain was generated which could grow only in the presence of exogenously supplied D-alanine. The extent of growth of the dal^-/dat^- *L. monocytogenes* mutant in mice could therefore be controlled by the amount and duration of D-alanine administration.

Another strategy of attenuating *L. monocytogenes* was developed by Dietrich et al. (109). These investigators used a deletion mutant of *L. monocytogenes* that lacks the entire lecithinase operon (Fig. 7.1), including the virulence-associated genes *act*A, *mpl*, and *plcB*. This strain can infect macrophages and replicate in the host cell cytosol but cannot spread to adjacent cells. This attenuated mutant was further weakened by addition of a plasmid containing the gene for lysis protein PLY118 of the listerial bacteriophage A118. PLY118 expression was controlled by the *actA* promoter, which is active when *L. monocytogenes* is in the host cell cytoplasm. Thus, this *L. monocytogenes* mutant escapes from the phagosome and then lyses when the PLY118 gene is expressed in the cytosol. Autolysis of the *L. monocytogenes* mutant apparently releases the plasmid DNA into the host cell cytoplasm, allowing the expression of the transgene by the host cell. The expression of three transgenes, the reporters green fluorescent protein and chloramphenicol acetyltransferase (CAT) and the H-2 K^b-restricted ovalbumin epitope (peptides 257–264), delivered in this manner was detected in an experimentally infected macrophage line by measuring activation of an epitope-specific $CD8^+$ T-cell hybridoma. Conceivably, this approach combines the adjuvancy of *L. monocytogenes* infection with the efficacy of DNA vaccination. It remains to be seen whether these autolytic attenuated mutants are as effective at protecting mice against replicating pathogens as *L. monocytogenes* recombinants derived from wild-type strains.

Epitope spreading, a phenomenon in which an immune response initially induced to specific epitopes eventually spreads to other epitopes not originally targeted, is apparently inconsistently induced by immunization with live recombinant *L. monocytogenes* vaccines. Experimental vaccines do exist that result in the generation of immune responses against alternative antigens expressed on the target cell but not on the immunogen. For example, s.c. immunization of mice with iron oxide beads coupled to ovalabumin induces protective antitumor immunity against B16 melanoma cells transfected with the ovalbumin gene. Mice that successfully resist challenge with ovalbumin-expressing B16 tumor cells were subsequently resistant to rechallenge with the parental B16 tumor cell line (131). By contrast, the protective antitumor immunity elicited by infection with *Listeria* recombinants appears to be specific for the target antigen expressed by *L. monocytogenes*, at least in the Renca tumor system (Z.-K. Pan and Y. Paterson, unpublished observations). Mice immunized against the model tumor antigen influenza nucleoprotein resisted challenge with Renca-NP tumor cells and were subsequently rechallenged with wild-type Renca or the syngeneic CT26-NP tumor cells. Whereas the mice were protected against growth of the CT26-NP tumor cells, which are antigenically unrelated to wild-type Renca cells, the Renca cell line lacking NP grew progressively in these mice which had already rejected a challenge of Renca-NP (Z.-K. Pan and Y. Paterson, unpublished observations). More recently, we have found that Lm-NP immunized mice challenged with CT26-NP tumor cells can sometimes resist a subsequent challenge with the parental CT26 tumor cells (Z.-K. Pan, L. M. Weiskirch and Y. Paterson, unpublished observations). Conceivably, it might be advantageous for a therapeutic vaccine to induce epitope spreading, since recognition of additional epitopes could increase the pool of potentially antigen-reactive T-cell clones and might prevent evasion of the immune response by loss or mutation of the targeted antigen. However, the phenomenon of epitope spreading was defined in models of autoimmunity and is associated with the pathology of pristane-induced arthritis and relapsing experimental autoimmune encephalomyelitis (132).

There are also inherent limitations to the strategy of immunizing against specific tumor- or pathogen-associated antigens. Immunogenic proteins recognized in the context of a wide variety of class I and II HLA molecules must be identified and, in the case of genetically engineered vaccines, the genes must be cloned. Because the possibility always exists that mutants could arise that express altered forms of the targeted antigens, or that have lost expression altogether, antigens chosen for immunization protocols should be essential for maintenance of the malignant phenotype of tumor cells or for the maintenance of virulence in pathogens. A rapidly growing number of immunogenic tumor antigens has already been identified, and some antigens are found on a large proportion of human cancers (133). Some of these tumor-associated antigens are oncogenic (e.g., 134,135), suggesting that their expression necessarily may be stable.

Finally, there may be vector-specific constraints on vaccine design. Secretion of foreign proteins by *L. monocytogenes* is apparently inhibited by acidic or hydrophobic regions (G. R. Gunn and Y. Paterson, unpublished observations); in designing recombinant vectors, we delete the corresponding coding regions from the transgene. In addition, expression of some proteins has substantially reduced listerial virulence. One such *L. monocytogenes* mutant secreted a protein containing a proline-rich region (G. R. Gunn and Y. Paterson, unpublished observations), which conceivably interferes with actin-mediated cell-to-cell spreading. To induce actin polymerization, the virulence factor ActA binds to the profilin-binding cellular protein vasodilator-stimulated phosphoprotein (VASP) (136); microinjection of oligoproline into *L. monocytogenes*-infected cells inhibits actin polymerization and bacterial motility (137). Transgene size also affects successful vaccine construction. The *L. monocytogenes* recombinants we have successfully generated contain transgenes of ≤1.3 kb. To the extent that this size constraint is due to limitations of the *L. monocytogenes* protein synthesis and secretion pathways, use of *L. monocytogenes* as a delivery vehicle for DNA (109) could circumvent this difficulty.

7.13 CONCLUSIONS

L. monocytogenes is a promising candidate therapeutic vaccine vector that naturally infects APCs, targets antigen delivery to both the class I MHC pathway of endogenous antigen presentation and also to the class II pathway of exogenous antigen presentation. At the same time, *L. monocytogenes*-induced cytokines are capable of not only enhancing antigen presentation function, but also inducing a Th1-type cytokine profile associated with cell-mediated immune responses.

The attractiveness of this live recombinant vaccine vector approach is that infection with *L. monocytogenes* induces a vigorous immune response of the same type that is considered important for the elimination of other intracellular pathogens, perhaps including HIV, and is also believed important for the eradication of tumors. It has been argued that it is "danger" signals which are most important for the generation of immune responses (138). Thus, the context in which antigens are encountered may be more important than their mere presence. *L. monocytogenes*, a pathogen with lethal capacity (at least in the absence of a functioning immune system), clearly is recognized as dangerous almost as soon as it is detected by the innate immune system. By using this vector to deliver antigen, we are, therefore, not only targeting the antigen to the appropriate pathways of antigen processing but also exploiting the innate immune system to provide the milieu of cytokines required to ensure that the antigen-specific response will be amplified. In this sense, *L. monocytogenes*, and indeed all bacterial vaccine vectors, may act as potent adjuvants as well as antigen delivery vehicles.

ACKNOWLEDGMENTS

The authors thank George R. Gunn III for help with the figures. L. M. W. was supported by National Institutes of Health training grant T32 CA09140.

7.14 REFERENCES

1. Townsend, A. R., J. Rothbard, F. M. Gotch, G. Bahadur, D. Wraith, and A. J. McMichael. 1986. The epitopes of influenza nucleoprotein recognized by cytotoxic T lymphocytes can be defined with short synthetic peptides. *Cell 44*:959.
2. Shimonkevitz, R., J. Kappler, P. Marrack, and H. Grey. 1983. Antigen recognition by H-2-restricted T cells. I. Cell-free antigen processing. *J. Exp. Med. 158*:303.
3. Braciale, T. J., and V. L. Braciale. 1991. Antigen presentation: structural themes and functional variations. *Immunol. Today 12*:124.
4. Monaco, J. J. 1995. Pathways for the processing and presentation of antigens to T cells. *J. Leukoc. Biol. 57*:543.
5. Carbone, F. R., and M. J. Bevan. 1990. Class I-restricted processing

and presentation of exogenous cell-associated antigen *in vivo. J. Exp. Med. 171*:377–387.

6. Kovacsovics-Bankowski, M., K. Clark, B. Benacerraf, and K. L. Rock. 1993. Efficient major histocompatibility complex class I presentation of exogenous antigen upon phagocytosis by macrophages. *Proc. Natl. Acad. Sci. USA 90*:4942.
7. Kovacsovics-Bankowski, M., and K. L. Rock. 1995. A phagosome-to-cytosol pathway for exogenous antigens presented on MHC class I molecules. *Science 267*:243.
8. Huang, A. Y., P. Golumbek, M. Ahmadzadeh, E. Jaffee, D. Pardoll, and H. Levitsky. 1994. Role of bone marrow-derived cells in presenting MHC class I-restricted tumor antigens. *Science 264*:961.
9. Mackaness, G. B. 1962. Cellular resistance to infection. *J. Exp. Med. 116*:381.
10. Dunne, D. W., D. Resnick, J. Greenberg, M. Krieger, and K. A. Joiner. 1994. The type I macrophage scavenger receptor binds to gram-positive bacteria and recognizes lipoteichoic acid. *Proc. Natl. Acad. Sci. USA 91*:1863.
11. Alvarez-Dominguez, C., E. Carrasco-Marin, and F. Leyva-Cobian. 1993. Role of complement component C1q in phagocytosis of *Listeria monocytogenes* by murine macrophage-like cell lines. *Infect. Immun. 61*:3664.
12. Chastellier, C., and P. Berche. 1994. Fate of *Listeria monocytogenes* in murine macrophages: evidence for simulataneous killing and survival of intracellular bacteria. *Infect. Immun. 62*:543.
13. Geoffroy, C., J. L. Gaillard, J. E. Alouf, and P. Berche. 1987. Purification, characterization and toxicity of the sulfhydryl-activated hemolysin listeriolysin O from *Listeria monocytogenes. Infect. Immun. 55*:1641.
14. Bielecki, J., P. Youngman, P. Connelley, and D. A. Portnoy. 1990. *Bacillus subtilis* expressing a haemolysin gene from *Listeria monocytogenes* can grow in mammalian cells. *Nature 345*:175.
15. Ikonomidis, G., Y. Paterson, F. J. Kos, and D. A. Portnoy. 1994. Delivery of a viral antigen to the class I processing and presentation pathway by *Listeria monocytogenes. J. Exp. Med. 180*:2209.
16. Hiltbold, E. M., S. A. Safley, and H. K. Ziegler. 1996. The presentation of class I and class II epitopes of listeriolysin O is regulated by intracellular localization and by intercellular spread of *Listeria monocytogenes. J. Immunol. 157*:1163.
17. Berche, P., J.-L. Gaillard, and P. J. Sansonetti. 1987. Intracellular growth of *Listeria monocytogenes* as a prerequisite for *in vivo* induction of T cell-mediated immunity. *J. Immunology 138*:2266.
18. Sheehan, B., C. Kocks, S. Dramsi, E. Gouin, A. D. Klarsfeld, J. Men-

gaud, and P. Cossart. 1994. Molecular and genetic determinants of the *Listeria monocytogenes* infectious process. *Curr. Top. Microbiol. Immunol. 192*:187.

19. Tilney, L. G., and D. A. Portnoy. 1989. Actin filaments and the growth, movement, and spread of the intracellular bacterial parasite, *Listeria monocytogenes. J. Cell Biol. 109*:1597.
20. van Dijk, H., F. M. Hofhuis, E. M. Berns, C. van der Meer, and J. M. Willers. 1980. Killed *Listeria monocytogenes* vaccine is protective in C3H/H3J mice without addition of adjuvants. *Nature 286*:713.
21. von Koenig, C. H., H. Finger, and H. Hof. 1982. Failure of killed *Listeria monocytogenes* vaccine to produce protective immunity. *Nature 297*:233.
22. Szalay, G., C. H. Ladel, and S. H. E. Kaufmann. 1995. Stimulation of protective $CD8^+$ T lymphocytes by vaccination with nonliving bacteria. *Proc. Natl. Acad. Sci. USA 92*:12389.
23. Goossens, P. L., G. Milon, P. Cossart, and M.-F. Saron. 1995. Attenuated *Listeria monocytogenes* as a live vector for induction of $CD8^+$ T cells *in vivo*: A study with the nucleoprotein of the lymphocytic choriomeningitis virus. *Int. Immunol. 7*:797.
24. Schwartz, R. H. 1992. Costimulation of T lymphocytes: the role of CD28, CTLA-4, and B7/BB1 in interleukin-2 production and immunotherapy. *Cell 71*:1065.
25. Freeman, G. J., J. G. Gribben, V. A. Boussiotis, J. W. Ng, V. A. Restivo, Jr., L. A. Lombard, G. S. Gray, and L. M. Nadler. Cloning of B7-2: a CTLA-4 counter-receptor that costimulates human T cell proliferation. *Science 262*:909.
26. Hathcock, K. S., G. Laszlo, H. B. Dickler, J. Bradshaw, P. Linsley, and R. J. Hodes. 1993. Identification of an alternative CTLA-4 ligand costimulatory for T cell activation. *Science 262*:905.
27. Harding, F. A., J. G. McArthur, J. A. Gross, D. H. Raulet, and J. P. Allison. 1992. CD28-mediated signalling co-stimulates murine T cells and prevents induction of anergy in T cell clones. *Nature 356*:607.
28. Jenkins, M. K., and J. G. Johnson. 1993. Molecules involved in T-cell costimulation. *Curr. Opin. Immunol. 5*:361.
29. Liu, Y. and C. A. Janeway Jr. 1992. Cells that present both specific ligand and costimulatory activity are the most efficient inducers of clonal expansion of normal CD4 T cells. *Proc. Natl. Acad. Sci. USA 89*:3845.
30. Dranoff, G., E. Jaffee, A. Lazenby, P. Golumbek, H. Levitsky, K. Brose, V. Jackson, H. Hamada, D. M. Pardoll, and R. C. Mulligan. 1993. Vaccination with irradiated tumor cells engineered to secrete murine granulocyte-macrophage colony-stimulating factor stimulates potent,

specific, and long-lasting antitumor immunity. *Proc. Natl. Acad. Sci. USA 90*:3539.

31. Morrissey, P. J., L. Bressler, L. S. Park, A. Alpert, and S. Gillis. 1987. Granulocyte-macrophage colony-stimulating factor augments the primary antibody response by enhancing the function of antigen-presenting cells. *J. Immunol. 139*:1113.
32. Witmer-Pack, M. D., W. Olivier, J. Valinsky, G. Schuler, and R. M. Steinman. 1987. Granulocyte/macrophage colony-stimulating factor is essential for the viability and function of cultured murine epidermal Langerhans cells. *J. Exp. Med. 166*:1484.
33. Fischer, H.-G., S. Frosch, K. Reske, and A. B. Reske-Kunz. 1988. Granulocyte-macrophage colony-stimulating factor activates macrophages derived from bone marrow cultures to synthesis of MHC class II molecules and to augmented antigen presentation function. *J. Immunol. 141*:3882.
34. Smith, P. D., C. L. Lamerson, H. L. Wong, L. M. Wahl, and S. M. Wahl. 1990. Granulocyte-macrophage colony-stimulating factor stimulates human monocyte accessory cell function. *J. Immunol. 144*:3829.
35. Larsen, C. P., S. C. Ritchie, R. Hendrix, P. S. Linsley, K. S. Hathcock, R. J. Hodes, R. P. Lowry, and T. C. Pearson. 1994. Regulation of immunostimulatory function and costimulatory molecule (B7-1 and B7-2) expression on murine dendritic cells. *J. Immunol. 152*:5208.
36. Sallusto, F. and A. Lanzavecchia. 1994. Efficient presentation of soluble antigen by cultured human dendritic cells is maintained by granulocyte/macrophage colony-stimulating factor plus interleukin 4 and downregulated by tumor necrosis factor α. *J. Exp. Med. 179*:1109.
37. Kaye, P. M. 1995. Costimulation and the regulation of antimicrobial immunity. *Immunol. Today 16*:423.
38. Celluzzi, C. M., J. I. Mayordomo, W. J. Storkus, M. T. Lotze, and L. D. Falo, Jr. 1996. Peptide-pulsed dendritic cells induce antigen-specific, CTL-mediated protective tumor immunity. *J. Exp. Med. 183*:283.
39. Condon, C., S. C. Watkins, C. M. Celluzzi, K. Thompson, and L. D. Falo, Jr. 1996. DNA-based immunization by *in vivo* transfection of dendritic cells. *Nature Med. 2*:1122.
40. Guzman, C. A., M. Rohde, T. Chakraborty, E. Domann, M. Hudel, J. Wehland, and K. N. Timmis. 1995. Interaction of *Listeria monocytogenes* with mouse dendritic cells. *Infect. Immun. 63*:3665.
41. Gong, J. L., K. M. McCarthy, R. A. Rogers, and E. E. Schneeberger. 1994. Interstitial lung macrophages interact with dendritic cells to present antigenic peptides derived from particulate antigen to T cells. *Immunol. 81*:343.
42. Scheicher, C., M. Mehlig, R. Zecher, and K. Reske. 1992. Dendritic

cells from mouse bone marrow: *in vitro* differentiation using low doses of recombinant granulocyte-macrophage colony-stimulating factor. *J. Immunol. Methods 154*:253.

43. Hanada, K.-I., R. Tsunoda, and H. Hamada. 1996. GM-CSF-induced *in vivo* expansion of splenic dendritic cells and their strong costimulation activity. *J. Leukoc. Biol. 60*:181.
44. Wagner, R. D., and C. J. Czuprynski. 1993. Cytokine mRNA expression in livers of mice infected with *Listeria monocytogenes. J. Leukoc. Biol. 53*:525.
45. Schluter, D., S. B. Oprisiu, S. Chahoud, D. Weiner, O. D. Wiestler, H. Hof, and M. Deckert-Schluter. 1995. Systemic immunization induces protective $CD4^+$ and $CD8^+$ T cell-mediated immune responses in murine *Listeria monocytogenes* meningoencephalitis. *Eur. J. Immunol. 25*:2284.
46. Klink, M., and W. Rudnicka. 1995. *Listeria monocytogenes* infection in pregnant mice: abnormalities in the function of non-adherent accessory light density dendritic cells. *FEMS Immunol. Med. Microbiol. 12*:143.
47. Guzman, C. A., E. Domann, M. Rohde, D. Bruder, A. Darji, S. Weiss, J. Wehland, T. Chakraborty, and K. N. Timmis. 1996. Apoptosis of mouse dendritic cells is triggered by listeriolysin, the major virulence determinant of *Listeria monocytogenes. Mol. Microbiol. 20*:119.
48. Kaye, P. M., N. J. Rogers, A. J. Curry, and J. C. Scott. 1994. Deficient expression of co-stimulatory molecules on *Leishmania*-infected macrophages. *Eur. J. Immunol. 24*:2850.
49. Boehm, U., T. Klamp, M. Groot, and J. C. Howard. 1997. Cellular responses to interferon-gamma. *Annu. Rev. Immunol. 15*:749.
50. Mosmann, T. R., H. Cherwinski, M. W. Bond, M. A. Giedlin, and R. L. Coffman. 1986. Two types of murine helper T cell clone. I. Definition according to profiles of lymphokine activities and secreted proteins. *J. Immunol. 136*:2348.
51. Kelso, A. 1995. Th1 and Th2 subsets: paradigms lost? *Immunol. Today 16*:374.
52. Mosmann, T. R., and R. L. Coffman. 1989. Th1 and Th2 cells: different patterns of lymphokine secretion lead to different functional properties. *Annu. Rev. Immunol. 7*:145.
53. Romagnani, S. 1995. Biology of human Th1 and Th2 cells. *J. Clin. Immunol. 15*:121.
54. Fitch, F. W., R. Stack, P. Fields, D. W. Lancki, and D. C. Cronin. 1995. Regulation of T lymphocyte subsets. *Ciba Found. Symp. 195*:68.
55. Trinchieri, G. 1993. Interleukin-12 and its role in the generation of TH1 cells. *Immunol. Today 14*:335.
56. Croft, M., L. Carter, S. L. Swain, and R. W. Dutton. 1994. Genera-

tion of polarized antigen specific CD8 effector populations: reciprocal action of interleukin (IL)-4 and IL-12 in promoting type 2 versus type 1 cytokine profiles. *J. Exp. Med. 180*:1715.

57. Locksley, R. M., F. P. Heinzel, M. D. Sadick, B. J. Holaday, and K. D. Gardner, Jr. 1987. Murine cutaneous leishmaniasis: susceptibility correlates with differential expansion of helper T-cell subsets. *Ann. Inst. Pasteur-Immunol. 138*:744.
58. Heinzel, F. P., M. D. Sadick, B. J. Holaday, R. L. Coffman, and R. M. Locksley. 1989. Reciprocal expression of interferon gamma or interleukin 4 during the resolution or progression of murine leishmaniasis. Evidence for expansion of distinct helper T cell subsets. *J. Exp. Med. 169*:59.
59. Scott, P., P. Natovitz, R. L. Coffman, E. Pearce, and A. Sher. 1988. Immunoregulation of cutaneous leishmaniasis. T cell lines that transfer protective immunity or exacerbation belong to different T helper subsets and respond to distinct parasite antigens. *J. Exp. Med. 168*:1675.
60. Heinzel, F. P., D. S. Schoenhaut, R. M. Rerko, L. E. Rosser, and M. K. Gately. 1993. Recombinant interleukin 12 cures mice infected with *Leishmania major. J. Exp. Med. 177*:1505.
61. Else, K. J., F. D. Finkelman, C. R. Maliszewski, and R. K. Grencis. 1994. Cytokine-mediated regulation of chronic intestinal helminth infection. *J. Exp. Med. 179*:347.
62. Finkelman, F. D., K. B. Madden, A. W. Cheever, I. M. Katona, S. C. Morris, M. K. Gately, B. R. Hubbard, W. C. Gause, and J. F. Urban, Jr. 1994. Effects of interleukin 12 on immune responses and host protection in mice infected with intestinal nematode parasites. *J. Exp. Med. 179*:1563.
63. Yagi, H., Y. Tokura, H. Wakita, F. Furukawa, and M. Takigawa. 1996. TCRV$\beta 7^+$ Th2 cells mediate UVB-induced suppression of murine contact photosensitivity by releasing IL-10. *J. Immunol. 156*:1824.
64. Nishigori, C., D. B. Yarosh, S. E. Ullrich, A. A. Vink, C. D. Bucana, L. Roza, and M. L. Kripke. 1996. Evidence that DNA damage triggers interleukin 10 cytokine production in UV-irradiated murine keratinocytes. *Proc. Natl. Acad. Sci. USA 93*:10354.
65. Gorelik, L., A. Prokhorova, and M. B. Mokyr. 1994. Low-dose melphalan-induced shift in the production of a Th2-type cytokine to a Th1-type cytokine in mice bearing a large MOPC-315 tumor. *Cancer Immunol. Immunother. 39*:117.
66. Liblau, R. S., S. M. Singer, and H. O. McDevitt. 1995. Th1 and Th2 $CD4^+$ T cells in the pathogenesis of organ-specific autoimmune diseases. *Immunol. Today 16*:34.
67. Hsieh, C.-S., S. E. Macatonia, C. S. Tripp, S. F. Wolf, A. O'Garra,

and K. M. Murphy. 1993. Development of TH1 $CD4^+$ T cells through IL-12 produced by *Listeria*-induced macrophages. *Science 260*:547.

68. Manetti, R., P. Parronchi, M. G. Giudizi, M.-P. Piccinni, E. Maggi, G. Trinchieri, and S. Romagnini. 1993. Natural killer cell stimulatory factor (interleukin 12 [IL-12]) induces T helper type 1 (Th1)-specific immune responses and inhibits the development of IL-4-producing Th cells. *J. Exp. Med. 177*:1199.
69. Scott, P. 1993. IL-12: initiation cytokine for cell-mediated immunity. *Science 260*:496.
70. Brunda, M. J., L. Luistro, R. R. Warrier, R. B. Wright, B. R. Hubbard, M. Murphy, S. F. Wolf, and M. K. Gately. 1993. Antitumor and antimetastatic activity of interleukin 12 against murine tumors. *J. Exp. Med. 178*:1223.
71. Nastala, C. L., H. D. Edington, T. G. McKinney, H. Tahara, M. A. Nalesnik, M. J. Brunda, M. K. Gately, S. F. Wolf, R. D. Schreiber, W. J. Storkus, and M. T. Lotze. 1994. Recombinant IL-12 administration induces tumor regression in association with IFN-γ production. *J. Immunol. 153*:1697.
72. Schafer, R., D. A. Portnoy, S. A. Brassell, and Y. Paterson. 1992. Induction of a cellular immune response to a foreign antigen by a recombinant *Listeria monocytogenes* vaccine. *J. Immunol. 149*:53.
73. Pan, Z.-K., G. Ikonomidis, D. Pardoll, and Y. Paterson. 1995b. Regression of established tumors in mice mediated by the oral administration of a recombinant *Listeria monocytogenes* vaccine. *Cancer Res. 55*:4776.
74. Paglia, P., I. Arioli, N. Frahm, T. Chakraborty, M. P. Colombo, and C. A. Guzman. 1997. The defined attenuated *Listeria monocytogenes* delta mp12 mutant is an effective oral vaccine carrier to trigger a long-lasting immune response against a mouse fibrosarcoma. *Eur. J. Immunol. 27*:1570.
75. Kaufmann, S. H. E. 1993. Immunity to intracellular bacteria. *Annu. Rev. Immunol. 11*:129.
76. Mengaud, J., H. Ohayon, P. Gouno, R.-M. Mege, and P. Cossart. 1996. E-cadherin is the receptor for internalin, a surface protein required for entry of *L. monocytogenes* into epithelial cells. *Cell 84*:923.
77. Drevets, D. A., R. T. Sawyer, T. A. Potter, and P. A. Campbell. 1995. *Listeria monocytogenes* infects human endothelial cells by two distinct mechanisms. *Infect. Immun. 63*:4268.
78. Gaillard, J.-L., P. Berche, C. Frehel, E. Gouin, and P. Cossart. 1991. Entry of *L. monocytogenes* into cells is mediated by internalin, a repeat protein reminiscent of surface antigens from gram-positive cocci. *Cell 65*:1127.

79. Marco, A. J., J. Altimara, N. Prats, S. Lopez, L. Dominguez, M. Domingo, and V. Briones. 1997. Penetration of *Listeria monocytogenes* in mice infected by the oral route. *Microbial Pathol. 23*:255.

80. Pron, B., C. Boumaila, F. Jaubert, S. Sarnacki, J.-P. Monnet, P. Berche, and J.-L. Gaillard. 1998. Comprehensive study of the intestinal stage of Listeriosis in a rat ligated ileal loop system. *Infect. Immun. 66*:747.

81. Roll, J. T., and C. J. Czuprynski. 1990. Hemolysin is required for extraintestinal dissemination of *Listeria monocytogenes* in intragastrically inoculated mice. *Infect. Immun. 58*:3147.

82. Nishikawa, S., T. Miura, S. Sasaki, and A. Nakane. 1996. The protective role of endogenous cytokines in host resistance against an intragastric infection with *Listeria monocytogenes* in mice. *FEMS Immunol. Med. Microbiol. 16*:291.

83. Conlan, J. W. 1997. Neutrophils and tumour necrosis factor-alpha are important for controlling early gastrointestinal stages of experimental murine listeriosis. *J. Med. Microbiol. 46*:239.

84. Unanue, E. R. 1997. Studies in listeriosis show the strong symbiosis between the innate cellular system and the T-cell response. *Immunol. Rev. 158*:11.

85. Miettinen, A., J. Husu, and J. Tuomi. 1990. Serum antibody response to *Listeria monocytogenes*, listerial excretion, and clinical characteristics in experimentally infected goats. *Clin. Microbiol. 28*:340.

86. Salamina, G., E. Dalle Donne, A. Niccolini, G. Poda, D. Cesaroni, M. Bucci, R. Fini, M. Maldini, A. Schuchat, B. Swaminathan, W. Bibb, J. Rocourt, N. Binkin, and S. Salmaso. 1996. A foodborne outbreak of gastroenteritis involving *Listeria monocytogenes. Epidemiol. Infect. 117*:429.

87. Greeningloh, R., A. Darji, J. Wehland, T. Chakraborty, and S. Weiss. 1997. Listeriolysin and IrpA are major protein targets of the human humoral response against *Listeria monocytogenes. Infect. Immun. 65*:3976.

88. Lingnau, A., T. Chakraborty, K. Niebuhr, E. Domann, and J. Wehland. 1996. Identification and purification of novel internalin-related proteins in *Listeria monocytogenes* and *Listeria ivanovii. Infect. Immun. 64*:1002.

89. Dramsi, S., P. Dehoux, M. Lebrun, P. L. Goossens, and P. Cossart. 1997. Identification of four new members of the internalin multigene family of *Listeria monocytogenes* EGD. *Infect. Immun. 65*:1615.

90. Salk, J., P. A. Bretscher, P. L. Salk, M. Clerici, and G. M. Shearer. 1993. A strategy for prophylactic vaccination against HIV. *Science 260*:1270.

91. Paul, W. E. 1995. Reexamining AIDS research priorities. *Science 267*:633.

92. Pardoll, D. M. 1996. Cancer vaccines: a road map for the next decade. *Curr. Opin. Immunol. 8*:619.

93. Shen, H., J. F. Miller, X. Fan, D. Kolwyck, R. Ahmed, and J. T. Harty. 1998. Compartmentalization of bacterial antigens: differential effects on priming of CD8 T cells and protective immunity. *Cell 92*:535.

94. Ikonomidis, G., D. A. Portnoy, W. Gerhard, and Y. Paterson. 1997. Influenza-specific immunity induced by recombinant *Listeria monocytogenes* vaccines. *Vaccines 15*:433.

95. Shen, H., M. K. Slifka, M. Matloubian, E. R. Jensen, R. Ahmed, and J. F. Miller. 1995. Recombinant *Listeria monocytogenes* as a live vaccine vehicle for the induction of protective anti-viral cell-mediated immunity. *Proc. Natl. Acad. Sci. USA 92*:3987.

96. Slifka, M. K., H. Shen, M. Matloubian, E. R. Jensen, J. F. Miller, and R. Ahmed. 1996. Antiviral cytotoxic T-cell memory by vaccination with recombinant *Listeria monocytogenes. J. Virol. 70*:2902.

97. Levy, J. A. 1993. Pathogenesis of human immunodeficiency virus infection. *Microbiol. Rev. 57*:183.

98. Clerici, M., and G. M. Shearer. 1993. A Th1 to Th2 switch is a critical step in the etiology of HIV infection. *Immunol. Today 14*:107.

99. Graziosi, C., G. Pantaleo, K. R. Gantt, J. P. Fortin, J. F. Demarest, O. J. Cohen, R. P. Sekaly, and A. S. Fauci. 1994. Lack of evidence for the dichotomy of Th1 and Th2 predominance in HIV-infected individuals. *Science 265*:248.

100. Mosmann, T. R. 1994. Cytokine patterns during the progression to AIDS. *Science 265*:193.

101. Klein, M. R., C. A. van Baalen, A. M. Holwerda, S. R. Kerkhof Garde, R. J. Bende, I. P. Keet, J. J. K. Eeftinck-Schattenkerk, A. D. Osterhaus, H. Schuitemaker, and F. Miedema. 1995. Kinetics of Gag-specific cytotoxic T lymphocyte responses during the clinical course of HIV-1 infection: a longitudinal analysis of rapid progressors and long-term asymptomatics. *J. Exp. Med. 181*:1365.

102. Barker, E., C. E. Mackewicz, and J. A. Levy. 1995. Effects of Th1 and Th2 cytokines on $CD8^+$ cell response against human immunodeficiency virus: implications for long-term survival. *Proc. Natl. Acad. Sci. USA 92*:11135.

103. Frankel, F. R., S. Hegde, J. Lieberman, and Y. Paterson. 1995. Induction of cell-mediated immune responses to human immunodeficiency virus type 1 Gag protein by using *Listeria monocytogenes* as a live vaccine vector. *J. Immunol. 155*:4775.

104. Bourgault, I., F. Chirat, A. Tartar, J. P. S. Levy, J. G. Guillet, and V. A. Simian. 1994. Immunodeficiency virus as a model for vaccina-

tion against HIV: induction in rhesus macaques of Gag- or Nef-specific cytotoxic T lymphocytes by lipopeptides. *J. Immunol.* *152*:2530.

105. Paul, W. E., and R. A. Seder. 1994. Lymphocyte responses and cytokines. *Cell* *76*:241.

106. Pan, Z.-K., G. Ikonomidis, A. Lazenby, D. Pardoll, and Y. Paterson. 1995. A recombinant *Listeria monocytogenes* vaccine expressing a model tumour antigen protects mice against lethal tumour cell challenge and causes regression of established tumours. *Nature Med.* *1*:471.

107. Lehmann, P. V., E. E. Sercarz, T. Forsthuber, C. M. Dayan, and G. Gammon. 1993. Determinant spreading and the dynamics of the autoimmune T cell repertoire. *Immunol. Today* *14*:203.

108. Jensen, E. R., R. Selvakumar, H. Shen, R. Ahmed, F. O. Wettstein, and J. F. Miller. 1997. Recombinant *Listeria monocytogenes* vaccination eliminates papillomavirus-induced tumors and prevents papilloma formation from viral DNA. *J. Virol.* *71*:8467.

109. Dietrich, G., A. Bubert, I. Gentschev, Z. Sokolovic, A. Simm, A. Catic, S. H. E. Kaufmann, J. Hess, A. A. Szalay, and W. Goebel. 1998. Delivery of antigen-encoding plasmid DNA into the cytosol of macrophages by attenuated suicide *Listeria monocytogenes. Nature Biotech.* *16*:181.

110. Domann, E., J. Wehland, M. Rohde, S. Pistor, M. Hartl, W. Goebel, M. Leimeister-Wachter, M. Wuenscher, and T. Chakraborty. 1992. A novel bacterial virulence gene in *Listeria monocytogenes* required for host cell microfilament interaction with homology to the proline-rich region of vinculin. *EMBO J.* *11*:1981.

111. Kocks, C., E. Gouin, M. Tabouret, P. Berche, H. Ohayon, and P. Cossart. 1992. L. monocytogenes-induced actin assembly requires the actA gene product, a surface protein. *Cell* *68*:521.

112. Rouquette, C., C. de Chastellier, S. Nair, and P. Berche. 1998. The ClpC ATPase of Listeria monocytogenes is a general stress protein required for virulence and promoting early bacterial escape from the phagosome of macrophages. *Mol. Microbiol.* *27*:1235.

113. Rouquette, C., M. T. Ripio, E. Pellegrini, J. M. Bolla, R. I. Tascon, J. A. Vazquez-Boland, and P. Berche. 1996. Identification of a ClpC ATPase required for stress tolerance and in vivo survival of *Listeria monocytogenes. Mol. Microbiol.* *21*:977.

114. Portnoy, D. A., T. Chakraborty, W. Goebel, and P. Cossart. 1992. Molecular determinants of *Listeria monocytogenes* pathogenesis. *Infect. Immun.* *60*:1263.

115. Leimeister-Wachter, M., E. Domann, and T. Chakraborty. 1992. The expression of virulence genes in *Listeria monocytogenes* is thermoregulated. *J. Bacteriol.* *174*:947.

116. Bockmann, R., C. Dickneite, B. Middendorf, W. Goebel, and Z.

Sokolovic. 1996. Specific binding of the *Listeria monocytogenes* transcriptional regulator PrfA to target sequences requires additional factor(s) and is influenced by iron. *Mol. Microbiol. 22*:643.

117. Poyart, C., E. Abachin, I. Razafimanantsoa, and P. Berche. 1993. The zinc metalloprotease of *Listeria monocytogenes* is required for maturation of phosphatidylcholine phospholipase C: direct evidence obtained by gene complementation. *Infect. Immun. 61*:1576.
118. Camilli, A., L. G. Tilney, and D. A. Portnoy. 1993. Dual roles of plcA in *Listeria monocytogenes* pathogenesis. *Mol. Microbiol. 8*:143.
119. Kohler, S., A. Bubert, M. Vogel, and W. Goebel. 1991. Expression of the iap gene coding for protein p60 of *Listeria monocytogenes* is controlled on the posttranscriptional level. *J. Bacteriol. 173*:4668.
120. Kuhn, M., and W. Goebel. 1989. Identification of an extracellular protein of *Listeria monocytogenes* possibly involved in intracellular uptake by mammalian cells. *Infect. Immun. 57*:55.
121. Wuenscher, M. D., S. Kohler, A. Bubert, U. Gerike, and W. Goebel. 1993. The iap gene of *Listeria monocytogenes* is essential for cell viability, and its gene product, p60, has bacteriolytic activity. *J. Bacteriol. 175*:3491.
122. Southwick, F. S., and D. L. Purich. 1996. Intracellular pathogenesis of Listeriosis. *N. Engl. J. Med. 334*:770.
123. Gellin, B. G., and C. V. Broome. 1989. Listeriosis. *JAMA 261*:1313.
124. Decker, C. F., G. L. Simon, R. A. DiGioia, and C. U. Tuazon. 1991. *Listeria monocytogenes* infections in patients with AIDS: report of five cases and review. *Rev. Infect. Dis. 13*:413.
125. de Vega, T., S. Echevarria, J. Crespo, E. Artinano, G. San Miguel, and F. Pons Romero. 1992. Acute hepatitis by *Listeria monocytogenes* in an HIV patient with chronic HBV hepatitis. *J. Clin. Gastroenterol. 15*:251.
126. Goossens, P. L., and G. Milon. 1992. Induction of protective $CD8^+$ T lymphocytes by an attenuated *Listeria monocytogenes actA* mutant. *Int. Immunol. 4*:1413.
127. Alexander, J. E., P. W. Andrew, D. Jones, and I. S. Roberts. 1993. Characterization of an aromatic amino acid-dependent *Listeria monocytogenes* mutant: attenuation, persistence, and ability to induce protective immunity in mice. *Infect. Immun. 61*:2245.
128. Chakraborty, T., F. Ebel, J. Wehland, J. Dufrenne, and S. Notermans. 1994. Naturally occurring virulence-attenuated isolates of *Listeria monocytogenes* capable of inducing long term protection against infection by virulent strains of homologous and heterologous serotypes. *FEMS Immunol. Med. Microbiol. 10*:1.
129. Barry, R. A., H. G. A. Bouwer, D. A. Portnoy, and D. J. Hinrichs. 1992. Pathogenicity and immunogenicity of *Listeria monocytogenes*

small-plaque mutants defective for intracellular growth and cell-to-cell spread. *Infect. Immun. 60*:16525.

130. Thompson, R. J., H. G. A. Bouwer, D. A. Portnoy, and F. R. Frankel. 1998. Pathogenicity and immunogenicity of a D-alanine-requiring strain of *Listeria monocytogenes. Infect. Immun. 66*:3552.
131. Falo, L. D., Jr., M. Kovacsovics-Bankowski, K. Thompson, and K. L. Rock. 1995. Targeting antigen into the phagocytic pathway *in vivo* induces protective tumour immunity. *Nature Med. 1*:649.
132. Elson, C. J., R. N. Barker, S. J. Thompson, and N. A. Williams. 1995. Immunologically ignorant autoreactive T cells, epitope spreading and repertoire limitation. *Immunol. Today 16*:71.
133. Robbins, P. F., and Y. Kawakami. 1996. Human tumor antigens recognized by T cells. *Curr. Opin. Immunol. 8*:628.
134. Tindle, R. W. 1996. Human papillomavirus vaccines for cervical cancer. *Curr. Opin. Immunol. 8*:643.
135. Disis, M. L., and M. A. Cheever. 1996. Oncogenic proteins as tumor antigens. *Curr. Opin. Immunol. 8*:637.
136. Chakraborty, T., F. Ebel, E. Domann, K. Niebuhr, B. Gerstel, S. Pistor, C. J. Temm-Grove, B. M. Jockusch, M. Reinhard, U. Walter, and J. Wehland. 1995. A focal adhesion factor directly linking intracellularly motile *Listeria monocytogenes* and *Listeria ivanovii* to the actin-based cytoskeleton of mammalian cells. *EMBO J. 14*:1314.
137. Southwick, F. S., and D. L. Purich. 1994. Arrest of Listeria movement in host cells by a bacterial ActA analogue: implications for actin-based motility. *Proc. Natl. Acad. Sci. USA 91*:5168.
138. Matzinger, P. 1994. Tolerance, danger, and the extended family. *Annu. Rev. Immunol. 12*:991.

INDEX